CRISIS
MANAGEMENT
IN ANESTHESIOLOGY

With Contributions By

Emily Ratner, M.D.
Assistant Professor
Department of Anesthesia
Stanford University School of Medicine
Stanford, California

Robert S. Holzman, M.D.
Assistant Professor
Department of Anesthesia
Harvard Medical School
Senior Associate in Anesthesia
Department of Anesthesia
Boston Children's Hospital
Boston, Massachusetts

CRISIS
MANAGEMENT
IN ANESTHESIOLOGY

David M. Gaba, M.D.

Associate Professor
Department of Anesthesia
Stanford University School of Medicine
Stanford, California
Staff Anesthesiologist
Anesthesiology Service
Palo Alto Department of Veterans Affairs
  Medical Center
Palo Alto, California

Kevin J. Fish, M.Sc., M.B., Ch.B., F.R.C.A., F.R.C.P.(C)

Professor
Department of Anesthesia
Stanford University School of Medicine
Stanford, California
Staff Anesthesiologist
Anesthesiology Service
Palo Alto Department of Veterans Affairs
  Medical Center
Palo Alto, California

Steven K. Howard, M.D.

Assistant Professor
Department of Anesthesia
Stanford University School of Medicine
Stanford, California
Staff Anesthesiologist
Anesthesiology Service
Palo Alto Department of Veterans Affairs
  Medical Center
Palo Alto, California

Churchill Livingstone
New York, Edinburgh, London, Melbourne, Madrid, Tokyo

Library of Congress Cataloging-in-Publication Data

Gaba, David M.
    Crisis management in anesthesiology / David M. Gaba, Kevin J.
  Fish, Steven K. Howard : with contribution by Emily Ratner, Robert
  S. Holzman.
      p.   cm.
  Includes bibliographical references and index.
  ISBN 0-443-08910-8
    1. Anesthesia—Complications. 2. Anesthesia—Decision making.
  3. Medical emergencies. 4. Surgical emergencies.   I. Fish, Kevin
  J. II. Howard, Steven K. III. Title.
    [DNLM: 1. Decision Making. 2. Anesthesiology—education.
  3. Emergency Medicine—education. WO 200 G112c 1994]
  RD82.5.G33 1994
  617.9'6041—dc20
  DNLM/DLC
  for Library of Congress   93-39076
                                       CIP

© Churchill Livingstone Inc. 1994

Distributed in the United Kingdom by Churchill Livingstone, Robert Stevenson House, 1–3 Baxter's Place, Leith Walk, Edinburgh EH1 3AF, and by associated companies, branches, and representatives throughout the world.

Accurate indications, adverse reactions, and dosage schedules for drugs are provided in this book, but it is possible that they may change. The reader is urged to review the package information data of the manufacturers of the medications mentioned.

The Publishers have made every effort to trace the copyright holders for borrowed material. If they have inadvertently overlooked any, they will be pleased to make the necessary arrangements at the first opportunity.

Copy Editor: *Bridgett Dickinson*
Production Supervisor: *Patricia McFadden*
Cover Design: *Paul Moran*

Printed in the United States of America

First published in 1994   7 6 5 4 3 2 1

Foreword

Managing critical events is one of the most challenging and important tasks required of the anesthetist. So, why is it that, until now, no one has written a book about the basic principles of how to do it? To be sure, there are plenty of books, articles, refresher course syllabuses, and audio and video tapes about how to perform every conceivable anesthesia task safely and about what is medically correct to do in response to a critical event. The operative word is *medically*. Plenty of advice is available about what is or is not medically sound, but almost no educational material, grounded in theory, is available that discusses the human aspects of crisis intervention. What are the general principles for managing such events? What is the generic approach, a "mental model," for thinking about and for responding to those rare situations that all anesthetists hope will never happen to them? These may be rare events, yet they are the reason anesthetists must train so long before being allowed to stand at the head of the table alone. Now there is a textbook that captures the essence of what it is hoped will become instinctive during that training. What is described in this innovative text should be required reading for anyone who administers anesthesia.

Why is this material so important? Anesthesia continues to be a unique speciality that demands of its practitioners something approaching perfection. The training is essentially an apprenticeship, during which it is expected that there will be enough challenges to practice, under close supervision, the management of problems that arise unexpectedly. But, of course, not all problems will be seen; in reality, very few will be experienced. In addition, there will probably not be too many really "exciting" opportunities to practice crisis management skills. When an event does happen, learning certainly occurs, but it does so without the benefit of a theoretical basis for teaching the general skills that will apply to the next event. It is unlikely that one event will have the same specific attributes as the last one, or probably any previous event experienced by that individual. That is why a general approach to crisis management, which takes skills that are common to management of many events, should be an important new component of anesthesia training.

The roots of *Crisis Management in Anesthesiology* derive from disciplines that are foreign to anesthesia and that are on the "soft" side of the research spectrum. Such interdisciplinary work is the hardest kind of research for an investigator to attempt because it carries the risk of not being recognized in any of the disciplines to which it relates. Journal reviewers get confused because this is not something with which they are familiar. It does not seem like the "science" they usually consider. The authors should be commended for taking the risk. It has been worth it.

It is not enough to read about crisis management. Reading provides only the foundation; practice is the teacher. This is one of the roles for courses using simulators of various kinds. *Crisis Management in Anesthesiology* is the textbook that should accompany such a course. Only time will tell whether the use of simulators and other similar technology will achieve a place in medical education. Even if medical economics constrains the use of such technology, this book will still stand by itself as a source for education and training about what none but the most thrill-seeking anesthetist *wants* to experience, but which every anesthetist *will* experience. This book, and the theoretical ground it lays in medicine, should make the probability of successful experiences much more likely.

Jeffrey B. Cooper, Ph.D.

Associate Clinical Professor
Department of Anesthesia
Harvard Medical School
Chairman
Department of Anesthesia
New England Deaconess Hospital
Boston, Massachusetts

Ellison C. Pierce, Jr., M.D.

Associate Professor
Department of Anesthesia
Harvard Medical School and Harvard–
MIT Division of Health Sciences and Technology
Director
Biomedical Engineering and Anesthesia Technology
Massachusetts General Hospital
Boston, Massachusetts

Preface

Who This Book Is For

This book is written for everyone who administers anesthesia. While we are aware of the political and economic conflicts between nurse anesthetists and anesthesiologists, these conflicts are totally irrelevant to the goals of this book. A central tenet of our teaching is that whoever is present with the patient during the anesthetic needs to be highly skilled at responding to crises, both as an individual and in concert with other members of the patient care team. Many of the lessons we teach concerning team leadership may be of most importance to the anesthesiologist, who is the nominal head of the anesthesia care team. However, we strongly emphasize that optimum management of crises requires coordinated input from *all* team members. In this book we use the generic term *anesthetist* to refer to either an anesthesiologist or a certified nurse anesthetist.

Crisis Management in Anesthesiology is aimed at both experienced practitioners and trainees. We contend that the concepts we present have not been adequately taught to anesthetists in the past, nor are they easily learned during everyday clinical work. Novices will want to learn them early to make them a part of their routine practices. Experts will need to constantly review and reinforce existing routines, just as pilots must recurrently train and practice their crisis management skills regardless of their years of flying experience.

What This Book Is About

Crisis Management in Anesthesiology focuses on different issues than those found in traditional medical or anesthesia textbooks. Whereas other books about anesthesia primarily deal with the patient's normal or abnormal physiology, or with the technical and clinical characteristics of drugs and equipment, this book focuses primarily on the *mind* of the anesthetist. Just as pharmacologists attempt to synthesize the "perfect" anesthetic drug, and just as engineers aim to build "fail-safe" devices, we strive to help anesthetists to optimize their own performance because that is the most crucial link in the chain of safe patient care.

This book is a guide to crisis management in anesthesia. The first two chapters analyze the expertise of the ideal anesthetist in terms of its component parts. This ideal anesthetist uses a repeated process of observation, decision, and action under the adaptive control of an "internal supervisor." Besides managing his or her own activities, the expert must manage those of a team of individuals working together on the patient's behalf. The material in these chapters is analogous to the didactic components of the Crew Resource Management programs that are now a regular part of airline pilot training.

The second section, the Catalog of Critical Events in Anesthesiology, is designed to assist the anesthetist in implementing another strategy used in aviation. The Catalog is a systematic compilation of emergency procedures for the kinds of crises encountered in clinical practice. Just as all pilots must learn to recognize and respond to a variety of emergency situations, we believe that anesthetists should do the same. The Catalog presents events of interest to anesthetists in a uniform, concise fashion designed to improve the recognition of and response to crises. It can be used as a study guide to allow the anesthetist to prepare in advance to recognize and manage crisis situations, as well as during the debriefing after a crisis as a reminder of information that could have been considered or actions that could have been performed. Finally, it can be used as a tool for interactive training in anesthesia crisis management using verbal simulation, role-playing, or realistic anesthesia simulators.

What This Book Is Not About

While crisis management in anesthesia is built on the foundation of a sound knowledge base and adequate technical skills, *Crisis Management in Anesthesiology* assumes that the reader is either already familiar with, or in the process of learning, the medical knowledge and technical skills necessary to practice anesthesia. It is not meant to be a reference text on anesthesia, nor is it a text on the pathophysiology of surgical patients or their specific *preoperative* evaluation and treatment. These topics are covered thoroughly in numerous other textbooks and reference works.

Perhaps most importantly, this book is *not* a "cookbook" of anesthesia. You will not find recipes for perfect anesthetics. The Catalog of Critical Events in Anesthesiology is a guidebook only. The Management section of each entry in the Catalog is purposefully *not* in the format of a decision tree or algorithm. We believe that patient care in the anesthesia environment is too complicated to give simple decision trees with distinct branch points. Such algorithms are also difficult to remember because of their branching structure. Therefore, our management guides are written as a hierarchical list of what to check or to do, roughly in the order that an experienced practitioner might do them.

In particular, we make no claim that following the management guide for any listed event will guarantee the resolution of a clinical problem or that it will forestall an adverse outcome for the patient. The material is intended only for the education of anesthetists. While we have tried to be comprehensive, we make no claim to be exhaustive. The lists of manifestations for each event contain those signs that we believe to be most important; they do not include every possible sign. Similarly, no management guide can take into account every combination of patient status and atypical circumstance.

We strongly encourage all anesthetists to deviate from the responses listed in the management sections of the Catalog entries whenever and *however* necessary to deal with a specific situation. We also strongly encourage anesthetists to adapt this Catalog to their own practices, based on their experiences with different drugs and techniques.

Who Are the Authors

You may be curious about our backgrounds and why we are qualified to write this unusual book. All of us are full-time academic anesthesiologists at Stanford University School of Medicine and the Palo Alto Department of Veterans Affairs Medical Center. David Gaba trained at Stanford and has been practicing anesthesia for 12 years. He is a licensed private pilot (PP-ASEL) and has a long-standing interest in aviation and spaceflight. Kevin Fish was trained in Britain and Canada, and has been practicing anesthesia for 22 years. Steven Howard also trained at Stanford, and has been practicing anesthesia for 4 years.

In addition to clinical teaching we have conducted considerable research on the human performance of anesthetists, delineating how individuals think as they conduct anesthesia (see Ch. 1 references). A considerable part of this work has used a realistic, "hands-on" simulator of anesthesia that our laboratory invented (Comprehensive Anesthesia Simulation Environment [CASE]). The material in *Crisis Management in Anesthesiology* grew out of a special course on Anesthesia Crisis Resource Management that we developed for use with the CASE simulator. This course has now been taught to more than 120 anesthesia residents, teaching faculty, private practitioners, and nurse anesthetists. Their comments and criticisms have been incorporated into this book.

We asked Robert Holzman and Emily Ratner to use their specific expertise in subspecialties of anesthesia to write the pediatric anesthesia and obstetric anesthesia chapters, respectively. We were also assisted in the early stages of the development of the Catalog of Critical Events in Anesthesiology by Frank Sarnquist, M.D. a Stanford faculty anesthesiologist with 23 years of academic and private practice experience.

David M. Gaba, M.D.
Kevin J. Fish, M.D.
Steven K. Howard, M.D.

Acknowledgments

Crisis Management in Anesthesiology would never have come about without the support of the Anesthesia Patient Safety Foundation (APSF). We are grateful to the APSF whose grant program funded both the original development of the Comprehensive Anesthesia Simulation Environment simulator and, later, the construction of the Anesthesia Crisis Resource Management (ACRM) course.

We owe a debt to the many residents of the Stanford University Department of Anesthesia who, as part of their training, wrote the earliest drafts of some of the entries in the Catalog. Collectively, their efforts gave us a place to start in the compilation of the Catalog and their grist for our editorial mill made the job considerably easier.

We would like to acknowledge a number of investigators in cognitive science and human factors whose work is discussed in this book. Although they are referenced in the text, mere academic citation cannot express the depth of our appreciation for the works they have published and their personal support for our efforts to apply them to the business of anesthesia. Jens Rasmussen is perhaps the founder of attempts to study the real world cognition of individuals and groups working in ill-structured domains. We owe much to his delineation of the multiple levels of mental activity occurring simultaneously in dynamic situations.

James Reason provided important insights to the underlying causes of errors and accidents. These are summarized in his book *Human Error* (Cambridge University Press, Cambridge, UK, 1990). Because these are very complicated topics and they are largely beyond the control of the individual anesthetist, our book does not fully address this area. We do cover these issues to some extent in our sections on "production pressure." In fact they probably deserve a book of their own for anesthetists.

David Woods provided us not only with an understanding of why anesthesia is so similar to other complex dynamic worlds, and what fixation errors are all about, but also with a wealth of other concepts that subtly molded our outlook.

Of all the models of dynamic decision making in the literature, Gary Klein's *Recognition-Primed Decision Making* (RPD) is the one that bears the closest resemblance to our own formulation (although in truth we were ignorant of his existing work as we proceeded). Klein, Orasanu, and Calderwood's recent book, *Decision Making in Action: Models and Methods* (Ablex Publishing, Norwood, NJ, 1993) has redefined decision making, emphasizing "naturalistic decision making" of real decision makers in complex, dynamic, and ill-structured domains. The RPD paradigm is now becoming widely accepted in aviation and in military command and control.

Daniel Gopher clarified for us the importance of the allocation of attention and the various strategies by which anesthetists might manipulate the work load of their situation.

Incidentally (although not by accident), Professors Rasmussen, Reason, Woods, and Gopher were all participants in the Conference on Human Error in Anesthesia (February, 1991) which was organized by two of us (DMG, SKH) as an experts' consensus meeting on the critical issues of human performance in our specialty. This Conference was also a spur to complete *Crisis Management in Anesthesiology*.

We would like to thank a number of individuals working on human factors in aviation whose work has directly or indirectly guided our approach to anesthesia crisis management. They include John Lauber, Ph.D., National Transportation Safety Board; H. Clayton Foushee, Ph.D., Federal Aviation Administration; Robert Helmreich, Ph.D., National Aeronautics and Space Administration/University of Texas Aerospace Crew Performance Project; Judith Orasanu, Ph.D., National Aeronautics and Space Administration, Aerospace Human Factors Research Division, and Rand McNally, M.D., American Airlines.

We would like to thank the many students and fellows whose work in our laboratory contributed to the genesis of this book, in particular: Abe DeAnda, Jr., M.D., John Williams, M.D., Thomas Lee, and George Yang. We are grateful to Clarita Domingo for secretarial assistance in preparing our ACRM course and the Catalog of Critical Events in Anesthesiology.

Finally, we acknowledge that our ability to produce this book was aided immensely by our close-knit band of colleagues dedicated to research and education in the Anesthesiology Service of the Palo Alto Department of Veterans Affairs Medical Center, a close affiliate of the Department of Anesthesia, Stanford University School of Medicine. We are indebted to the Department of Veterans Affairs for providing the environment and the time in which to write this book.

David M. Gaba, M.D.
Kevin J. Fish, M.D.
Steven K. Howard, M.D.

Contents

SECTION I
Basic Principles of Crisis Management in Anesthesiology

"Hours of boredom, moments of terror." For most physicians outside of anesthesia, this saying captures the essence of the work experience of anesthetists. It is largely the occasional moments of terror, not the routine hours of boredom, that define our role in the operating room and the mental attitudes required to perform our job successfully. This is one aspect of anesthesia that sets our field (and a few related ones such as intensive care and emergency room medicine) apart from most other branches of medical care, certainly apart from primary or chronic care. Another aspect is the direct physical involvement of the anesthetist in the tasks of patient care. This includes the performance of invasive procedures, the administration of rapidly acting, potentially lethal medications, and the operation of increasingly complex devices. In all likelihood, the emphasis on direct action and the aura of danger lurking just below the surface are key factors that attracted many of us into this line of work.

Surprisingly, beyond the American Society of Anesthesiologists' enshrined motto of "Vigilance," little attention has been paid to how anesthetists go about, or should go about, working in a setting in which moments of terror do in fact occur. The practice of anesthesia is a complicated collection of mental and physical activities attuned more to the *efficient* care of routine cases than it is to the handling of life-threatening crises. What constitutes "expertise" in anesthesia is only now beginning to be explored. How newcomers to anesthesia become skilled practitioners is largely unknown. The systems of educating and training both anesthesiologists and certified nurse anesthetists have assumed that merely by selecting intelligent and motivated individuals to undergo training in anesthesia, they have *guaranteed* that trainees will be able to transform their own mental abilities into those of the ideal anesthetist, solely on the basis of abstract scientific lessons and the routine daily tasks of the operating room. They assume that crisis prevention and crisis management skills will emerge naturally through learning the basic science of anesthesia, pharmacology, and physiology or through repeated exposure to clinical experiences (by "osmosis"). These modalities are supplemented by a smattering of morbidity and mortality conferences and occasional continuing medical education lectures.

The standard assumption that every anesthetist who successfully completes a training program is a capable crisis manager has rarely been challenged. We are now discovering that the initial training and continuing education of anesthetists often leaves substantial gaps in the ability of some anesthetists to deal with crises. When a crisis does present itself—a patient suffers an unexpected cardiac arrest or a surgical catastrophe occurs—it is obvious to everyone who works in an operating room that some anesthetists cope better than others. These anesthetists take more steps to prevent a crisis, and they are better prepared when they occur. They are the ones who can bring order from chaos. They take command and know what to do and how to ensure that it gets done. They are the people that most of us would choose to administer "our" anesthetic if we needed it. The skills that distinguish these expert crisis managers go beyond the traditional aspects of medical, scientific, and technical knowledge. Why are some anesthetists seemingly better suited than others to manage the "moments of terror" that are so much a part

1

of our world? Is it strictly an unlearnable aspect of the individual's personality? Conversely, if some are not well suited to handle crises, where does the fault lie?

In this book we contend that crisis management involves skills that can be identified and taught. Why has the anesthesia community been slow to realize this fact? Medicine, in general, has been attached to a view of the physician as a pensive provider of healing arts based on careful applications of personal skill and, in the last 100 years, scientific knowledge. This view works well enough for relatively static branches of medicine in which careful reflection and an extended doctor-patient relationship are the dominant aspects of care. Yet we believe that this view has prevented the training process of anesthetists from addressing the real dominant aspects of *our* work: dynamism, time pressure, intensity, complexity, uncertainty, and risk. In our opinion, to understand the anesthetist better we must turn away from research on learning and decision making in medicine and look at the experience of other human activities that share the key aspects of our domain.

Dynamism, time pressure, complexity, uncertainty, and risk are seen in such activities as aviation, spaceflight, process control (nuclear power and chemical manufacturing), shipping, military command, and fire fighting. Aviation offers considerable parallels with anesthesia, and in fact pilots share our aphorism, "hours of boredom, moments of terror." Especially in aviation, cognitive psychologists and human factor engineers have been actively trying to pinpoint the elements of optimal performance and to design work routines and training strategies to improve the abilities of both new and existing personnel. Several successful strategies to improve air crew performance and safety in aviation have not been adequately matched in anesthesia. They include

1. Use of written checklists to help prevent crises from occurring
2. Use of established procedures (both memorized and written) in responding to crises
3. Training in decision making and crew coordination for cockpit (and cabin) crews
4. Systematic practice in the handling of crisis situations, including the use of part-task trainers and full-mission realistic simulators

We believe that anesthetists should adopt many of these strategies to improve their performance and to enhance patient safety.

Finally, we would like to share with you our philosophy of anesthesia practice, which underlies this book. *You* are responsible for giving the best possible care to your patients. Although perfect performance is unachievable, you should strive to approach it. Honing your understanding of medicine, physiology, and anesthesia technology is an essential step. Sharpening your diagnostic and technical skills is another. You must realize, however, that the real world in which you work will make it difficult to translate these skills into optimal patient care. Experience alone will not guarantee good performance, nor can it make you immune to the types of errors that plague all humans in complex, dynamic domains. Production pressures, distractions, and the intensity of cases will challenge your best intentions. An important beginning is to admit that crises *will* occur in spite of, or even because of, your own best efforts. Approach each case as if it is a disaster waiting to happen, and plan as best as you can to prevent it. Make explicit provisions for the failure of elements in the anesthetic or surgical plans. Prepare yourself to recognize and manage *all* the crises that you could face regardless of how they might be triggered. Utilize your institution's quality assurance programs to adapt your practice as required, based on your own experiences and those of others. As you review your performance and that of your colleagues, try to avoid becoming fixated solely on the medical and technical aspects of how a crisis was managed; consider also the teamwork aspects and the way in which the "larger system" helped or hindered patient care. Seek to change those aspects of the situation that impeded optimum management.

Reading about crisis management is not enough. As with pilots, military personnel, athletes, and musicians, actual practice of the skills is important. Our Anesthesia Crisis Resource Management course teaches the material on crisis management found in this book, but its centerpiece is a session in the Comprehensive Anesthesia Simulation Enviroment (CASE) simulator. During the simulations the anesthetists practice handling a variety of challenging scenarios in a real operating room equipped with actual clinical equipment and staffed by nurses and surgeons with whom the anesthetists must interact. The team's performance in the simulation scenarios is recorded on videotape, which then becomes the focus of a 2-hour debriefing session of review and critique with an expert instructor. The simulation sessions and debriefings are powerful learning experiences.[1] As anesthesia simulators become more common, more anesthetists will be able to train in crisis management in this way.

Even if you do not have access to a simulator, you can practice these skills through role-playing or verbal simulation. Each oral examination of the American Board of Anesthesiologists involves an exercise in case management, which usually includes one or more crises. Similar exercises can be conducted between pairs of anesthetists. Finally, you can prepare for crises on your own by systematically reviewing, aloud, what you would do in a variety of problem situations. Many pilots and astronauts have described doing this at home, even to the extent of touching the controls on a paper mockup as they would use the controls in the cockpit, in order to prepare themselves for the simulator exercises and the actual flights that truly put them to the test. Your responsibility to your patients demands the same commitment.

Chapters 1 and 2 begin with a comprehensive look at a theory of decision making and crisis management in anesthesia. Chapter 1 provides a theoretical background on the psychology of the anesthetist during routine patient care and during crisis management. Chapter 2 provides concrete advice on how to forestall crises and how to manage the situation should they arise. The material in these chapters is analogous to the didactic components of the Crew Resource Management programs that are now a regular part of the training of airline pilots. The material is general in scope and can apply to virtually any perioperative situation.

Reference

1. Howard SK, Gaba DM, Fish KJ et al: Anesthesia crisis resource management training: teaching anesthesiologists to handle critical incidents. Aviat Space Environ Med 63:763, 1992

Chapter One

Theory of Dynamic Decision Making
and Crisis Management

Decision Making and Crisis Management

This book is about decision making and crisis management in anesthesia. What is a *crisis?* It is "a time of great danger or trouble whose outcome decides whether possible bad consequences will follow."[1] For our purposes the time of great danger is typically a brief, intense event or sequence of events that offer a clear and present danger to the patient. Almost by definition, a crisis requires an active response to prevent injury to the patient; it is unlikely to resolve on its own.

Skilled crisis management in anesthesia is no mystery. It demands that the anesthetist, while under stress and time pressure, *optimally* implement standard techniques of diagnosis and treatment to the patient. Medical knowledge and skills are essential components of the decisions and actions performed during crises, but they are not enough. To actually make things happen quickly and safely for patient management, the anesthetist must manage the entire *situation,* including the environment, the equipment, and the patient care team. These management skills involve aspects of cognitive and social psychology and even sociology and anthropology. These fields may seem foreign to the anesthetist, but they provide insights into the expertise of the experienced practitioner, the inadequacies of the novice, and the pitfalls that face every anesthetist. In this chapter we delineate the underlying conceptual foundations of crisis management. These concepts provide an important background both for Chapter 2 (Principles of Anesthesia Crisis Resource Management), which gives practical guidance on how to be a better crisis manager, and for the remainder of this book (Section II: Catalog of Critical Events in Anesthesiology), which gives specific preparation for the recognition and management of a large variety of crisis situations.

Anesthesiology, by Its Nature, Involves Crises

Why is a book on medical crisis management addressed to anesthetists? What makes anesthesiology and a few other medical domains (such as intensive care medicine and surgery) different from most other medical fields, including the bulk of internal medicine and pediatrics? The answer, to a large extent, is that the clinical environment of anesthesiology is dynamic, and this dynamism interacts very strongly with the complexity of the environment.[2] The combination of complexity and dynamism makes crises much more likely to occur and more difficult to deal with; thus, the expert anesthetist must be skilled in their management. Following the work of Woods,[3] we address the aspects of anesthesia that make it a "complex, dynamic world." Such aspects are that it is event-driven and dynamic; complex and tightly coupled; uncertain; and risky.

Event-Driven and Dynamic

The anesthetized patient's state changes continuously. With some exceptions (such as during induction of anesthesia), what happens *during* anesthesia is heavily determined by events outside the anesthetist's control. Although preventive measures can reduce the likelihood of certain events, others cannot be avoided even in principle because they are inevitable side effects of procedures that must be carried out owing to medical necessity (e.g., surgical blood loss). These unpredictable and dynamic events drive the concerns of the anesthetist in equal measure with the predictable, preplanned aspects of the case.

Complex and Tightly Coupled

In technological systems, complexity stems from a large number of interconnected components. The patient is the main "system" of interest to the anesthetist. Patients are intrinsically very complex, and they contain many components, the underlying functions of which are imperfectly understood. Unlike industrial or aviation systems, patients are not designed, built, or tested by humans, nor do they come with an operator's manual.

Some physiologic systems are buffered from changes in others, while certain core components, such as oxygen delivery and blood flow, are *tightly coupled* together and interact strongly.[4,5] Anesthesia ablates some protective and compensatory physiologic mechanisms and will force the patient's systems to become more tightly coupled. The patient's physiology may also become tightly coupled to external systems such as ventilators or infusions of hemodynamically active drugs.

Although the medical equipment connected to the patient is not as complex as that found in aircraft or spacecraft, it consists of a proliferation of independent devices with multiple, nonstandardized interconnections. Devices are often designed in isolation, so that interactions between devices, or between the equipment and the human operator, may not be adequately addressed in the design phase. These factors increase the complexity of the domain.

Uncertain

The patient as a system contains inherent uncertainties. The medical world knows very little about the underlying causes of specific physiologic events, although the general physiologic principles involved can be described. The true state of the patient cannot usually be measured directly but must be inferred from ambiguous patterns of clinical observations and data from electronic monitors. These data are imperfect because, unlike industrial systems (which are designed and built with sensors in key areas to measure the most important variables), separate, predominantly noninvasive methods are used to measure the variables that are easiest to monitor. Most physiologic functions are observed indirectly through weak signals available at the body surface and thus are prone to various sorts of electrical and mechanical interference. Even the invasive measurements are vulnerable to artifacts and uncertainties of interpretation.

Even if the anesthetist could know the exact patient state, the response of the patient to interventions is extremely variable. Even in "normal" patients, genetic or acquired differences in reflex sensitivity, pharmacokinetics, or pharmacodynamics can yield a wide range of responses to a given dose of drug or to a routine action (e.g., laryngoscopy). In diseased or traumatized patients, or in the presence of acute abnormalities, these responses may be markedly abnormal, and patients may "overreact" or "underreact" to otherwise appropriate actions.

Risky

The decisions and actions taken by anesthetists can contribute to the outcome of the patient. Even for elective surgery the risk of catastrophe is ever-present. Death, brain damage, or other permanent injury are the end-results of many pathways that can begin with fairly innocuous triggering events. Each intervention, even if appropriate, is associated with side effects, some of which are themselves catastrophic. Furthermore, many risks cannot be avoided. Unlike a commercial flight, which can be delayed or aborted if a problem occurs, immediate surgery may be necessary to treat a medical problem that is itself life-threatening. Balancing the risks of the anesthesia and surgery versus the risk of the underlying surgical disease is often extremely difficult.

Models of Crisis Management Must Come from Nonmedical Domains

Where are anesthetists to look for models of how to manage crises? Crisis management is not taught in medical school and it is not a hallmark of most other medical specialties. While crises do occur in surgery, intensive care, emergency room care (including trauma management), and invasive cardiology, none of these fields has addressed the teaching of crisis management systematically. For parallels we must turn to other complex dynamic worlds such as aviation and nuclear power. These industries have directly addressed issues of optimal crisis management performance by the humans "in the loop." In the case of military aviation, the need to optimize human performance systematically has been evident since before World War II and has continued steadily, spurred by the very cogent desire of pilots to stay alive in the air. Commercial aviation learned much from military aviation, and the last 15 years have seen intensified efforts concerning human performance issues in aircrews and air traffic controllers. For nuclear power it was largely the accident at Three Mile Island (and later the Chernobyl catastrophe) that demonstrated the importance of human factors in safe performance. For over a decade all these industries have recognized that maximizing safety and productivity requires an understanding of individual and group cognitive psychology aimed at changing organizational structure, equipment design, operational protocols, and crew training. For example, in 1979 a thorough analysis[6] of 60 airline accidents, including data from cockpit voice and flight data recorders, disclosed lethal decision making errors by individual crew members or inadequate teamwork by crews. These findings were confirmed in detailed simulator studies of flight crews.[7] As a result of these investigations of crew performance, the aviation industry has embraced a training philosophy of cockpit (now called "crew") resource management (CRM).[6,8,9] In CRM training, crews are instructed not only in the "nuts and bolts" of managing crises such as engine fires, but also in how to manage their individual and collective resources to work together optimally as a team. While there is no proof that such training actually improves flight safety, such training courses have now been adopted by most U.S. (and many non-U.S.) commercial air carriers. This book presents a similar perspective on crisis management for anesthetists.

How Do Crises Arise?

A crisis is often perceived as sudden in onset and rapid in development, but, at least in retrospect, one can usually identify an evolution of the crisis from underlying triggering events.

Figure 1-1 illustrates this process. In this model underlying factors lead to specific *triggering events,* which initiate a *problem.* A problem is defined as an abnormal situation that requires the attention of the anesthetist, but is unlikely by itself to harm the patient. Problems can then evolve and, if not detected and corrected by the anesthetist, they may lead to an *adverse outcome* for the patient. We consider this process in detail.

Problems Often Result from Latent Underlying Conditions

The events that trigger problems do not occur at random. They emerge from three sets of underlying conditions: (1) *latent errors,* (2) *predisposing factors,* and (3) *psychological precursors.*

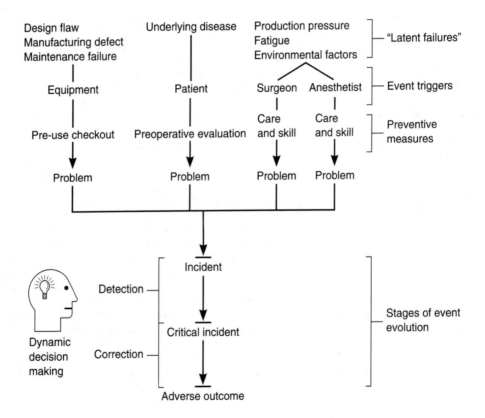

Fig. 1-1. The process by which problems are triggered and then evolve during anesthesia. Interrupting this process can be accomplished by preventive measures or by dynamic detection and correction of the evolving event.

Latent Errors

Latent errors, as described by Reason,[10] are

...errors whose adverse consequences may lie dormant within the system for a long time, only becoming evident when they combine with other factors to breach the system's defenses. [They are] most likely to be spawned by those whose activities are removed in both time and space from the direct control interface: designers, high-level decision makers, construction workers, managers, and maintenance personnel.

Such latent errors exist in all complex systems. Reason describes them as "resident pathogens," which, like microorganisms in the body, remain under control until sets of local circumstances "combine with these resident pathogens in subtle and often unlikely ways to thwart the system's defenses and bring about its catastrophic breakdown"[10] (Fig. 1-2).

In anesthesia, latent errors can result from administrative decisions regarding scheduling of cases, assignment of personnel to staff them, and the priorities given to such things as rapid turnover between cases. They can also result from the design of anesthesia equipment and its user interfaces. Manufacturing defects and failures of routine maintenance are also latent errors.

Predisposing Factors

The external environment constitutes predisposing factors. In aviation the major predisposing factor is weather; in anesthesia they are the patient's underlying diseases and the nature of

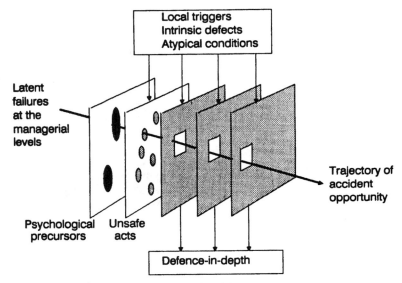

Fig. 1-2. Reason's model of accident causation. Accidents (adverse outcomes) require a combination of latent failures, psychological precursors, event triggers, and failures in several layers of the system's "defense-in-depth." This model is functionally equivalent to that shown in Figure 1-1. (From Reason,[10] with permission.)

the surgery. These will each affect the likelihood of problems arising de novo or in combination with the actions of the anesthetist and the surgeon. The underlying diseases often can be controlled or their effects planned for, but in most circumstances they cannot be eliminated before anesthesia is begun.

Psychological Precursors

The final set of underlying features consists of latent psychological precursors, which predispose the anesthetist or surgeon to commit an unsafe act that triggers a problem. The primary psychological precursors are traditionally referred to as *performance shaping factors,* and include such things as fatigue, boredom, illness, drugs (both prescription drugs and drugs of abuse), and environmental factors such as noise and illumination. These are discussed in detail in a number of review articles,[11-14] and some general strategies to deal with performance shaping factors are discussed in Chapter 2.

Triggering Events

With or without latent underlying conditions, each problem is initiated through one or more triggering events. Historically, anesthetists have been most concerned about events that they create themselves, such as esophageal intubation or drug swaps, but these are relatively rare compared with those events that are triggered in other ways. The triggering events come from (1) the patient, (2) the surgery, (3) the anesthesia, and (4) the equipment.

The Patient

Many problems occur de novo owing to the underlying medical pathology of the patient and independently of any precipitating action. For example, studies of myocardial ischemia in the perioperative period[15-17] demonstrate that ischemia often occurs without any significant change in hemodynamic status.

The Surgery

Surgical stimulus alone is a profound trigger of many physiologic responses, including hypertension, tachycardia, laryngospasm, and bronchospasm. Problems linked to the patient's medical pathology may be precipitated by routine actions of the surgeon. Also, unplanned events such as surgical compression of organs or transection of vital structures can rapidly evolve into serious problems.

The Anesthesia

Induction and maintenance of anesthesia can precipitate problems in patients even in the absence of significant underlying medical disease. Actions or errors on the part of the anesthetist can directly jeopardize the patient, as when central venous cannulation causes a pneumothorax. An operation may require standard but complex maneuvers that may trigger problems, such as turning the patient to the prone position. Especially in patients under general anesthesia and with neuromuscular blockade, the body's own protective mechanisms are blunted or obliterated, making the patient more vulnerable to our actions.

The Equipment

General anesthesia is maintained and the patient's vital functions are monitored by using electromechanical equipment. Should this equipment fail, the patient can suffer irrevocable harm. However, it is very rare for an equipment malfunction, *by itself,* to harm the patient immediately. Examples of this might include electrocution, fires, and airway overpressure events. More typically, an equipment failure stops a life support or monitoring function, which can in theory be performed in another way if the failure is identified and the necessary backup systems are available and functional. Equipment problems often *contribute* to difficulties in handling other problems, either because they usurp the attention of the anesthetist or because the treatment of the main problem requires the use of equipment that itself has failed.

Prevention of Problems

It would seem that eliminating the latent factors that predispose to the occurrence of problems would be an effective strategy to improve patient safety.[10] However, since most of the latent factors affecting anesthesia are the result of a complex evolution of medical economics in combination with historical and political factors, changing them is a difficult, slow, and frustrating process. In addition to latent factors, there are many external circumstances that cannot be controlled. Therefore, the most effective strategy for preventing problems is targeted at individual cases. The anesthetist makes specific checks for triggering factors and makes corrections as necessary. These checks include (1) the patient, (2) the surgeon and anesthetist, and (3) the equipment.

The Patient

The anesthetist begins by using traditional forms of medical decision making in preoperative evaluation of the patient and in planning the anesthetic. During this evaluation the anesthetist considers the patient's medical status and the urgency of the surgery and whether any further treatment can make the patient a better risk. This is a crucial opportunity for the anesthetist to prevent adverse outcomes for the patient. If surgery can proceed, there may still be additional preventive measures that should be implemented to deal with specific medical conditions (e.g., cricoid pressure when the patient's stomach is full) or to prepare for specific surgical procedures (e.g., use of a double lumen tube for thoracic surgery). In Chapter 2 we emphasize the necessity of developing a sound anesthetic plan for the patient that takes each of these measures into account. In many cases, however, there are competing goals, which will prevent a perfect plan from being developed. The optimum plan in such cases must be a compromise between the various risks and benefits.

The Surgeon and Anesthetist

Surgeons and anesthetists have a duty to perform their jobs with appropriate care and skill. They must honestly determine whether their own ability, fitness, and preparation match those demanded by the planned procedure. In Chapter 2 we discuss in detail how anesthetists can deal with possible deteriorations in their performance so as to prevent harm to the patient.

The Equipment

A thorough pre-use checkout of critical life-support equipment is considered mandatory before every anesthetic. In addition, the anesthetist should ensure that appropriate backup equipment is available for all life-critical functions.

Production Pressure

Production pressure[4,5,12,14] is the internal or external pressure on the anesthetist to keep the operating room schedule moving along speedily, with few cancellations and minimum time between cases. When anesthetists succumb to these pressures, they may fail to perform adequate preoperative evaluation and planning or fail to perform adequate pre-use checkout of equipment. Even when preoperative evaluation does take place, overt or covert pressure from surgeons (or others) to proceed with elective cases despite the existence of serious or uncontrolled medical problems can cause anesthetists to do things that they believe to be unsafe.

We recently conducted a randomized survey of California anesthesiologists concerning their experience with production pressures. We found that 49% of respondents had witnessed an event in which patient safety was compromised owing to pressure on the anesthesiologist. Moreover, 32% reported strong to intense pressure from surgeons to proceed with a case they wished to cancel; 36% reported strong to intense internal pressure to "get along with surgeons"; and 45% reported strong pressures to avoid delaying cases. Significantly, 20% agreed with the statement, "If I cancel a case, I might jeopardize working with that surgeon at a later date." The economic pressures are obvious.

Production pressure also leads to *haste* by the anesthetist, which is another psychological precursor to the commission of unsafe acts. In the survey, 20% of respondents answered "sometimes" to the statement, "I have altered my normal practices in order to speed the start of surgery," while 4% answered "often" to this statement, and 20% of respondents rated pressure by surgeons to *hasten* anesthetic preparation or induction as strong or intense.

Problems Will Inevitably Occur
Despite Attempts to Prevent Them

Despite attempts to prevent the occurrence of problems during anesthesia, experience shows that problems of varying severity occur in a large fraction of cases. The exact frequency of problems is not known very accurately. Existing studies probably have underestimated the occurrence of problems because they depended on written reports by the anesthetists of what occurred during the case rather than on real-time, objective recording of the events. Several research groups (including our own) are in the process of videotaping actual clinical care; perhaps these studies will give a better estimate. Despite their limitations, two studies offer some data concerning the frequency of problem events.

In the Multicenter Study of General Anesthesia,[18] 17,201 patients received general anesthesia under specific protocols with random stratification to receive one of four anesthetic techniques (each of the three common volatile anesthetic agents or narcotics plus nitrous oxide). The anesthetists observed the patients for the occurrence of any of a large variety of carefully defined perioperative outcomes, which were adverse events ranging from minor events such as sore throat or hypotension (i.e., systolic blood pressure reduced by more than 20% from baseline) to serious events such as myocardial infarction or death. Based on our definition of a "problem," most of the outcomes measured in this study would constitute a perioperative problem that could evolve to harm the patient. There were 34,926 observed outcomes in the 17,201 patients. Clearly, some patients had more than one outcome while others had none, but 86% of patients had at least one undesirable outcome. Although most events were minor and caused no injury to the patient, over 5% of patients had one or more *severe* events requiring "significant therapy, with or without full recovery." This incidence is probably a lower limit for severe events because the entry criteria of the study excluded critically ill patients and emergency cases in which evolving problems of a severe nature might be even more likely to occur.

In another study by Cooper et al,[19] "impact events," which were "undesirable, unexpected, and could cause at least moderate morbidity," occurred in 18% of patients either in the operating room or in the postanesthesia recovery unit and 3 percent of all cases involved a "serious" event. These too are probably lower limits, since for technical reasons the study excluded patients electively destined for an intensive care unit.

On extrapolating from both of these studies, it seems that at least 20% of cases involve a problem event requiring intervention by the anesthesiologist, while around 5% of cases involve a potentially catastrophic event. The actual frequency of problems may be higher in practice settings with greater than average case complexity. Incidentally, the frequency of serious events in anesthesia is considerably greater than that in aviation by at least several orders of magnitude, since there are about 28,000 commercial flights per day (Aircraft Owners and Pilots Association 1993 Fact Card, Frederick, MD) and there are very few serious incidents or accidents, although the exact number is unknown. The total *accident* rate from *all causes* for commercial flights is 1.2 per 100,000 departures; air carrier accidents with one or more fatalities occur at a rate of 0.36 per 100,000 departures.

How Do Problems *Evolve* into Adverse Outcomes?

Once a problem occurs, there are various possibilities for its future evolution, as shown schematically in Figure 1-3. The problem may be self-limited or may continue to exist without any threat to the patient. It can increase in severity. It can trigger new problems (cross-triggering) within the patient or within the anesthesia/surgery system; the new problems may be more threatening than the original problem. Multiple small problems in several different subsystems can together create a more serious situation than any one of them alone (combination). A problem triggered by one factor may interfere with the management of problems triggered by others (triggered failure of recovery), or it may distract the anesthetist's attention from other, more serious problems.

While there are no universally accepted criteria for categorizing the states of evolution of a perioperative problem, we term the next state an *incident*—a problem that will not resolve on its own and is likely to continue evolving. A *critical* incident is an incident that can *directly* cause an adverse patient outcome. Further information on the nature of critical incidents comes from studies[20-22] performed by Cooper and colleagues at the Massachusetts General Hospital in Boston. These studies pioneered the investigation of incident pathways and have collected data both retrospectively and prospectively on critical incidents, which they defined as

... a human error or equipment failure that could have led (if not discovered or corrected in time) or did lead to an undesirable outcome ranging from length of hospital stay [or increased stay in a recovery room or intensive care unit] to death.

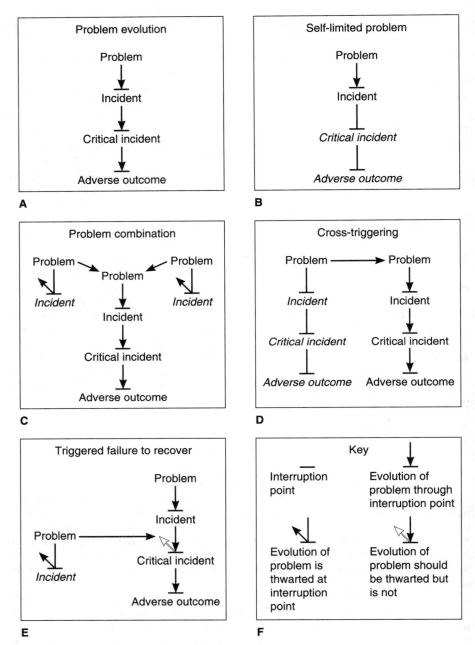

Fig. 1-3. Schematic depiction of five examples of possible pathways for problem evolution and interaction. **(A)** Problem evolution: a single problem evolves into an adverse outcome. **(B)** Self-limited problem: a problem evolves into an incident but fails to evolve into a critical incident *in the absence of any intervention*. **(C)** Problem combination: two typically minor problems combine to trigger a more serious problem. **(D)** Cross-triggering: a problem fails to evolve but triggers a new problem, which does evolve into an adverse outcome. **(E)** Triggered failure to recover: one usually minor problem makes it impossible to interrupt the evolution of another problem. **(F)** Key to symbols.

Each event was categorized as to its primary cause: human error, equipment failure, disconnection (a special type of equipment failure), or other. For human errors a distinction was made between technical errors in performing appropriate actions and judgmental errors in which the actions occurred as planned but were inappropriate. In addition to these categorizations, the authors collected information on a variety of "circumstances that conceivably could have contributed to the occurrence of an error or to a failure to promptly detect an error"; these were termed *associated factors*.

Table 1-1 shows the distribution of the 25 most frequent critical incidents reported in these studies. Note that the true incidence of such events is unknown because the denominator of total cases from which these events were taken is not known. While the distribution of events

Table 1-1. Most Frequent Critical Incidents

Incident Description	Number of Incidents
Breathing circuit disconnection during mechanical ventilation	57
Syringe swap	50
Gas flow control technical error	41
Loss of gas supply	32
Intravenous line disconnection	24
Vaporizer off unintentionally	22
Drug ampule swap	21
Drug overdose (syringe, judgmental)	20
Drug overdose (vaporizer, technical)	20
Breathing circuit leak	19
Unintentional extubation	18
Misplaced endotracheal tube	18
Breathing circuit misconnection	18
Inadequate fluid replacement	15
Premature extubation	15
Ventilator malfunction	15
Misuse of blood pressure monitor	15
Breathing circuit control technical error	15
Wrong choice of airway management technique	13
Laryngoscope malfunction	12
Wrong intravenous line used	12
Hypoventilation (human error only)	11
Drug overdose (vaporizer, judgmental)	9
Drug overdose (syringe, technical)	8
Wrong choice of drug	7
Total	507

(From Cooper et al,[22] with permission.)

may have changed somewhat since the original studies in the late 1970s and mid-1980s, critical incident studies have been repeated in many settings and countries since the original reports of Cooper et al, with similar results.[23-25]

Table 1-2 gives the kinds of associated factors that were found for these critical incidents. As we shall see, these are familiar themes, which provide concrete examples of the latent factors, and the frequency of "failure to check" as an associated factor reinforces our previous discussion of measures to avoid equipment failures.

The Anesthetist Is Responsible for Detecting and Correcting Problems Early in Their Evolution

Discussions of the anesthetist's role in patient safety usually focus on problems triggered by the anesthetist. In truth, the source of a problem is irrelevant; the anesthetist's job is to intervene whenever necessary to alleviate injury to the patient. Clearly, problems that evolve rapidly or whose manifestations are particularly severe incur the gravest danger, but any problem that is not self-limited and that begins to evolve along the pathway to an adverse outcome constitutes a crisis.

Table 1-2. Associated Factors in Critical Incidents

Associated Factor	*Number of Incidents*
Failure to check	223
First experience with situation	208
Inadequate total experience	201
Inattention or carelessness	166
Haste encouraged by situation	131
Unfamiliarity with equipment or device	126
Visual restriction	83
Inadequate familiarity with anesthetic technique	79
Other distractive simultaneous anesthesia activities	71
Teaching in progress	60
Excessive dependency on other personnel	60
Unfamiliarity with surgical procedure	59
Lack of sleep/fatigue	55
Supervisor not present enough	52
Failure to follow personal routine	41
Inadequate supervision	34
Conflicting equipment designs	34
Unfamiliarity with drug	32
Failure to follow institutional practice	31

(From Cooper et al,[22] with permission.)

The primary weapon of crisis management is the *detection* and *correction* of evolving problems, incidents, critical incidents, and adverse outcomes. Reason[10] also described the multiple points of interruption of evolving incidents as "defense-in-depth." As shown in Figure 1-2, adverse outcomes only occur when an incident is triggered as described above, *and* it evolves into a critical incident, *and* the defense-in-depth fails. Ideally the defenses succeed before an adverse outcome occurs, but even if patient injury occurs, the anesthetist must still be involved in mitigating the severity of the injury. Major adverse outcomes (death or permanent injury) following surgery are rare for healthy patients, and complex life-saving surgery can be performed even for patients at high risk. Therefore, anesthetists and the rest of the surgical team are usually, but not always, successful in detecting problems and intervening to correct them prior to patient injury. Understanding this process, which is at the heart of crisis management in anesthesia, is the subject of the rest of this chapter.

Anesthetists Make Complex Decisions During Intraoperative Patient Care

This process of crisis management through the detection and correction of evolving events involves a specialized type of *dynamic decision making.* We will look at the cognitive psychology of individuals and groups as it concerns decision making in anesthesiology. Some of this material is a result of direct extrapolations to anesthesiology from laboratory research in cognitive psychology or from applied research in other complex dynamic worlds. Other parts of it stem from studies on the behavior of anesthesiologists in our laboratory and other laboratories and from our own systematic examination of and introspection on the nature of our work. Our intent in this chapter is to provide you with an introduction to the psychological issues involved in optimal performance by anesthetists.

Decision making in anesthesiology simultaneously involves both the typical decisions of routine care and the nonroutine decisions made during the management of problems or crises. For any given case the anesthetist executes a variety of tasks, including checking equipment, establishing appropriate vascular access, inducing and maintaining anesthesia, securing the airway, positioning the patient, administering drugs as needed, terminating the anesthetic, and either awakening the patient or transporting the patient to the intensive care unit or postanesthesia recovery unit while still anesthetized. In addition, the anesthetist must perform tasks for the surgeon, maintain a clean work space, and interact with the operating room personnel.

How is it possible to do so many things simultaneously in a complex and dynamic environment? The secret involves aspects of information processing that are now well known to cognitive scientists and computer scientists. They are

Parallel processing
   Working at different levels of mental activity
   Performing more than one task simultaneously
Multitasking or multiplexing
   Performing one task at a time, but switching rapidly from one set to another
Iteration
   Performing a sequence of actions repetitively

We will show how expert performance in anesthesia involves these features in a repeated "loop" of observation, decision, action, and re-evaluation. An important feature of this loop is that there is little or no distinction between diagnostic and therapeutic activities.

Decision Making Involves Multiple Levels of Mental Activity

Following the work of Rasmussen,[26,27] we have divided the anesthetist's mental activities into several levels at which the anesthetist is able to operate nearly simultaneously using parallel processing and multitasking. At the *sensorimotor* level, activities involving sensory perception or motor actions take place with minimal conscious control; they are smooth, practiced, and highly integrated patterns of behavior. At the *procedural* level the anesthetist performs regular *subroutines* in a familiar work situation, subroutines that have been derived from previous work episodes. The level of *abstract reasoning* is used primarily in unfamiliar situations for which no well-practiced expertise or subroutine is available from previous encounters.

Anesthetists Must Dynamically Adapt Their Own Thought Processes

We have extended Rasmussen's model by the addition of two levels of mental activity. *Supervisory control* is concerned with dynamic allocation of the anesthetist's finite attention to routine and nonroutine actions, to multiple problems, and to all five cognitive levels. *Resource management* occurs at the highest level of mental activity and deals with the command and control of all available resources. These two levels involve dynamic adaptation of the anesthetist's own thought processes. This ability to "think about thinking" in order to strategically control one's own mental activities, called *metacognition* by psychologists,[28,29] is a very important part of successful anesthesia crisis management.

A Comprehensive Model of Dynamic Decision Making and Crisis Management

On the basis of these concepts we have developed a model (Fig. 1-4) of the thought processes of anesthetists as they administer anesthesia and respond to intraoperative problems. The model is consistent with those developed for other complex dynamic domains.[10,27,30] It involves parallel processing and multitasking at multiple levels of mental activity, with a primary loop of observation, decision, action, and re-evaluation. In the following section we describe this model in detail in order to depict the fundamental psychological elements of expert anesthesia care. The model provides a conceptual framework and a vocabulary for more precisely describing, analyzing, and categorizing the behavior of anesthetists during actual events.

Observation

Management of dynamic situations depends on the anesthetist's responses to many sources of rapidly changing information. These include clinical observation of the patient; a multitude of displays from electronic monitors; visual inspection of the surgical field, the activities of nurses, and suction cannisters and sponges; normal and abnormal sounds of the patient and equipment; and reports of laboratory test results or radiographic interpretations. The attention capacity of the human mind can only attend closely to one or two items at a time. The anesthetist's mental process of supervisory control must decide what information to attend to and how frequently to observe it. Just as pilots flying on instruments must develop a continuous

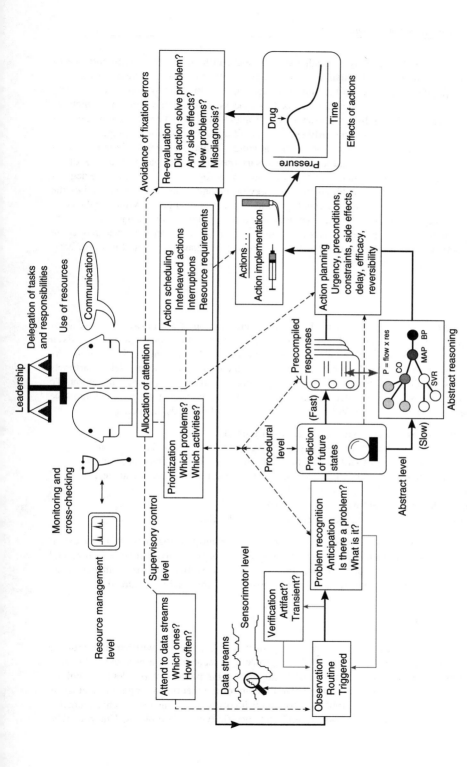

Fig 1-4. Our model of the anesthetist's complex process of intraoperative decision making. As described fully in the text, there are five levels of mental activity. There is a primary loop (heavy black arrows) of *observation, decision, action,* and *re-evaluation*. This loop is controlled by higher levels of supervisory control (allocation of attention) and resource management. P, pressure; res, resistance; CO, cardiac output; SVR, systemic vascular resistance; MAP, mean arterial pressure; BP, blood pressure.

scanning pattern for their displays, anesthetists are taught in their training the importance of scanning their environment. The main difficulty in both domains is to fully interpret the data, not just scan the displays, while still retaining enough capacity to maintain control of a variety of other important tasks (the technical term for this process is *situation awareness,* which we describe in more detail later). In fact, the anesthetist's attention is such a scarce resource that its allocation is extremely important in nearly every aspect of dynamic decision making.

Vigilance is defined as the capacity to *sustain* attention. It plays a crucial role in the observation and detection of problems and thus is a necessary prerequisite for meaningful care of the patient. (It is the motto of the American Society of Anesthesiologists.) Vigilance can be degraded by the performance-shaping factors mentioned previously, and it can be overwhelmed by the sheer amount of information and the rapidity with which it is changing. While vigilance is *essential,* it alone is not enough to preserve patient safety. It is thus a *necessary, but not sufficient, component* of decision making and crisis management. The vigilant observer may err in making observations or in the many steps beyond observation that are required to make decisions and manage crises successfully.

Verification

In the operating room environment the available information is not always reliable. Most monitoring is noninvasive and indirect and is therefore prone to *artifacts* (false data). Even direct clinical observations such as vision or auscultation can be ambiguous. Brief *transients* (true data of short duration), which will quickly correct themselves, can occur. Neither artifacts nor transients should be interpreted as indicating a problem requiring precipitous action. To prevent them from skewing the decision making process, many critical observations must be verified before they are acted on. Verification uses a variety of methods, including

Repeating the observation or observing the short-term trend
Observing an existing redundant channel (e.g., invasive arterial pressure and cuff pressure)
Correlating multiple related variables (e.g., heart rate, heart rhythm, and blood pressure)
Activating a new monitoring modality (e.g., placement of a pulmonary artery catheter)
Recalibrating an instrument or testing its function
Replacing an entire instrument with a backup device
Asking for a second opinion from other anesthetists or technicians

Knowing when and how to verify data is another important metacognitive skill. For example, the anesthetist must decide under what conditions it is useful to invest time, attention, and energy in establishing a new data stream, such as placing a pulmonary artery catheter in the middle of a case, as opposed to relying on more indirect data streams that are already in place.

Problem Recognition

After making and verifying observations, the next step is to decide whether they indicate that the patient's course is "on track" or that a problem is occurring. If a problem is found, a decision must be made as to its nature and importance. This process of problem recognition (also known as *situation assessment*) is a central feature of the theories of cognition that apply to complex dynamic worlds.[10,30] Problem recognition involves matching sets of environmental cues (data) to patterns that are known to represent specific types of problems. Unfortunately, given the high uncertainty seen in anesthesia, the available data streams do not always disclose the existence of a problem, and even when a problem is detected, the cues often do not specify its nature or cause. Therefore, one part of supervisory control involves determining what to do when a clear-cut match or "diagnosis" cannot be made. Anesthetists, like other dynamic decision makers, use approximation strategies to handle these ambiguous situations; psychologists describe these strategies as *heuristics*. One heuristic is to categorize what is happening as one of several generic problems, each of which encompasses many different underlying conditions. Another is to gamble on a single diagnosis (*frequency gambling*[31]), initially choosing the single most frequent candidate event. In preparing for a case, the anesthetist may adjust a mental index of suspicion for recognizing certain specific problems anticipated for that particular patient or surgical procedure. The anesthetist must also decide whether a single underlying diagnosis explains all the data or whether they could be due to multiple causes.[32] This decision is important because excessive attempts to refine the diagnosis can be very costly in terms of allocation of attention.

Use of heuristics is typical of expert anesthetists and often results in considerable time saving in dealing with problems. Like all heuristics, these approaches are two-edged swords. As we will see in the section on re-evaluation of data, both frequency gambling and inappropriate allocation of attention solely to expected problems can seriously derail problem solving when these gambles do not pay off.

Prediction of Future States

Problems must be assessed in terms of their significance for the future states of the patient. Predicting future states[33] based on the occurrence of seemingly trivial problems is a major part of the anticipatory behaviors that characterize expert crisis managers. Those problems that are already critical or that can be predicted to evolve into critical incidents receive the highest priority. Prediction of future states also influences action planning by defining the time frame available for required actions.

Precompiled Responses and Abstract Reasoning

Having recognized a problem, how does the expert anesthetist respond? The classical paradigm of decision making[34] involves a careful comparison of the evidence with various causal hypotheses that could explain it. This is then followed by a careful analysis of all possible actions and solutions to the problem. This approach, while powerful, is relatively slow and does not work well with ambiguous or scanty evidence. Many perioperative problems faced by anesthetists require quick action to prevent a rapid cascade to a catastrophic adverse outcome, and solution of these problems through formal deductive reasoning from first principles is just too slow.

The initial responses of experts to most perioperative events arise from precompiled rules or response plans for dealing with the specific type of event.[10,26,27,31] One model refers to this process as "recognition-primed decision making."[30] In the hands of an experienced practitioner precompiled responses to common problems are retrieved and executed rapidly. During precase planning the experienced anesthetist mentally rearranges and recompiles these responses on the basis of the patient's condition, the surgical procedure, and the problems to be expected. These responses usually are acquired through personal experience alone, although a few that involve major catastrophes (e.g., Advanced Cardiac Life Support) have been explicitly codified and taught systematically. We have demonstrated that the use of optimum response procedures is extremely variable, even among experts. For this reason, we developed the Catalog of Critical Events During Anesthesiology (Chs. 3 through 11) to allow anesthetists to study and practice optimized routines for handling a large variety of events.

On the other hand, even optimized responses are destined to fail when the problem is not due to the suspected etiology or when it does not respond to the usual actions. For this reason (among others), performing anesthesia purely by precompiled "cookbook" procedures is not desirable. Even when quick action must be taken, careful reasoning about the problem using fundamental medical knowledge does take place. This may involve a search for high-level analogies[10] (e.g., "this case is similar to that one last week, except that...") or true deductive reasoning from the deep knowledge base and careful analysis of all possible solutions. When we have studied anesthetists managing simulated crises, they appeared to respond primarily with precompiled plans while linking their course of action to abstract medical concepts.[35,36] Whether this represents merely "self-explanation" or "justification" or true abstract reasoning is unclear, in part because the particular simulated crises they faced did not *require* novel abstract solutions. At this time we do not know the degree to which abstract reasoning is involved in anesthesia crisis management.

Coordination of Activities via Supervisory Control

The anesthesiologist's attention must be divided between many cognitive functions and between many tasks and must often be devoted to more than one problem. In fact, during actual cases we have analyzed the tasks performed by both novice and experienced anesthetists and the mental work load these tasks imposed.[37-39] Not only is there a plethora of tasks, but these tasks can periodically generate enough mental work load to degrade the anesthetist's ability to respond to other events. On the basis of the simulator research, on the work load studies, and on the observation of real anesthesia care, we believe that anesthetists' abilities to modulate their own thinking (metacognition) through supervisory control and resource management are the key components of crisis management.

One aspect of this modulation is the active management of work load. Rather than being totally at the mercy of periods of rising work load the anesthetist takes active steps to prepare for them. Gopher (Position paper, Conference on Human Error in Anesthesia, 1991) and Schneider and Detweiler[40] describe a variety of strategies for work load management.

Distributing work load over time: The expert prepares for future tasks when the current load is low ("preloading") and will delay or shed low-priority tasks when the work load is high. Also, the supervisory controller multiplexes tasks over time as described below.

Distributing work load over resources: When work load cannot be distributed over time and when additional noncompeting resources are available, task loads can be distributed to them. Some resources are internal to the individual anesthetist. For example, a single anesthetist *can* simultaneously ventilate by hand, assess the cardiac rhythm, and discuss patient care with the surgeon. The single anesthetist *cannot* simultaneously insert an intravenous line and ventilate the patient by hand. If performed at the same time, these two tasks must be distributed to different individuals. The anesthetist coordinates this distribution of tasks and supervises their proper execution at the resource management level.

Changing the nature of the task: Many tasks are not fixed; they can be executed to different standards of performance. As these standards are loosened, the work load required to perform them is reduced. For example, during periods of massive blood loss the anesthetist will focus primarily on administering blood and fluids and on monitoring the blood pressure. In such cases less critical tasks such as writing on the anesthesia record will be foregone (off-loaded) to lessen the work load. The acceptable norms of blood pressure will also be widened.

The "supervisory controller" in the mind allocates the scarce resource of *attention* during multitasking. For the anesthetist this supervisory controller must determine how frequently different data streams are observed, what priorities are given to routine tasks versus potential or actual problems, and how to schedule actions so that the necessary attention and motor resources will be available to execute them. Such intensive demands on the anesthetist's attention could easily swamp the available mental resources. Therefore, the ideal anesthetist strikes a balance between acting quickly on every small perturbation (which takes a lot of attention) and adopting a more conservative "wait and see" attitude. This balance must be constantly shifted between these extremes as the situation changes. However, we have observed that during true crisis situations some practitioners show a great reluctance to switch from "business as usual" to "emergency mode" even when serious problems are detected. Erring too far in the direction of "wait and see" can be particularly catastrophic.

Supervisory control and resource management also involve the optimum planning of *actions* and the scheduling of their efficient execution. At any given time there are multiple things to do, each of which is intrinsically appropriate; yet they cannot all be done at once. Each action must be interleaved with the myriad of other activities that are ongoing. The expert anesthetist considers many factors in planning and adapting optimum action sequences, including

Preconditions necessary for carrying out the actions (e.g., it is impossible to measure a thermodilution cardiac output if there is no pulmonary artery catheter in place)
Constraints on the proposed actions (e.g., it is impossible to check the pupils when the head is fully draped in the surgical field)
Side effects of the proposed actions
Rapidity and ease of implementing the actions
Certainty of success of the actions
Reversibility of the actions and the cost of being wrong
Cost of the actions in terms of attention and resources

Experts in other complex dynamic domains (specifically tank commanders and fire chiefs) have been observed to conduct a mental simulation of the actions they are contemplating to determine whether there are hidden flaws in their plans.[41] Although this practice would make sense for anesthetists, we have not yet observed them doing it, perhaps because they are able to execute their actions incrementally, dynamically changing their plans.

Action Implementation

A particular hallmark of anesthesiology is that the decision maker does not just write orders but is involved directly in the implementation of actions. Executing these actions requires substantial attention and may in fact impair the anesthetist's physical ability to perform other activities (e.g., when an action requires a sterile procedure). In performing actions a variety of errors of execution, termed *slips*, may occur. These are actions that do not occur as planned, such as turning the wrong switch or making a syringe swap. Norman[42] has categorized errors of this type as

Capture error: A common action taking over from the one intended (e.g., a "force of habit")
Description error: Performing the correct action on the wrong target (e.g., flipping the wrong switch)
Memory error: Forgetting an item in a sequence
Sequence error: Performing an action out of sequence from other actions
Mode error: Actions appropriate for one mode of operation but incorrect in another mode, (thus, the BAG/VENTILATOR selector valve on the breathing circuit selects one of two modes of ventilation; failure to activate the ventilator when in the VENTILATOR mode can be catastrophic)

Some of the risks due to slips in anesthesia have been addressed through the use of *engineered safety devices*, which physically prevent incorrect actions. For example, newer anesthesia machines have interlocks that physically prevent the simultaneous administration of more than one volatile anesthetic agent. Other interlocks physically prevent the selection of a gas mixture containing less than 21% oxygen.

Current designs of medical equipment do not always make it easy for anesthetists to implement the actions they have chosen. These complex issues of human-machine interaction are beyond the scope of this book, but they are being addressed by a number of investigators.[43–47]

Re-evaluation

Successful dynamic problem solving under uncertainty requires the supervisory control level to initiate frequent re-evaluation of the situation. The initial diagnosis and situation assessment can be incorrect, especially when the available cues do not precisely identify a problem. Even actions that are appropriate to the problem are not always successful and sometimes cause serious side effects. Furthermore, there is often more than one problem to deal with at a time. Only by frequently reassessing the situation can the anesthetist adapt to dynamically changing circumstances. The re-evaluation process returns the anesthetist to the "observation" step, but with specific assessments in mind:

> Did the actions have any effect (e.g., did the drug reach the patient)?
> Is the problem getting better, or is it getting worse?
> Are there any side effects resulting from previous actions?
> Are there any other problems or new problems that were missed before?
> Was the initial situation assessment or diagnosis correct?

As we described previously, the process of continually updating the situation assessment and of monitoring the efficacy of chosen actions is termed *situation awareness*, a concept that has been used extensively in aviation.[33, 48–50]

Fixation Errors

Faulty re-evaluation, inadequate plan adaptation, and loss of situation awareness can each result in a type of human error termed a *fixation error*.[51,52] This type of error is extremely common in dynamic situations. Fixation errors were prominent among the performance failures observed by our laboratory's studies of anesthesiologists' responses to simulated critical incidents[35,36,53] and occurred among both novice residents and experienced practitioners. Similar results were found by Schwid and O'Donnell[54] using a computer-screen-only anesthesia simulator. In this study certain fixation errors prevented anesthesiologists from correctly managing lethal situations (e.g., anaphylaxis).

Incorrect initial diagnoses are to be expected given the complexity and uncertainty of the data available to the anesthetist. What makes a fixation error is the *persistent* failure to revise a diagnosis or plan in the face of readily available evidence that suggests a revision is necessary. There are three main types of fixation error[51,52] that should be carefully understood, namely

This and only this

The persistent failure to revise a diagnosis or plan despite plentiful evidence to the contrary

The available evidence interpreted to fit the initial diagnosis

Attention allocated to a minor aspect of a major problem

Everything but this

The persistent failure to *commit* to the definitive treatment of a major problem

An extended search for information made without ever addressing potentially catastrophic conditions

Everything's OK

The persistent belief that no problem is occurring in spite of plentiful evidence that it is

Abnormalities attributed to artifacts or transients

Failure to declare an emergency or accept help when facing a major crisis

Resource Management

The concept of resource management is borrowed directly from the domain of aviation. It encompasses the ability of the anesthetist to command and control *all* the resources at hand in order to execute the anesthesia as planned and to respond to problems that arise. This is, in essence, the ability to translate the *knowledge* of what needs to be done into effective team *activity* in the complex and ill-structured *real world* of the operating room. It is not enough for the anesthetist to know what to do or even to be able to do each task alone. The anesthetist can only accomplish so much in a given time, and there are some tasks that must be performed by others (e.g., laboratory tests, radiography). When the task load exceeds the resources available, the anesthetist must mobilize help and distribute the tasks among those present. Many issues concerning optimum teamwork are not yet well understood, although the study of teamwork is currently a very active area of research by cognitive scientists and experts in many complex and dyanamic worlds.[55] But research in aviation *has* already demonstrated that effective resource management is an important component of teamwork by the cockpit crew.[6,8,29,56–58] The hallmarks of resource management derived from these studies are

Prioritization of tasks

Distribution of work load

Communication

Mobilization and use of all available resources

Monitoring and cross-checking; utilization of all available data

Our simulator studies[35,36,53,59] of anesthesiologists responding to critical incidents showed that even when they recognized a problem and had decided on medically reasonable actions, their resource management skills were often very weak. We consider these skills to be so important that they form a major component of the principles of anesthesia crisis resource management described in Chapter 2.

The Model of Decision Making Maps the Pathways for Poor Crisis Management

Why is it important to understand these abstract ideas of cognitive science? What good is this material to the practicing anesthetist? This model of the anesthetist's thought processes

Table 1-3. Examples of Mapping Intraoperative Occurrences to the Model of Dynamic Decision Making

Example Occurrence	*Possible Failures in Components of Dynamic Decision Making*
Decreasing blood pressure not noticed	Poor allocation of attention, perhaps due to distractions or excessive work load Vigilance failure, perhaps due to fatigue or boredom Human-machine interaction problem
Decreasing pressure noticed but not believed to be true	Verification failure "Cry wolf" syndrome, fixation error of "Everything's OK"
Hypotension assumed to be true but not to be a problem	Failure in problem recognition or situation assessment Fixation error of "Everything's OK"
Hypotension noted to be a problem but not of high priority	Failure in prioritization
Hypotension thought to be important but no action taken	Failure in precompiled responses (lacking) Failure of abstract reasoning to support precompiled responses
Actions taken grossly ineffective or time-wasting	Poor action planning Fixation error of "Everything but this" (failure of commitment)
Actual cause of hypotension (e.g., pulmonary overpressure) different from that initially assumed (e.g., hypovolemia)	Failure of re-evaluation Failure to use all available data Fixation error of "This and only this"
Good diagnosis, good plans, ineffective team performance	Failure of resource management

should help the anesthetist identify successful and unsuccessful case management behaviors. Table 1-3 gives examples of how the model of decision making maps occurrences to possible underlying mental failures. Each element of both successful and unsuccessful crisis management has its roots not in the peculiar failures of a few aberrant practitioners but rather in the intrinsic nature of the psychology of dynamic decision making under time pressure and stress. An important step in improving patient care is the careful evaluation of the various aspects of human performance that can be improved by changes in the selection and training of anesthetists, by continued education of practitioners, or by alterations in operational systems and policies.

In Chapter 2 we take some of the lessons that we have learned from analyzing the behavior of anesthetists and apply them to a set of specific principles of anesthesia crisis resource management. We draw from our model of decision making and concentrate on the levels of supervisory control and resource management. We give specific advice on how to avoid the various pitfalls in dynamic decision making. These principles, if integrated into anesthetists' practices, should bring them closer to the ideal as crisis managers.

References

1. Webster's New World Dictionary. 3rd College Ed. Simon & Schuster, New York, 1988
2. Gaba DM: Dynamic decision-making in anesthesiology: cognitive models and training approaches. p. 122. In Evans DA, Patel VL (eds): Advanced Models of Cognition for Medical Training and Practice. Springer-Verlag, Berlin, 1992
3. Woods DD: Coping with complexity: the psychology of human behavior in complex systems. p. 128. In Goodstein LP, Andersen HB, Olsen SE (eds): Tasks, Errors, and Mental Models. Taylor & Francis, London, 1988
4. Perrow C: Normal Accidents. Basic Books, New York, 1984
5. Gaba DM, Maxwell M, DeAnda A: Anesthetic mishaps: breaking the chain of accident evolution. Anesthesiology 66:670, 1987
6. Jensen RS, Biegelski CS: Cockpit resource management. p. 176. In Jensen RS (ed): Aviation Psychology. Gower Technical, Aldershot, UK, 1989
7. Ruffell-Smith HP: A simulator study of the interaction of pilot workload with errors, vigilance, and decisions. National Aeronautics and Space Administration, Washington, DC, 1979
8. Orlady HW, Foushee HC: Cockpit resource management training. NASA Conference Publication 2455. National Aeronautics and Space Administration, Washington, DC, 1987
9. Helmreich RL, Wilhelm JA, Gregorich SE, Chidester TR: Preliminary results from the evaluation of cockpit resource management training: performance ratings of flight crews. Aviat Space Environ Med 61:576, 1990
10. Reason JT: Human Error. Cambridge University Press, Cambridge, 1990
11. Paget JBR, Lambert TF, Sridhar K: Factors affecting an anaesthetist's work: some findings on vigilance and performance. Anaesth Intensive Care 9:359, 1981
12. Gaba DM: Human error in anesthetic mishaps. Int Anesthesiol Clin 27:137, 1989
13. Weinger MB, Englund CE: Ergonomic and human factors affecting anesthetic vigilance and monitoring performance in the operating room environment. Anesthesiology 73:995, 1990
14. Gaba DM: Human performance issues in anesthesia patient safety. Probl Anesth 5:329, 1991
15. Slogoff S, Keats AS: Does perioperative myocardial ischemia lead to postoperative myocardial infarction? Anesthesiology 62:107, 1985
16. Slogoff S, Keats AS: Further observations on perioperative myocardial ischemia. Anesthesiology 65:539, 1986
17. Knight AA, Hollenberg M, London MJ et al: Perioperative myocardial ischemia: importance of preoperative ischemic pattern. Anesthesiology 68:681, 1988

18. Forrest JB, Cahalan MK, Rehder K: Multicenter study of general anesthesia. II. Results. Anesthesiology 72:262, 1990
19. Cooper JB, Cullen DJ, Nemeskal R et al: Effects of information feedback and pulse oximetry on the incidence of anesthesia complications. Anesthesiology 67:686, 1987
20. Cooper JB, Newbower RS, Long CD, McPeek B: Preventable anesthesia mishaps: a study of human factors. Anesthesiology 49:399, 1978
21. Cooper JB, Long CD, Newbower RS, Philip JH: Critical incidents associated with intraoperative exchanges of anesthesia personnel. Anesthesiology 56:456, 1982
22. Cooper JB, Newbower RS, Kitz RJ: An analysis of major errors and equipment failures in anesthesia management: considerations for prevention and detection. Anesthesiology 60:34, 1984
23. Utting JE, Gray TC, Shelley FC: Human misadventure in anaesthesia. Can Anaesth Soc J 26:472, 1979
24. Craig J, Wilson ME: A survey of anaesthetic misadventures. Anaesthesia 36:933, 1981
25. Chopra V, Bovill JG, Spierdijk J: Accidents, near accidents and complications during anaesthesia. A retrospective analysis of a 10-year period in a teaching hospital. Anaesthesia 45:3, 1990
26. Rasmussen J: Skills, rules, and knowledge: signals, signs, and symbols, and other distinctions in human performance models. IEEE Trans Syst Man Cybernet SMC 13:257, 1983
27. Rasmussen J: Information processing and human-machine interaction: an approach to cognitive engineering. Elsevier Science, New York, 1986
28. Orasanu J: Shared mental models and crew decision making. Princeton University Cognitive Science Laboratory, Princeton University, Princeton, NJ, 1990
29. Orasanu JM: Decision making in the cockpit. p. 137. In Wiener E, Kanki B, Helmreich R (eds): Cockpit Resource Management. Academic Press, New York, 1993
30. Klein GA: Recognition-primed decisions. Adv Man Machine Syst Res 5:47, 1989
31. Reason J: Generic error-modeling system (GEMS): a cognitive framework for locating common human error forms. p. 63. In Rasmussen J, Duncan K, Leplat J (eds): New Technology and Human Error. Wiley, Chichester, UK, 1987
32. Woods DD, Roth EM, Pople H Jr: Cognitive environment simulation: an artificial intelligence system for human performance assessement. U.S. Nuclear Regulatory Commission, Washington, DC, 1987
33. Sarter NB, Woods DD: Situation awareness: a critical but ill-defined phenomenon. Int J Aviat Psychol 1:45, 1991
34. Orasanu J, Connolly T: The reinvention of decision making. p. 3. In Klein G, Orasanu J, Calderwood R (eds): Decision Making in Action: Models and Methods. Ablex Publishing, Norwood, NJ, 1993
35. Gaba DM, DeAnda A: The response of anesthesia trainees to simulated critical incidents. Anesth Analg 68:444, 1989
36. DeAnda A, Gaba DM: The role of experience in the response to simulated critical incidents. Anesth Analg 72:308, 1991
37. Dallen L, Nguyen L, Zornow M et al: Task analysis/workload of anesthetists performing general anesthesia, abstracted. Anesthesiology 73:A498, 1990
38. Gaba DM, Herndon OW, Zornow MH et al: Task analysis, vigilance, and workload in novice residents, abstracted. Anesthesiology 75:A1060, 1991
39. Herndon O,Weinger M, Paulus M et al: Analysis of the task of administering anesthesia: additional objective measures, abstracted. Anesthesiology 75:A47, 1991
40. Schneider W, Detweiler M: The role of practice in dual-task performance: toward workload modeling in a connectionist/control architecture. Hum Factors 30:539, 1988
41. Klein GA, Calderwood R, Macgregor D: Critical decision method for eliciting knowledge. IEEE Trans Syst Man Cybernet SMC 19:462, 1989
42. Norman DA: Categorization of action slips. Psychol Rev 88:1, 1981
43. Norman DA: The Psychology of Everyday Things. Basic Books, New York, 1988
44. Cook RI, Woods DD, McDonald JS, Potter S: Human factors standards for operating room equipment: do they work? Does it matter?, abstracted. Anesthesiology 71:A335, 1989
45. Woods DD, Cook RI, Sarter N, McDonald JS: Mental models of anesthesia equipment operation: implications for patient safety, abstracted. Anesthesiology 71:A983, 1989

46. Cook RI, Woods DD, McDonald JS: Human Performance in Anesthesia: A Corpus of Cases. Cognitive Systems Engineering Laboratory, Department of Industrial and Systems Engineering, Ohio State University, Columbus, Ohio, 1991

47. Cook RI, Woods DD, Howie MB: Unintentional delivery of vasoactive drugs with an electromechanical infusion device. J Cardiothorac Anesth 6:238, 1991

48. Endsley MR: Design and evaluation for situation awareness enhancement. p. 97. In Proceedings of the Human Factors Society Thirty-second Annual Meeting. Human Factors Society, Santa Monica, 1988

49. Tenney YJ, Adams MJ, Pew RW et al: A principled approach to the measurement of situation awareness in commercial aviation (NASA Contractor Report 4451). National Aeronautics and Space Administration, Washington, DC, 1992

50. Gaba DM, Howard SK, Small S: Situation awareness in anesthesiology. Submitted to Human Fact (Feb 1993)

51. DeKeyser V, Woods DD, Masson M, Van Daele A: Fixation errors in dynamic and complex systems: descriptive forms, psychological mechanisms, potential countermeasures. Technical Report for NATO Division of Scientific Affairs, Brussels, Belgium, 1988

52. DeKeyser V, Woods DD: Fixation errors: failures to revise situation assessment in dynamic and risky systems. p. 231. In Colombo AG, Bustamante AS (eds): Systems Reliability Assessment. Kluwer Academic Publishers, Dordrecht, Germany, 1990

53. DeAnda A, Gaba DM: Unplanned incidents during comprehensive anesthesia simulation. Anesth Analg 71:77, 1990

54. Schwid HA, O'Donnell D: Anesthesiologists' management of simulated critical incidents. Anesthesiology 76:495, 1992

55. Swezey RW, Salas E: Teams: Their Training and Performance. Ablex Publishing, Norwood, NJ, 1992

56. Foushee HC, Helmreich RL: Group interaction and flight crew performance. p. 189. In Wiener EL, Nagel DC (eds): Human Factors in Aviation. Academic Press, San Diego, 1988

57. Helmreich RL: Theory underlying CRM training: psychological issues in flight crew performance and crew coordination. p. 15. In Orlady HW, Foushee HC (eds): Cockpit Resource Management Training (NASA Conference Publication 2455). National Aeronautics and Space Administration, Washington, DC, 1986

58. Orasanu J, Salas E: Team decision making in complex environments. p. 327. In Klein G, Orasanu J, Calderwood R (eds): Decision Making in Action: Models and Methods. Ablex Publishing, Norwood, NJ, 1993

59. Howard SK, Gaba DM, Fish KJ et al: Anesthesia crisis resource management training: teaching anesthesiologists to handle critical incidents. Aviat Space Environ Med 63:763, 1992

Chapter Two
Principles of Anesthesia Crisis Resource Management

Resource Management Is a Crucial Skill for Anesthetists

Successful conduct of anesthesia depends on more than just having the requisite medical knowledge and technical skills. These must be translated into effective *management* of the situations that arise using the cognitive knowledge and skills discussed in Chapter 1. In this chapter we turn those abstract concepts into a set of practical principles to guide you in improving or refreshing your case management skills. These principles should be useful for any anesthesia case, but they are particularly important in difficult or complex cases and in other "crisis" situations. The principles revolve around the identification and optimal use of a variety of *resources* that are available in the operating room.

What Are *Resources*?

Your work environment contains many individuals and many things that you must coordinate to manage the patient optimally. Some resources are obvious, such as the anesthesia machine; others are not very obvious, such as use of the scrub nurse to perform manual ventilation during a major catastrophe. You are very unlikely to identify all the relevant resources in the heat of the moment unless you have given them some serious thought beforehand.

Resources can be categorized as self, operating room personnel, equipment, cognitive aids, external resources, and plans. We discuss each of these in detail below.

Self

Your professional knowledge and skills are your most important resource because they enable you to take direct action to protect the patient or to supervise the use of the other resources at your disposal. However, like all resources, the self-resource is neither omnipotent nor inexhaustible. Many factors will limit your ability to care for the patient optimally. As discussed in the previous chapter, your *attention* is a scarce resource, and you must learn to use it wisely. A significant part of these principles of crisis management will address ways in which you can best divide your attention between the various tasks at hand and between the various problems you face.

Remember too, that as a human your performance is not constant. It will vary both over the course of a day and from day to day, and it is affected by many performance-shaping factors such as fatigue, stress, illness, and medication. Fortunately, good anesthesia practice does not typically demand peak human performance, but *any* case could call on more personal reserves than you have available.

The responsibility for providing good patient care is yours. You should be sensitive to any degradation of yourself as a resource, whether you detect it yourself or are told about it by others. You must respond appropriately to changes in your performance status; a patient should never suffer for your decision to "tough it out." No one will thank you for going ahead with a case if you cannot do your job properly and a catastrophe then ensues.

What can you do if you find that your performance is lagging? Under some circumstances, if you are ill, sleepy, or preoccupied with a personal matter, you may need to postpone the case or insist that someone replace you. The organizational structure of your practice should provide for such situations. If your ability is less severely degraded, you may still need to mobilize additional resources to maintain adequate performance levels. You could, for example, ask a colleague to assist you with particularly difficult parts of a case, or you could alert the circulating nurse to be ready to help you more than usual. You might also set the alarm limits on your monitors more stringently than you otherwise would and raise their audio volume to alert you to potential problems at an earlier stage. For impairments linked to your overall level of arousal (such as fatigue or illness) you might act in ways that raise your arousal level, such as standing throughout the case or conversing with operating room personnel.

Hazardous Attitudes and Production Pressure

Your *attitudes* are an important component of your abilities. They can affect your performance just as strongly as physiologic performance-shaping factors. Psychologists studying judgment in aviators have identified five attitude types as being particularly *hazardous,* and they have developed specific antidote thoughts for each hazardous attitude[1] (Table 2-1). Aviation psychologists instruct pilots to actually verbalize the antidote thought whenever they find themselves thinking in a hazardous way.

Table 2-1. Examples of Hazardous Attitudes and Their Antidotes

Hazardous Attitude	*Antidote*
Antiauthority: "Don't tell me what to do. The policies are for someone else."	"Follow the rules. They are usually right."
Impulsivity: "Do something quickly—anything!"	"Not so fast. Think first."
Invulnerability: "It won't happen to me. It's just a routine case."	"It *could* happen to me. Even routine cases develop serious problems."
Macho: "I'll show you I can do it. I can intubate anybody."	"Taking chances is foolish. Plan for failure."
Resignation: "What's the use? It's out of my hands. It's up to the surgeon."	"I'm not helpless. I can make a difference. There is always something else to try that might help."

(Adapted from Aeronautical Decision Making,[1] with permission.)

The invulnerability and macho attitudes are particularly hazardous for anesthetists. The belief that a catastrophe "cannot happen to me" and that your expert performance allows you to do anything can make you cavalier about planning and executing patient care. It can alter your thresholds for believing abnormal data or for recognizing problems, thereby leading to the fixation error of "everything's OK."

Hazardous attitudes are compounded by production pressures to do more cases in less time with fewer cancellations and with less opportunity for preoperative evaluation. The economic and social realities of practice can cause these pressures to become *internalized* by anesthetists, who then develop hazardous attitudes they might otherwise have resisted. For example, the surgeon would no longer need to overtly push you to go ahead with a case that should be cancelled if you have already altered your own approach to conform to the surgeon's wishes. Of course, there will be valid reasons to go ahead with a questionable case when medical urgency demands it. Under these conditions the usual protocols for elective case management must be adapted. In the final analysis *you* must ensure that the patient's benefit is the primary criterion in such decisions, and you should establish a bottom line of safe planning, pre-use checkout of equipment, and patient preparation beyond which you will not be pushed. For example, it is dangerous to bring a patient from a critical care area (such as an emergency room) to an operating room in which the equipment has not been checked for faults. Once again, even if surgeons and administrators have pressured you to proceed, they will *not* thank you if the patient suffers, nor will they come to your defense during litigation.

To simplify these decisions you may wish to develop written consensus guidelines in conjunction with your colleagues in anesthesia, surgery, medicine, and pediatrics. This approach would be analogous to pre-established "go / no go" mission rules used for manned spaceflights, which are intended to take the decision away from the pressures of the "heat of the moment." The guidelines could address the appropriate workup for patients with various medical conditions in different surgical urgency categories and could also incorporate recommendations for resolving disputes concerning the risks and benefits of proposed surgery.[2] Nearly two-thirds of the anesthesiologists responding to our survey of California anesthesiologists thought that such guidelines could yield improvements in patient safety.

Operating Room Personnel

The other members of the operating room team are also important resources. The surgeon and anesthetist share responsibility for the patient, but it is the surgery that actually provides definitive benefits to the patient. The surgeon may know the patient well and may be able to give you important information about underlying medical or surgical conditions that could not be obtained from the patient or from the chart. Most surgeons are also more capable than you are to perform many important technical procedures that might be needed to manage a crisis.

Nursing and technical staff each have a duty to safeguard the patient by using the specialized knowledge and skills within their defined scope of knowledge. Making effective use of them as resources, while not exceeding their limits, is essential to achieving good outcomes. As we shall see, *every* person in the operating room can help you manage a complex situation.

Equipment

Anesthesia care in the industrial world requires considerable equipment, including gas delivery systems, ventilators, infusion pumps, and monitors. Clinical observation and direct manipulation of the patient are important skills for anesthetists, but they are not enough for optimal practice. The optimum will occur when *every* piece of information, *every* action, and *every* piece of equipment is used to its best advantage. In order to achieve this goal the anesthetist must

Ensure that the relevant routine equipment is present, is appropriately maintained, and is working properly
Ensure that critical backup equipment is immediately available
Know how to operate the basic functions of each piece of equipment and know the operating characteristics of the device in both normal and abnormal circumstances
Be careful not to make errors in using the equipment and to correct those errors that do occur

In commercial aviation, pilots are type rated and can only fly aircraft of the type for which they are certified. For example a captain type rated only for a Boeing 737 cannot act in any cockpit crew capacity on a Boeing 727 regardless of the number of hours of total flying experience. Furthermore, aircrews receive extensive training in the operation of the aircraft's systems. Both the literature[3] and our own experience as clinicians and teachers suggest that many anesthetists are not well versed in the operation of their equipment. These devices are the tools of our trade, and knowing how to use them is just as important as, if not more important than, knowing about physiology and pharmacology. It is your responsibility to acquire this knowledge and skill. The operation of many devices is not intuitive, and there are often hidden pitfalls in their operation that can lead to a failure to function properly. While many investigators (including ourselves) are attempting to address these difficulties, they will never be solved completely, which makes it all the more important for you to be well versed in the individual operational features of your equipment.

Cognitive Aids

There are a variety of written and mechanical aids[4] immediately at hand to help you think during patient care. They relieve you of having to memorize every piece of information that might be needed for all possible cases. The medical record, for example, contains a wealth of information about the patient's current and past medical history, as well as the results of laboratory and radiologic tests. Your anesthetic record is another important source of information, especially if you have not been present for the entire case. Recognize that your memory is imperfect. Never be afraid to double-check your recollection of important data with the written source. Additional case information may also be obtained from the data stored as trends within the monitoring equipment in use.

The extensive range of pharmaceuticals used by anesthetists is supported by a variety of aids. The labels on drug ampules and syringes are important cognitive cues. Using ampules or vials with labels that meet legibility standards and using standardized printed syringe labels may reduce the likelihood of medication errors in the operating room.[5]

Each drug also comes with a package insert containing extensive information on the drug's characteristics. These are compiled in the widely available *Physicians' Desk Reference* (Medical Economics Data, Montvale, NJ). Many anesthetists also use written tables and lists that contain information on the preparation of drug infusions and their appropriate dose ranges. Calculators and computers can be used to compute dosing regimens or to control infusion pumps directly.

Manuals, checklists, and written protocols are also available to guide the checkout and operation of equipment. There are a few protocols for the management of events such as malignant hyperthermia. However, the use of such aids in anesthesia is minimal compared with that in aviation. The Catalog of Critical Events in Anesthesiology (Section II) can also be used as a cognitive aid during case management. Reference works and handbooks contain a wealth of useful information on the medical and anesthetic management of virtually every type of condition.

Where such aids are not currently available we encourage you to design and produce your own to help you optimize your ability to manage crisis situations.

External Resources

In most centers in which surgery is performed (hospitals and stand-alone outpatient surgery centers) there are many *external* resources available to assist you in preventing or managing adverse events (this may not be true in physician offices). These resources include laboratory services, blood bank, radiology, consulting physicians (most commonly used for crisis management are cardiologists and neurologists), engineers, risk managers, and administrators. You must consider in advance how you will mobilize these resources. Where are resources physically located? What communication systems exist and how do you use them?

Regional and national resources also exist. A good example is the malignant hyperthermia (MH) hotline (209-634-4917), which can provide expert advice in the management of patients with suspected MH susceptibility or with full-blown MH. Other external resources include the telephone technical support offered by poison control centers and by many manufacturers of drugs and equipment. The Manufacturers' Index section of the *Physicians' Desk Reference* lists these numbers for most drug manufacturers.

All physicians can now obtain computer access to the National Library of Medicine's MED-LINE index, providing an instantaneous search capability of the world's medical literature. Any medical librarian should be able to conduct a search on your behalf or to assist you in obtaining an account.

Plans

Resources can be mobilized and used "on the fly," but the best use of resources requires advance planning. The plans themselves become key resources, since they enable you to manipulate the situation more quickly. Appropriate plans come in three forms: *global plans* for resource mobilization in a specific work <u>environment</u>; an *anesthetic plan* for dealing with the particular problems of a specific <u>patient</u>; and generalized *emergency procedures* for the management of <u>critical incidents</u>. A good program of quality assurance (also known as quality improvement or total quality management) is of enormous value to all forms of planning. It is the mechanism by which knowledge of past adverse events can be translated into changes in practice that minimize their recurrence.

Global plans should incorporate a detailed knowledge of each environment in which you care for patients, whether it is an operating room, a postanesthesia care unit, or a remote setting such as a magnetic resonance imaging suite. The equipment and external resources available in each setting may differ, and you will *not* be able to use them effectively unless you plan in advance. Know the contents of your anesthesia carts, including emergency use items such as flashlights, resuscitation drugs, and pressure infusion sets. Know the location and operating characteristics of emergency equipment. Learn to operate the available defibrillators. Examine the contents of the crash carts to assure yourself that you will have what you need to resuscitate a patient. Know what other equipment exists and where it is located, such as spare oxygen cylinders and regulators, MH kits, equipment to manage the difficult airway, spare flashlights, fire extinguishers, and battery-powered monitors. Think about the location of critical external resources such as satellite laboratories or pharmacy stations so that you can instruct runners how to get back and forth. Know how to call for help and how to call a "code" in the event of a cardiac arrest or other major emergency. Every facility has its own procedures and code alert language. Find out who will respond to a code both day and night. If you are not sure whom to contact, call the facility's telephone operator (usually dial 0), or if necessary, dial 911 (in the United States) to reach the dispatcher for paramedic, police, and fire departments.

Construction of the Anesthetic Plan

Preoperative evaluation of the patient and construction of a suitable anesthetic plan is an important task that you perform to prevent the occurrence of events that can evolve into adverse outcomes. The plan delineates how you will conduct the anesthetic, how you will deal with the problems you are likely to face, and what other resources you must mobilize to meet the anesthetic goals for the case. A sound plan matches the anesthetic technique to the patient's disease state, the technical requirements of surgery (e.g., position of the patient), the anesthesia equipment available, and the skills of the anesthetist. It also includes specific backup procedures and contingency plans to be used if the original plans fail. Faulty plans tend to occur when underlying disease states either go undetected or are ignored because of inadequate data gathering during preoperative evaluation. Poor planning may also result from the invulnerability type of hazardous attitude. A faulty anesthetic plan will expose the patient to risk even if it is carried out perfectly.

Generalized Emergency Procedures

Systematically prepared emergency procedures are used in virtually all complex dynamic work environments, not because the operators are ignorant, but because experience has shown that even well-trained, intelligent people need support during rapidly changing problem situations. Every licensed pilot (including the purely recreational pilot) is taught specific emergency procedures for a variety of contingencies. In the case of large commercial aircraft the emergency procedure manuals are quite extensive. Pilots are expected to memorize certain critical portions of each procedure and then to rely on the manual (and *not* on their memory) for the rest of the procedure. Airline pilots practice these procedures regularly during simulator-based recurrent training programs.

The situation in anesthesiology has been considerably different. The responses to only a few extremely severe events (e.g., cardiopulmonary resuscitation, MH) are taught in a formal fashion. For the most part, anesthesiologists are expected to learn responses to adverse events solely by experiencing them. Each teaching anesthetist may have a favorite "clinical pearl" concerning emergency responses to hand down to trainees, but few pass these on consistently. For most practitioners serious adverse events are uncommon, and even those responses that were once second nature are soon forgotten for lack of use. It is for this reason that we created the Catalog of Critical Events in Anesthesiology for this volume (Chs. 3 through 11).

Briefings

For planning to be most effective it should ensure the coordination of all members of the patient care team. Every anesthetist is part of an operating room team, which involves surgeons, nurses, and various other technical personnel. Aspects of the surgical procedure, such as the desired patient position and the extent of planned dissection may alter the plan; if these are not clearly defined on the surgical schedule, the surgeons must be consulted. If predictable problems might necessitate changing plans or aborting the procedure, this should be specifically discussed in advance with the surgical team. Many anesthetists also work as part of an anesthesia care team, whether made up of certified registered nurse anesthetists and anesthesiologists or of residents and faculty. For these teams it is equally imperative that the members agree on a plan before starting the anesthesia. When a case is routine and the team members are familiar with each other, this agreement may be achieved with few if any words. When a case is complex, when team members are inexperienced, or when they are unfamiliar with each other, the plan should be reviewed in detail. In these briefings it is important to consider appropriate contingency plans and who will determine when to switch from the initial plan to a backup one.

Case Management Behaviors

The discussion of resources should help you *prepare* to provide good anesthesia care at any time. We now turn to the question of how to act optimally *during* intraoperative patient management. Every strategy that you might choose is a two-edged sword, ideal for some situations but inadequate for others. Optimal care therefore requires constantly balancing and adapting your behavior to the changing situation.

Anticipation

We have stressed the need to anticipate the requirements of a case in advance. One aspect of this is to have a high index of suspicion for the medical problems that you might expect to encounter because of a patient's underlying diseases. You should look for these and make advance preparations to treat them. However, the risk of this strategy is that other problems that mimic the one you expect may in fact occur. It is important to keep an open mind and to make sure that you consider other possibilities (see discussion of re-evaluation below in the section on Crisis Management).

Throughout the case you need to maintain awareness of every change that occurs in your environment. As mentioned in Chapter 1, pilots call this "situation awareness"; another term is "staying ahead of the game." You can easily fall behind if the situation changes radically or quickly or if you fail to devote sufficient resources to meet the changes. When you find yourself getting seriously behind the events of a case, regardless of the reason, you *must* either slow down the progress of the case (e.g., ask the surgeon to hold off from significant actions while you catch up) or mobilize additional resources (see Call for Help below in the section on Crisis Management) so that you can catch up and get ahead.

Vigilance

The model of decision making in Chapter 1 indicates that vigilant observation of the patient is the necessary (although insufficient) starting point for expert case management. In discussing the self-resource we mentioned several performance-shaping factors and hazardous attitudes that can globally degrade your vigilance. There are two other factors that can specifically degrade your vigilance whenever they exist in a case: one is *distractions*, the other is a *high task load*.

Distractions of various kinds occur during every case. They include activities important to other operating room personnel, such as surgeons taking photographs, nurses counting instruments, or the intensive care unit calling to ask for the surgeon's instructions on a patient's care.

You should not give in to pressure to surrender your attention to the patient in order to assist in these activities. For example, if there is a phone at the anesthesia workstation, it should not be used routinely for phone calls that are not important to you. Nurses or clerks can transcribe laboratory results or relay messages between the surgeons and the intensive care unit.

Distractions can also include music, social conversation, and jokes. Each of these activities is appropriate under the right circumstances. They can make the work environment more pleasant and promote the development of team spirit, but they can also seriously lessen your ability to detect and correct problems. Tenney et al[6] have described how interruptions and distractions are prime contributors to the evolution of small problems into major catastrophes. Therefore, *you* must take charge of modulating these activities so that they do not become distracting. If the music is too loud, insist that the volume be reduced or that it be turned off. When a crisis occurs, *all* distractions should be eliminated or reduced as much as possible.

Allocation of Attention During Varying Task Loads

Allocation of attention is a dynamic process through which you must constantly prioritize the tasks requiring your attention. You should handle critical items quickly and leave the less critical problems for when you have ensured the stability of the patient. On the other hand, you *should* deal with minor problems when the task load is low because they might otherwise evolve to something more significant. You can also use times when the work load is low to prepare for upcoming high work load periods, such as emergence from anesthesia or termination of cardiopulmonary bypass.

It is important to maintain vigilant assessment of the patient even while you continue to carry out a myriad of routine tasks and to interact with students, teachers, subordinates, or supervisors. If you suspect that a problem is developing, allocate your attention primarily to problem recognition and patient evaluation until you prove to yourself that all is well. Whatever tasks occupy the operating room team, at least one individual must be watching the patient's condition at all times. The task load can quickly become excessive, making you so busy that it will be *impossible* to maintain vigilant situational awareness. If you find yourself in this situation, you must mobilize additional resources to help you carry out the needed tasks and watch the patient. A frightening example from aviation is that an airliner once crashed because all of the cockpit crew were preoccupied with a faulty indicator light for nose gear deployment, and they failed to notice that the autopilot had become disengaged—in other words, no one was flying the plane.[7]

Routine tasks can be very distracting. Rotating the operating table (especially 180 degrees) or repositioning the patient on the table (e.g., prone or lateral) is particularly difficult. During and after these tasks it is not uncommon to miss the signs of developing problems or to make errors such as failing to activate the ventilator. You can avoid losing vigilance at these times in several ways:

Assign the task to other personnel so that you are free to monitor the patient's condition; conversely, you can assign one person to watch the patient while you are busy with the task
Stop the task periodically to make routine checks
Use a checklist after the task is completed to review the patient's condition and to ensure that all necessary tasks have been performed

Use All Available Information

Considerable controversy has been generated since the early 1970s concerning the relative merits of direct clinical observation and acumen versus the use of electronic and mechanical monitoring devices. This is a false dichotomy; *neither* clinical observation nor any single monitor currently in use gives the entire picture. The goal is to utilize *all* the information at hand to help you care for the patient. The challenge is to learn how to integrate data from every possible source, giving each datum its appropriate weight toward a decision.

Similarly, it is important to pay attention to the activities of surgeons and nurses. Demand to know what is going on if something unusual appears to be happening with the surgery. Comments and concerns of other team members may not be addressed to you but may give early warning of an impending problem or provide critical information on how the problem can or cannot be solved.

The Burden of Proof Is on YOU to Ensure That the Patient Is Safe

Every type of observation has possible artifacts. Alarms from electronic monitors often occur repeatedly but falsely.[8] A "cry wolf" syndrome can develop in which the anesthetist *assumes* that an alarm is false, even when it is really true. Alarm sounds are typically distracting, and they seem to trigger a "make it stop" response in anesthetists, whose first (and sometimes only) move is to turn off the alarm.[9] This assumption can lead to catastrophe for the patient. When a monitor alarm sounds or when a question of patient safety is raised by your own observations or those of others, the burden of proof is on you to *first* determine that the patient is safe, and *then* to deal with any technical problems. Your evaluation of the patient can include checking alternate electronic monitors, but you should always remember to check the patient using all your senses, including visual inspection, auscultation, and feeling the pulse. Some anesthetists describe their overall practice style as always assuming that the patient might be in trouble, and then continuously proving to themselves that the patient is really safe.

Crisis Management

Although crises typically evolve from smaller problems (see Ch. 1), it is not uncommon to be suddenly faced with a serious event. Perhaps you missed the early indications of a problem, perhaps you took over a case from someone without a sufficient briefing, or perhaps the surgeon has just done something that has profoundly affected the patient. When a serious problem presents suddenly, highly practiced emergency procedures must be used. We present a basic protocol, analogous to the ABCs of cardiopulmonary resuscitation, and suggest that it be memorized (see list p. 40). It should be implemented whenever a potentially catastrophic event is detected. Once underway, it can be modified or elements can be rescinded if necessary. Its use will allow you to retrieve more specific critical incident protocols, such as those included in this book, and to use your own knowledge and experience to produce an optimum plan for handling the underlying problem.

Take Command as Team Leader

We believe that in most operating room crises the senior anesthetist involved in the case will be best equipped to manage the situation and should take command. A more experienced team

---

Protocol for the Initial Response to a Serious Event

<u>INITIATE IMMEDIATE LIFE-SUPPORT MEASURES</u>

Turn off all anesthetics in use (double-check)

Increase the oxygen concentration to 100% and verify that it approaches 100%

Maintain oxygenation at all costs. If in doubt about the ventilation system or oxygen supply use a backup system or oxygen source

Ensure that the patient has a pulse and that the blood pressure is acceptable. Commence ACLS if there is no pressure or pulse. Double-check vasodilator infusions. Support the circulation with fluids and vasopressors as necessary.

---

member, even if junior in rank to the rest of the team, can assume the leadership role, but make certain that the team understands who is in charge. What does it mean to be a leader? It is primarily a matter of *deciding* what needs to be done, *prioritizing* the necessary tasks, and *assigning* them to specific individuals. In order to fulfill these leadership functions the anesthetist must have good technical knowledge and skills and must remain calm and organized. The leader's command authority is vital to maintaining control of the situation, but control should be accomplished with full participation of the team. The leader should be the clearinghouse for information and suggestions from other team members. When junior members of the team have vital information or are in a better position to manage the crisis, they need to convey that fact assertively to the team leader. The American Airlines Crew Resource Management (CRM) course incorporates a saying that covers these situations: "Authority with participation, assertiveness with respect" (personal communication, Rand McNally, M.D., CRM instructor, American Airlines, 1991).

Declare an Emergency Early Rather than Late

Clinicians sometimes delay in making the switch from "business as usual" to crisis management, even as a situation worsens. Often this represents denial that a catastrophe is really occurring (the fixation error of "everything's OK"), and it may also reflect fears of upsetting the surgeons, altering the operating room routine, or appearing weak and incompetent. Declaring an emergency mobilizes needed resources, and quickly communicates to the team that a crisis is at hand. There is a risk in declaring an emergency prematurely or too frequently—too many false alarms will make the team less likely to believe you in the future (the "cry wolf" syndrome again). But the risk of *not* responding quickly to an emergency usually far exceeds the risk of doing so. The leader can vary the level of urgency as necessary and the declaration can always be cancelled if the problem resolves.

Good Communication Makes a Good Team

Communication between team members is crucial in a crisis. It is the glue that molds separate individuals into a powerful team. The leader must communicate the appropriate sense of urgency for a situation without inducing panic. You should notify the surgeons and nurses of ongoing problems and convey to them concisely the nature of the problem, what you need them to do (or not do), and your immediate plans. Order them to suspend or abort the surgery if necessary. Conversely, you should be prepared to help the surgeons or nurses in any reasonable way when they encounter problems as long as you can also maintain safe assessment of the patient and control of the anesthetic course.

Good team communication is a complex skill. We have observed many instances of poor communication between team members in both real and simulated operating room settings. The following are some principles of good communication that you should practice to become a more effective team leader:

Do not raise your voice unless absolutely necessary. However, you may need to ask for silence forcefully, so that you can be heard as the leader

State your commands or requests as clearly and as precisely as possible

Avoid making statements into thin air (e.g., "I need a lidocaine drip"). Whenever possible address statements or questions to a specific person and be sure that they know you are speaking to them

Close the communication loop. Provide and request acknowledgments of critical communications. Pilots are *required* by law to "read back" clearances such as "cleared for takeoff." Operating room personnel can and should do the same. Verify ambiguous messages; if you are not sure what someone said, clarify it with that person

Foster an atmosphere of open exchange among all operating room personnel. Listen to what other people have to say regardless of their job description or status. They may *know* something important about the patient or the situation that you do not. If you are in charge, you must decide whether their information needs to be acted on, but you cannot make that decision if you are not aware of it. Others may *detect* errors that you or other team members have made, thus saving you from significant mistakes and helping you to recover from errors

Concentrate on <u>what</u> is right for the patient, rather than on <u>who</u> is right. Should conflict occur between team members, you can sort out the interpersonal issues at another time. The patient is depending on you to work together

Distribute the Work Load

When a crisis occurs, the leader must distribute the work load across all the resources at hand. A common scene in an operating room crisis is to have a handful of people seriously overworked while others stand around with nothing useful to do. You must exercise your leadership by assigning specific tasks to individuals according to their skills. In general, the most experienced individuals should perform the most critical tasks. A major crisis is not a good time for medical students, interns, or new anesthesia residents to practice intubation or line placement. Whenever possible the leader should remain free to observe the patient and monitors and to direct the team. The team leader should only become involved in manual tasks if specific expertise is *necessary* to ensure their correct and timely completion.

You should look for overloads and failures in your performance or that of the team. If someone is becoming overloaded, allocate more help to their task or take away some tasks previously assigned to them. If a task is not getting done by one individual, ask someone else to try, either along with or in place of the first individual. If *you* are becoming overloaded, you will have to distribute more tasks to others, if possible, or restrict your own attention only to the most critical items.

Call for Help

During any major crisis there will be more tasks than can be handled by the typical operating room team even if all members work to their maximum ability. Thus it is very important to call for help. You should determine whether personnel with special skills are needed and mobilize them immediately. You will need to know in advance whom you will call, how you will contact them, and how you will use the help that arrives. In a major operating room facility, the assistance needed may be instantly at hand. However, in smaller facilities, at night, and on weekends or holidays there may be little help available. If necessary you may need to call for help from the emergency room or from the intensive care unit or even to call a hospital-wide "code." If you ask for outside assistance, make sure that the staff of the surgical suite know what is going on so that they can direct the help to your location rather than turning them away at the door!

Know How to Utilize the Help Available from Every Member of the Team

Anesthetists and Surgeons

Other anesthetists and surgeons have a knowledge and skill base similar to yours, so you can use them to perform or supervise critical tasks, for second opinions on difficult decisions, and as a check of your own accuracy and completeness. Most surgeons are better equipped than you to carry out critical procedures such as performing a tracheostomy or insertion of a chest tube. However, some surgeons, especially very specialized physicians such as ophthalmologists, may have less skill at these procedures than you do. You need to take these aspects of the situation into account as you plan for the next steps of an evolving crisis.

Nurses and Technicians

Skilled nonanesthetist personnel (nurses, anesthesia technicians) can be used for tasks within their scope of training, such as taking manual blood pressures, ventilating by hand, setting up lines and equipment, and making specific observations of the patient or monitors under your direction. They also are likely to know where to find drugs and equipment. Try to avoid sending all your skilled personnel out of the room for minor tasks when you may need them to help you manage something more critical.

Nonmedical Personnel

Even personnel with no medical training, such as orderlies and housekeepers, can be used for important tasks under your direction. They can pump blood, obtain supplies, remove trash, or help you move the patient. They can also be employed as runners to external resources such as the blood bank, laboratory, or pharmacy. If you use them as runners, make sure that they know where to go and that they have clear messages to convey or specific instructions on what to bring back to you.

Optimize Your Actions

As you begin to take action in response to a crisis, it will be important to structure your activities in an optimal fashion. If the patient's condition is deteriorating, you should quickly perform "generic" actions that buy time for more definitive ones. The initial life-support protocol is one example. In a crisis, escalate *rapidly* to therapies that have a high chance of success if the more routine therapies fail. Never assume that the next action *will* solve the problem. You must constantly be thinking of what to do next in case your current actions cannot be implemented or do not succeed. Think through the consequences of major *irreversible* actions, such as extubation or neuromuscular blockade, *before* initiating them. Once these bridges are burned, it may be difficult to recover.

Repeatedly Assess and Re-evaluate the Situation

In Chapter 1 we emphasize the importance of repeated re-evaluation of the patient. No crisis manager can be certain of success at any stage in the event. It is crucial to keep thinking ahead. Do not *assume* that anything about the situation is certain—double-check all important items. Anesthetic overdoses, syringe or ampule swaps, and hypoventilation or hypoxia are frequent causes of acute events. Mentally review all the actions that you have taken in the preceding few minutes. Force yourself to look at the vaporizers and any vasoactive infusions even if you believe that they were not in use.

After initiating critical life-support measures and stabilizing the patient's condition, you can stand back and use abstract reasoning. Think about the causal chain of the problem; try to understand the underlying causes and see that they are addressed. Remember that *any* single data source may be erroneous; cross-check redundant data streams to verify important data. Make sure that *all* available data are used, including the surgeon's observations, laboratory data, radiographs, and historical information from the patient's current and old charts.

Fixation Errors

The defining aspect of fixation errors is that they *persist* over time. Therefore, continuous re-evaluation should prevent them. The following are some practical suggestions for preventing the different types of fixation errors:

For: *"This and only this"*
The very act of repeated re-evaluation using all available data is the best antidote to this fixation. Cross-checking of data sources and constant questioning of one's mental model will usually disclose the invalidating evidence

For: *"Everything but this"*
The question of commitment is a difficult one. At what point do you quit collecting information and "go for it" on the most serious likely occurrence? There is no magic answer, but you should err on the side of providing definitive treatment for any suspected problem that requires it, especially if the risks of treatment are low in comparison with those of the problem (e.g., MH)

For: *"Everything's OK"*
Remember that the burden of proof is on you. For every abnormality you must assume that the patient is *not OK* until you satisfy yourself otherwise. Similarly, you must assume that any abnormality represents the worse possible diagnosis until you can determine what is actually going on

Documentation of Crises

Your primary task is always to *attend to the patient first*. Never let record keeping prevent you from taking care of the patient. However, good documentation of a crisis is important to its overall management. It will help you determine what happened and how to avoid further complications throughout the remainder of the case. Your documentation will be critical for meaningful quality assurance and in defending against possible litigation.

Retrospective recording of vital signs and your actions is appropriate when your attention must be devoted to patient care. Accurate records can be reconstructed from hard-copy trend plots, data logs of monitors, or records kept by nurses. Therefore, it is extremely helpful to activate electronic and human recorders at the first sign of a crisis. Do not turn off any monitors until you have made a hard-copy print out of all trend plots and data logs; otherwise their electronic memories may become erased. If you are not sure how to make hard copies, put a sign on the equipment instructing operating room staff to leave the monitor alone and find someone else to assist you who is more familiar with the equipment.

If enough skilled staff are available during an event, assign one of them the task of being timekeeper and recorder. Make sure that they receive all relevant details about drugs administered and laboratory data (including the time each specimen is sent). Following the event, reconcile the time on all clocks that were used (including the clocks within the monitors).

Never alter the record. If it contains an error that could influence some aspect of the patient's future care, you can note the corrections in a subsequent entry. If absolutely necessary for clarity, you may put a light line through the erroneous entry that maintains its legibility. You should date and time every entry you make in the chart, and it is especially important to sign or initial any changes you have made.

Follow-Up After a Major Crisis

Stay Involved in the Patient's Care

After a serious perioperative event your responsibility to your patient does not end when the patient is transferred to a ward or to an intensive care unit. In such situations it is even more important than usual for you to stay involved in the care of the patient. Make sure that appropriate consultations are obtained as needed to diagnose or manage the patient, to establish a prognosis, or to begin rehabilitation. The opinions and statements of surgeons or consultants may not always be correct. Keep in touch with the consultants and review their notes. Ensure that they are appropriately informed and do not allow any misinformation, speculation, or erroneous conclusions written by consultants to go unchallenged in the record.

Use Your Institution's Follow-up Protocol

Many institutions have a formal protocol for dealing with serious anesthesia-related events. The appendix at the end of this chapter is a copy of the protocol used by the Harvard Medical School's Department of Anesthesia. A complete description of the protocol by its authors has recently been published.[10] As we have already described, the first item of this protocol is to attend to the patient. The next step is to contact the department's or division's designated supervising official, who may be the clinical director or the chief of the department. This supervising official becomes the incident supervisor and coordinates the administrative response to the event. For example, the incident supervisor would contact the institution's risk manager and the anesthesia equipment manager (or biomedical engineering service). The Harvard protocol further provides that the clinical director or department chairman will designate a follow-up supervisor to coordinate the longer-term activities in response to the event.

A second important feature of the protocol is the necessity of impounding any equipment possibly at fault. It is tragic enough to have equipment failure contribute to the injury of one patient, but sequential injuries to multiple patients have been known to occur. Make sure that the next patient does not also suffer. Even if it is unlikely that equipment failures played any role in the event, the Harvard protocol recommends a routine inspection before it is returned to service. If there is any question of equipment failure, the equipment should be stored in a secure location and labeled "Do Not Disturb," and it should not be altered or manipulated in any way. Resist the impulse to experiment with the equipment to determine whether a fault occurred; you might impede discovery of the real cause.

You may also have a responsibility to report the failure to the manufacturer and (in the United States) to the Food and Drug Administration (FDA) under the Safe Medical Devices Reporting Act. The risk manager or biomedical engineering service of your institution should be able to help you to determine whether and how to make such a report.

If there is any suspicion of a drug problem, ampule swap, or syringe swap, you should impound all syringes, ampules, vials, sharps containers, and trash. It may be necessary to examine the vials, ampules, or syringes used or even to have assays of their contents conducted. If any error or contamination of a drug is found, you may need to inform the FDA.

The Medical Record and Quality Assurance

You should ensure that the medical record is complete, including an appropriate summary of the event. Make sure that the record truthfully reflects what happened; to the best of your ability reconstruct it objectively. Record the *facts* of the case as you know them, not speculation or interpretation. When you contact your insurance carrier, your attorney may ask you to write a separate summary of the event. Be careful not to speculate about the events with other personnel except in accordance with standard practices of patient care and quality assurance. These conversations may be discoverable in litigation, and any ill-considered speculations about what might have happened may later create difficulties in defending your actions.

After any salient event you should complete your department's standard quality assurance report and attach a copy of the anesthesia record and any summaries that you have put in the chart. This will ensure that you and your colleagues can thoroughly review the events of the case in the appropriate quality assurance forum. Make sure that all quality assurance materials are appropriately labeled "Confidential Quality Assurance Document."

There is some controversy about what to do with hard-copy printouts and strip charts from monitors; should they be placed in the patient's chart, attached to the quality assurance report, kept elsewhere, or discarded? If printouts are placed in some charts and not others, serious questions could be raised about how the decision to place the printouts was made. If the printouts are attached to the quality assurance report, they may not be admissable in court to support your case without releasing the entire quality assurance file on the case. Discarding the printouts will impede the quality assurance process in determining what happened and what, if any, changes are needed to avoid similar events in the future. You should consult with risk managers and attorneys before adopting an institutional or departmental policy.

Speak with the Patient's Family

Whenever a serious crisis has occurred in the operating room and there is any chance that the patient has suffered an adverse outcome, it will be necessary to inform the patient's family or guardian. Bacon[11,12] has given some practical advice on how best to do this. Ideally, you and the surgeon should speak to the family together. Practically speaking, this is often not possible since you are likely to be involved in stabilizing or transporting the patient long after at least one of the surgeons is free. You should still speak to the family even if others have already done so. In some institutions a risk manager may be available to assist you in informing the family.

When discussing the case with the family, outline what steps are currently being taken to care for the patient. Once again, tell the family the *facts* of the case as you know them, not speculation as to what might have happened. You can correct any misconceptions that the family may have by your explanation of the facts, but try not to make your explanations too complex. You should make yourself available to the family on subsequent occasions if they ask to meet with you, but you may wish to contact your insurer, attorney, or risk manager for assistance before such a meeting. Do not share confidential quality assurance documents or information with family members; these documents are confidential, and they exist solely for the purpose of evaluating and improving patient care.

Stress Management for the Anesthetist
After a Perioperative Catastrophe

Caring for a patient who suffers a perioperative catastrophe can be extremely stressful. In some cases the stress can degrade your performance capabilities, and it can adversely affect both your mental and physical health. Syndromes analogous to post-traumatic stress disorder can develop.[11-13] After encountering a major catastrophe you may not be capable of immediately moving on to the next case. You will be busy with follow-up activities, and you may be preoccupied with reviewing the previous case, searching for any error or for a meaningful lesson for the future. You should ask someone else to complete the rest of your assigned cases. Remember that the next patient should receive your full attention.

Some aspects of postevent stress management and support have been reviewed by Bacon.[11,12] He advocates the use of a program called Critical Incident Stress Debriefing, which was originally described by Mitchell[13] for use with emergency workers following major disasters. Support services for anesthetists and other operating room personnel who have been involved in an operating room catastrophe are often available within the anesthesia department under the aegis of the department chief or within the institution through the medical staff office or risk manager. Your insurer or attorney may also be able to assist you in seeking professional advice should you require it.

References

1. Aeronautical Decision Making. Advisory Circular Number 60-22. Federal Aviation Administration, Washington, DC, 1991
2. Gaba DM, Maxwell M, DeAnda A: Anesthetic mishaps: breaking the chain of accident evolution. Anesthesiology 66:670, 1987
3. Buffington CW, Ramanathan S, Turndorf H: Detection of anesthesia machine faults. Anesth Analg 63:79, 1984
4. Norman DA: Turn Signals Are the Facial Expressions of Automobiles. Addison-Wesley, Reading, MA, 1992
5. Rendall-Baker L: Better labels will cut drug errors. Anesth Patient Safety Newsletter 2:29, 1987
6. Tenney YJ, Adams MJ, Pew RW et al: A principled approach to the measurement of situation awareness in commercial aviation (NASA Contractor Report 4451). National Aeronautics and Space Administration, Washington, DC, 1992
7. Aircraft Accident Report NTSB-AAR-73-14: Eastern Air Lines, Inc. L1011, N310EA. National Transportation Safety Board, Washington, DC, 1973
8. Kestin IG, Miller BR, Lockhart CH: Auditory alarms during anesthesia monitoring. Anesthesiology 69:106, 1988
9. Quinn M: A philosophy of alarms. p. 169. In Gravenstein JS, Newbower RS, Ream AK et al (eds): The Automated Anesthesia Record and Alarm Systems. Butterworths, Boston, 1987
10. Cooper JB, Cullen DJ, Eichhorn JH et al: Administrative guidelines for response to an adverse anesthesia event. J Clin Anesth 5:79, 1993
11. Bacon AK: Death on the table. Anaesthesia 44:245, 1989
12. Bacon AK: Major anaesthetic mishaps—handling the aftermath. Curr Anaesth Crit Care 1:253, 1990
13. Mitchell JT: When disaster strikes...the critical incident stress debriefing process. J Emerg Med 9:36, 1983

Appendix

Guidelines for Action Following an Adverse Anesthesia Event*

Department of Anaesthesia, Harvard Medical School
Approved February 13, 1989

Objectives: To limit patient injury from a specific adverse event associated with anesthesia and to ensure that the causes of the events are identified so that a recurrence can be prevented.

Protocol: When a patient has died or has been injured from causes suspected to be related to anesthesia management, the following actions should be taken.

Immediate

1. *The primary anesthetist/anesthesiologist should concentrate on continuing patient care.* The primary anesthetist/anesthesiologist should notify a physician responsible for supervision of anesthesia activities in the relevant patient care area (e.g., anesthesia clinical director, anesthesia operating room administrator, team leader) as soon as possible (at least before the anesthetist transfers direct responsibility for that patient). The person so contacted will direct the process of immediate prevention of recurrence (if necessary), events documentation, and continued investigation or will delegate responsibility to someone other than the primary anesthetist/anesthesiologist. The individual performing these tasks is designated as the incident supervisor.

   Rationale: Information vital to reconstructing events may be accidentally discarded. The highest priority for the primary caregivers must be the care of the patient, so responsibility for administrative and investigative activities must be assigned to others. Typically, an anesthesiologist supervising a primary anesthetist/anesthesiologist should not be the incident supervisor. However, out of normal working hours, a primary or supervising anesthesiologist may choose to act as incident supervisor and may exercise discretion in calling for assistance or advice.

2. *Anesthesia equipment or supplies associated with the case, whether thought to be materially involved or not, should be sequestered before subsequent use. Nothing must be altered or discarded.* The primary anesthetist/anesthesiologist or incident supervisor shall immediately contact the hospital individual responsible for management of anesthesia equipment and supplies (equipment supervisor). The equipment supervisor or a designee of this person shall supervise the impound of involved supplies and equipment (including the anesthesia machine) in consultation with the hospital risk manager. A preliminary decision to continue use of urgently needed equipment may be made, following a safety inspection, at the discretion of the incident supervisor in consultation with the hospital risk manager.

   Rationale: Equipment or supplies involved in the event may be accidentally altered or discarded, preventing determination of cause.

---

*From Cooper JB et al,[10] with permission.

3. *The incident supervisor or attending anesthesiologist should contact the hospital risk manager immediately following the anesthetic for additional administrative support.*

   Rationale: Individual caregivers will rarely be experienced in dealing with an adverse occurrence. The risk manager can advise on the ways to communicate information to the patient or to the patient's family in a way that is forthright and comforting but that does not unintentionally alarm, misinform, or render judgment.

4. *The primary anesthetist/anesthesiologist and other individuals involved must document relevant information about the incident.*

   a. The primary anesthetist/anesthesiologist, after discussion with the incident supervisor, must write on the patient's medical record relevant information about what happened and what actions were taken. No erasures should be made or information obscured on the record. If a correction is necessary, the original should be lightly crossed out and changes initialed and dated. Additions to and explanations of notations on the record can be made, for example, to explain issues in which professional judgment was involved.

   b. The primary anesthetist/anesthesiologist must complete and file an incident report as soon as practicable.

   c. *Other individuals* involved in the incident should document their observations soon after the event. The documentation should be returned to the hospital patient care assessment coordinator or other appropriately designated individual.

   d. When writing about the events:
      1) State only the facts as you know them.
      2) Do not make judgments about causality or responsibility.
      3) Do not use judgmental terms or phrases.

5. *Give the highest priority to continued involvement in follow-up care of the patient.*

   a. Consult early and frequently with the surgeon.

   b. Immediately call on other consultants who may help improve long-term care or recovery.

Follow-up Investigations

1. The clinical director and/or department chairman shall be informed of each adverse event and will designate who shall supervise the event follow-up and investigation beyond the immediate actions. The follow-up supervisor shall

   a. Notify the individuals involved of their responsibilities as defined in this document.

   b. Be responsible for ensuring that procedures are followed to the extent necessary, reasonable, and possible.

   c. Maintain communication with those who are providing continuing anesthesia care and provide guidance and advice as needed.

   d. Ensure that information regarding the adverse event is communicated through the proper channels to the departmental quality assurance program.

2. The need to maintain equipment sequestration shall be determined by the incident follow-up supervisor and the individual responsible for managing anesthesia technology.

   a. If it is unlikely that the equipment was related to the event, the equipment can be returned to service after routine inspection.

   b. If it is possible that the equipment was related to the event, the following procedures should be implemented and supervised by the individual responsible for managing anesthesia technology or that person's designee:

      1) Store the equipment in a secure location. Label it DO NOT DISTURB.
      2) Document its physical condition and notable features as received and record its identification (e.g., serial number).
      3) Do not alter or inspect the equipment in any way that could affect further investigation.
      4) Conduct a thorough inspection of the equipment in the presence of the primary anesthetist/anesthesiologist, the insurance carrier, hospital risk manager, equipment manufacturers, or any of their designees.

3. If an equipment problem or failure is discovered or strongly suspected, the equipment supervisor, after consultation with the hospital risk manager, shall consider contacting the Food and Drug Administration (FDA) (via the Device Experience Network at 800-638-6725) and/or the Emergency Care Research Institute (ECRI) if it is believed necessary to warn other users. Alternatively, the manufacturer can communicate that information to the appropriate authorities, which may be required by law depending on the circumstances.

   Under the Safe Medical Devices Act, the hospital may be required to report the event to the manufacturer and FDA if a serious injury or death occurred.

4. Continue to verify and document medical care provided to the patient following the event.

Summary of Responsibilities for Adverse Event Protocol

Primary anesthetist/anesthesiologist: Concentrate on continuing care; notify anesthesia operating room administrator (or attending first if resident or certified registered nurse anesthetist); do NOT discard supplies or apparatus or tamper with equipment; document events in the patient's record; do NOT alter the record; stay involved with follow-up care; contact consultants as needed; submit a follow-up report; document continuing care in the patient's record.

Incident supervisor (e.g., anesthesia clinical director, operating room administrator, team leader): Advise primary anesthetist/anesthesiologist and other personnel involved; verify close contact with the surgeon and other consultants; contact the hospital risk manager; contact manager for anesthesia equipment or alternate.

Department chairman or clinical director: Directly supervise or delegate responsibility for incident investigation.

Anesthesia equipment manager or alternate: Ensure impounding of equipment, if necessary, and determine appropriate disposition of equipment; if pharmaceuticals or supplies were involved that may create hazard to other patients, contact pharmacy, materials management, nursing, or other departments; supervise continuing investigation of equipment or supplies-related issues; contact FDA, ECRI, or manufacturer if appropriate.

Follow-up supervisor: Notify the individuals involved of their responsibilities as defined in this document; be responsible for ensuring that procedures are followed to the extent necessary, reasonable, and possible; maintain communication with those who are providing continuing anesthesia care, and provide guidance and advice as needed; ensure that information regarding the adverse event is communicated through the proper channels to the department quality assurance program.

Catalog of Critical Events in Anesthesiology

The following chapters contain the Catalog of Critical Events in Anesthesiology. As described in detail in the Preface and in Chapters 1 and 2, this Catalog is intended to fill a gap in the training of anesthetists. Our aim is to provide a comprehensive (although not exhaustive) compilation of approaches to both common and uncommon emergency situations that can arise in the perioperative period. This is intended to make it easy to learn or review systematically how to recognize them and how to respond if they occur.

The first chapter deals with "generic" events, most of which describe a *manifestation* that may be caused by a variety of potentially serious underlying events. The generic events are listed in a separate chapter because they initially require no information other than the existence of that manifestation. For example, the generic event Hypotension (Event 7) presents an approach to deal with a common but potentially serious manifestation that can result from many different causes. The generic event covers the initial diagnostic and therapeutic approach to the problem and then cross-references the other events that represent specific pathophysiologic occurrences. Thus, the event Pulmonary Embolism (Event 18) is one specific, albeit unusual, cause of hypotension.

Each of the next four chapters groups together events related to a single organ system (cardiovascular, pulmonary, metabolic, neurologic), since there is considerable similarity of the manifestations and responses appropriate to each system. Following the chapters devoted to organ systems is a chapter involving equipment failures, many of which concern the anesthesia machine and the breathing circuit. Finally, there are three chapters covering events of special interest in subspecialty areas of anesthesia practice (cardiac, obstetric, and pediatric anesthesia). Of course, many events in the rest of the Catalog will be of interest to specialists in these areas, but the unique occurrences faced in their environments are grouped separately.

We developed a special format for the events in the Catalog to provide a uniform, concise framework for describing them to anesthetists. As this Catalog is intended to be a guidebook, not a reference text, we have not included the vast amount of explanatory and reference material that is available on each of these topics. What we do provide is the *essential material* that we believe is needed to prepare for handling specific perioperative crisis situations. Below we explain the format and headings used for each event in the Catalog.

Event

The name of the event.

Definition

The definition of the event and any common variants.

Etiology

The underlying cause(s) of the event. There is often more than one possible causal pathway for each defined event.

Typical Situations

The perioperative situations in which the event is most likely to occur. In these situations the anesthetist should be especially alert to encounter the event. If the likelihood of its occurrence is high enough, specific steps may need to be taken to prevent its occurrence or to obtain the special equipment or personnel needed to treat it if it should occur.

Prevention

The actions that can make the occurrence of the event less likely or that will make it easier to treat.

Manifestations

The ways in which the event could manifest itself. These include clinical observations, monitored variables, and laboratory data. Not every manifestation will be evident for any given occurrence of the event. Some manifestations typically are seen early in the course of the event; others will only be seen late in its evolution. The manifestations are listed in their approximate order of frequency and/or importance.

Similar Events

Other events whose manifestations can be similar to the manifestiations of this event. For some of these alternate diagnoses there are specific manifestiations that clearly distinguish them from this event.

Management

Guidelines on what to do if this event occurs, or if there is significant suspicion that it has occurred. The suggested management is described approximately in the order that an experienced practitioner might respond. The items listed in bold are the initial responses that we believe to be most important. The items following may be necessary for comprehensive management of the event but are not as critical.

We have chosen to produce these hierarchical guides rather than rigid algorithms or flow charts because the many permutations and combinations of real situations and real patients are too complex to allow the specification of definitive independent pathways of action.

Note: Every situation is different. It may be necessary to deviate from guidelines because of the specifics of a situation.

Remember these Aspects of Anesthesia Crisis Resource Management that
Apply to Every Case:
Ensure adequate oxygenation at all costs
Support the circulation as necessary
Call for help early rather than late
Tackle the most critical problems first

Complications

Specific complications of the event, which may occur either owing to progression of the event itself or as complications of treatment.

Suggested Readings

Relevant literature related to the event. We have tried to give the most useful references for each event, wherever possible citing easily accessible materials (the journals *Anesthesiology* and *Anesthesia and Analgesia*, *American Society of Anesthesiologists Refresher Course Lectures*, and standard textbooks). We have referenced less readily available sources whenever they are significantly better than other materials.

Note: No literature is cited as a definitive work. On occasion our opinions may differ in some respects from those stated in the references we cite. Readers are strongly encouraged to read all available material on each topic and to decide for themselves on the applicability of this work to their practice of anesthesia.

The following is a glossary of the abbreviations used in Chapters 3 through 11.

ABBREVIATIONS

A-a	Alveolar-arterial
ABG(s)	Arterial blood gas(es)
ACE	Angiotensin-converting enzyme
ACLS	Advanced Cardiac Life Support
ACT	Activated clotting time
AHA	American Heart Association
AIDS	Acquired immunodeficiency syndrome
aPTT	Activated partial thromboplastin time
ARDS	Adult respiratory distress syndrome
ASTM	American Society for Testing and Materials
AV	Atrioventricular
bpm	Beats per minute
BUN	Blood urea nitrogen
Ca^{2+}	Calcium ion
CABG	Coronary artery bypass graft
CAD	Coronary artery disease
CHF	Congestive heart failure
CK	Creatine kinase (synonomous with CPK)
Cl^-	Chloride ion
CNS	Central nervous system
CO_2	Carbon dioxide
COPD	Chronic obstructive pulmonary disease
CPAP	Continuous positive airway pressure
CPB	Cardiopulmonary bypass
CPK	Creatine phosphokinase (synonymous with CK)
CPR	Cardiopulmonary resuscitation
CSF	Cerebrospinal fluid
CT	Computed tomography
CVP	Central venous pressure
D_5W	Dextrose 5% in water
DIC	Disseminated intravascular coagulation
DISS	Diameter Index Safety System
DKA	Diabetic ketoacidosis
ECG	Electrocardiography
EEG	Electroencephalography
EMD	Electromechanical dissociation
ENT	Ear, nose, and throat
ETT	Endotracheal tube
FFP	Fresh frozen plasma
FiO_2	Inspired oxygen concentration
GI	Gastrointestinal
H^+	Hydrogen ion
HCO_3^-	Bicarbonate ion
H_2O	Water
HELLP	Syndrome of hemolysis, elevated liver function tests, low platelets

Hg	Mercury
IABP	Intra-aortic balloon pump
ICP	Intracranial pressure
ICU	Intensive care unit
Ig	Immunoglobulin
IVC	Inferior vena cava
K^+	Potassium ion
LR	Lactated Ringer's
LVAD	Left ventricular assist device
MAO	Monoamine oxidase
MAP	Mean arterial pressure
Mg^{2+}	Magnesium ion
$MgSO_4$	Magnesium sulfate
MH	Malignant hyperthermia
MRI	Magnetic resonance imaging
N_2	Nitrogen
N_2O	Nitrous oxide
Na^+	Sodium ion
$NaHCO_3$	Sodium bicarbonate
NIBP	Noninvasive blood pressure
NS	Normal saline
NSAID	Nonsteroidal anti-inflammatory drug
NTG	Nitroglycerin
O_2	Oxygen
PA	Pulmonary artery
PACU	Postanesthesia care unit
PALS	Pediatric advanced life support
pCO_2	Partial pressure of carbon dioxide
PCWP	Pulmonary capillary wedge pressure
PEEP	Positive end-expiratory pressure
pH	$-\log [\,H^+\,]$
PIP	Peak inspiratory pressure
pO_2	Partial pressure of oxygen
PO_4^{3-}	Phosphate
PRBCs	Packed red blood cells
PT	Prothrombin time
PTCA	Percutaneous transluminal coronary angioplasty
PTT	Partial thromboplastin time
PVC	Premature ventricular contraction
RBCs	Red blood cells
Rh	Rhesus blood group
SCI	Spinal cord injury
SIADH	Syndrome of inappropriate antidiuretic hormone secretion
SVR	Systemic vascular resistance
T(numeral)	Thoracic (level) dermatomal level of regional blockade
TEE	Transesophageal echocardiography
TIA	Transient ischemic attack
TURP	Transurethral resection of the prostate
V/Q	Ventilation/perfusion

Chapter Three
Generic Events

1 ACUTE HEMORRHAGE

Definition

Acute hemorrhage is the acute loss of a large volume of blood during a surgical procedure and can be either overt or covert:

Overt
   Can be visualized in the surgical field, on sponges, or in the suction containers
Covert
   No outward sign of bleeding (e.g., retroperitoneal or intrapleural hemorrhage, blood loss hidden in drapes)

Etiology

Bleeding from sizable blood vessel (artery or vein). May be result of surgical manipulation or trauma or may occur de novo
May be related to disorders of coagulation or therapeutic anticoagulation

Typical Situations

Vascular, cardiac, or thoracic surgery
Coagulopathy
Major trauma
Covert hemorrhage is more likely where the surgical field is obscured by drapes or is distant from the anesthetist
Acute hemorrhage may be a delayed complication of an earlier injury or invasive procedure
Retroperitoneal surgery or injury
Obstetric emergencies (see Event 72, *Obstetric Hemorrhage*)

Prevention

Identify and correct coagulopathy early, including monitoring of PT/PTT during warfarin or heparin therapy, or monitoring of ACT during intraoperative anticoagulation
Identify, institute prophylaxis for, and treat other potential bleeding sites (e.g., GI tract ulcers in ICU patients, long bone or pelvic fractures following major trauma)
Insert the largest possible IV catheter if you anticipate having to administer blood during a case

E V E N T 1

Manifestations

Overt

Blood in the surgical field

Blood on surgical sponges, on the drapes, and on the floor

Suction noise

Accumulation of blood in suction containers

Change in vital signs (fall in arterial pressure and filling pressures, rise in pulse rate)

Surgeon's comments (e.g., "Have you given any blood yet?")

Covert

Unexplained fall in arterial pressure, CVP, or PA pressure and/or rise in pulse rate

Fall in mixed venous O_2 (if monitored), especially in surgery where covert blood loss is possible

Increase in fluid requirements above what is expected

Little or transient blood pressure response to administration of an IV fluid bolus

Little or transient blood pressure response to vasopressor

Excessive response to vasodilator or anesthetic agents

Unexplained fall in urine output or hematocrit (a late sign)

Expanding abdomen or thigh, flank discoloration

Decreased oxygenation, increased PIP if hemothorax

Similar Events

Anesthetic or vasodilator overdose (see Event 62, *Volatile Anesthetic Overdose*)

Anaphylaxis (see Event 11, *Anaphylaxis and Anaphylactoid Reactions*)

Progressively inadequate volume replacement

Occlusion of venous return by compression of the vena cava by the gravid uterus, surgical packing, or retraction

Pneumothorax (see Event 28, *Pneumothorax*)

Pulmonary embolism (see Event 18, *Pulmonary Embolism*)

Cardiac tamponade (see Event 16, *Pericardial Tamponade*)

Inappropriate diuretic therapy

Tachyarrhythmias

Management

Inform surgeons of the problem

Keep them informed of its severity

If the abdomen is open, the surgeon can cannulate a large intra-abdominal vein for rapid transfusion or can cannulate the aorta directly for an arterial line

Clamping of the aorta below the diaphragm may be essential for resuscitation of the patient (especially in major trauma or gunshot wounds below the diaphragm)

Check and verify blood pressure

Treat severe hypotension with IV bolus of vasopressor/inotrope

Use ephedrine, 5–50 mg; epinephrine, 10–100 µg; or phenylephrine, 50–200 µg

Repeat as necessary to maintain an acceptable blood pressure

Rapidly restore circulating blood volume

Use blood, colloid, or crystalloid to replace circulating blood volume

If blood loss is sudden but may soon be controlled, hold off giving blood and continue to give crystalloid until bleeding is stopped

A pressurized bag of saline or colloid will run much faster than a unit of PRBCs through a small peripheral IV access

Dilute PRBCs with saline to increase speed with which they can be infused

Use an additional small-pore filter to avoid occluding the IV-giving set filter with debris

Use fluid warmer as soon as possible to heat all fluids administered; monitor body temperature

Increase F$_IO_2$, reduce/eliminate volatile agents and N$_2$O

Increase total gas flow to rapidly equilibrate breathing circuit

Replace volatile anesthetic as tolerated with narcotics, scopolamine, midazolam

CALL FOR HELP if major fluid resuscitation is necessary

If possible, the PRIMARY ANESTHESIOLOGIST should monitor patient and surgical status and direct activities of operating room personnel

Additional personnel can check and hang blood units and assist in administering blood products

Set up rapid transfusion device if available. If overtly lost blood is not contaminated, have a cell saver unit set up for autotransfusion of RBCs. This will occupy one person full time

Ensure adequate IV access

Minimum of one 16-gauge IV line, preferably more. In the case of severe blood loss place at least one very large-bore IV line (such as 8.5 French PA catheter introducer) in a suitable peripheral or central vein. Use large-bore rapid transfusion IV tubing if available

If IV access is difficult, change a small IV cannula to a large IV cannula by using the Seldinger technique

Check IV site to make sure IV line does not infiltrate

Obtain adequate supplies of IV fluid (colloid or crystalloid)

NOTIFY BLOOD BANK, get sufficient blood in the room

Order of preference for blood transfusion

Type-specific cross-matched unit

Type-specific partially cross-matched unit

Type-specific screened unit

Type-specific not screened unit

O-negative unit (universal donor)

Do NOT switch to type-specific blood after more than 2–3 units of O-negative whole blood or after 4–5 units of O-negative PRBCs

Watch the blood pressure and heart rate response to volume infusion for improvement of hemodynamic status

Follow CVP and/or PA pressure, if already available, to guide fluid replacement. Otherwise, get assistance to place CVP or PA catheter

Monitor hematocrit, electrolytes, and ABGs at regular intervals, no more than 30 minutes apart

Keep track of surgical events

Watch out for clamps on vessels carrying your fluids

If using induced hypotension (e.g., neurovascular surgery), maintain hypotension to reduce bleeding but ensure adequate circulating blood volume

Ask surgeons to control bleeding as soon as possible to allow effective fluid resuscitation

Complications

Myocardial ischemia, arrhythmias, cardiac arrest
Hypocalcemia
Hypothermia
Irreversible shock
Allergic/anaphylactic reaction to blood
Coagulopathy/DIC
Volume overload from overshoot of fluid resuscitation
ARDS
Transfusion-related viral infection
    Hepatitis
    Human immunodeficiency virus (AIDS)
Renal failure
Hyperkalemia

Suggested Readings

Miller RD: Transfusion therapy. p. 1467. In: Anesthesia. 3rd Ed. Churchill Livingstone, New York, 1990
Vincent JL: Fluids for resuscitation. Br J Anaesth 64:185, 1991

---

2 CARDIAC ARREST

Definition

Cardiac arrest is the abrupt cessation of effective mechanical activity of the heart and, in the spontaneously ventilating patient, cessation of effective ventilation.

Etiology

Ventricular tachyarrhythmias
Lack of sinus node activity or complete AV block without intervening escape rhythm
Complete absence of cardiac electrical activity (asystole)
Lack of cardiac mechanical activity in response to cardiac electrical stimulation (electro-mechanical dissociation)

Typical Situations

Patients with a history of arrhythmias
Patients with major trauma, acute hypovolemia, or shock
Following a primary respiratory arrest
Difficult intubation (see Event 3, *Difficult Tracheal Intubation*) or ventilation
Hypoxemia (see Event 8, *Hypoxemia*)
Hypercarbia (see Event 27, *Hypercarbia*)
Bradycardia during epidural or spinal anesthesia (see Event 13, *Sinus Bradycardia*)

Drug toxicity
Acute vagal reflexes (see Event 13, *Sinus Bradycardia*)
Direct myocardial contact with the electrocautery
Pulmonary embolism (see Event 18, *Pulmonary Embolism*)
Pericardial tamponade (see Event 16, *Pericardial Tamponade*)
Tension pneumothorax (see Event 28, *Pneumothorax*)

Prevention

Treat serious chronic arrhythmias with appropriate antiarrhythmic therapy, continue treatment
   through surgery
Avoid surgery and anesthesia after recent myocardial infarction
Place a pacemaker prophylactically for patients with high-grade AV block (transvenous or transcutaneous) or sinus bradycardia (transcutaneous or transesophageal). Test pacemaker capture prior to surgery
Use vagolytic pretreatment in patients or procedures at high risk of increased vagal tone
Treat with vagolytics early if bradycardia develops during anesthesia (especially regional anesthesia)

Manifestations

No arterial flow
      Absence of peripheral pulses
      Absence of pulse oximeter waveform
      Cuff blood pressure unmeasurable
      Invasive arterial pressure has no pulsations, MAP less than 20 mm Hg without CPR
Abnormal rhythm on ECG (*Note:* if EMD, rhythm may appear normal)
Absence of heart tones via auscultation
Fall in end-tidal CO_2
Cyanosis, blood in wound becomes dark
Vomiting/regurgitation of gastric contents
Loss of consciousness of awake patient, often followed by short seizure
Cessation of respiration in spontaneously ventilating patient

Similar Events

Profound hypotension (see Event 7, *Hypotension*)
Artifacts on monitoring devices
      ECG
      Pulse oximeter
      Blood pressure measurement systems (NIBP or invasive)

Management

Treat the patient, not the monitor
Verify that there is no pulsatile flow
      Palpate the carotid, femoral, or other pulse (the surgeon may also have easy access to
         palpable pulses)

Check NIBP and ECG monitors and leads

Auscultate heart tones

Notify surgeons and other operating room personnel **immediately** of the cardiac arrest

Call for help

Call operating room or hospital "code"

Request crash cart and defibrillator

Start chart recorder(s)

Turn off all anesthetics, administer 100% O$_2$ at high flow rate

Begin Basic Life Support

Airway

Secure airway, mask-ventilate, and intubate the patient as soon as possible if not already intubated

Breathing

Ventilate by hand at 12 breaths/min until intubated

When intubated, mechanical ventilation can be initiated

Circulation

Instruct surgeon, nurse, or colleague to begin chest compressions

80–100 bpm in adults, compression/ventilation ratio of 5:1

Watch for proper chest compression technique or fatigue of the person performing chest compressions

Diagnose and treat arrhythmias

Use ECG monitor or strip chart ECG machine if available

If not, place the defibrillator paddles on the chest wall for a "quick look"

Ventricular arrhythmias

Defibrillate up to three times in rapid sequence, increasing energy of countershock (200, 300, 360 J), and stopping each time to check for a pulse

Administer epinephrine IV push, 1 mg, repeat q3–5min

Attempt defibrillation, 360 J, 30–60 seconds after epinephrine

Administer lidocaine IV, 1–1.5 mg/kg

Attempt defibrillation, 360 J, 30–60 seconds after lidocaine

Continue with the above algorithm—consider bretylium, escalating doses of epinephrine

Use ABGs to guide acid-base management

Asystole/bradycardias

Epinephrine IV push, 1 mg, repeat q3–5min

Atropine IV push, 1 mg, repeat q3–5min

Isoproterenol, 1–3 µg/min infusion

Consider immediate pacing by transcutaneous route (the currently recommended route in the AHA guidelines) or transvenous route. For asystole, pacing must be initiated early if it is to be effective

EMD

Epinephrine IV push, 1 mg, repeat with escalating doses q3–5min

Calcium chloride IV push, 1 g (also effective for hyperkalemia)

If profound bradycardia, treat with atropine IV, 1 mg bolus

Consider the etiology of the arrest—review drugs administered, and actions or therapeutic maneuvers performed prior to the arrest. Correct any obvious underlying causes such as volatile anesthetic overdose, airway obstruction, hypo- or hyperkalemia

Secure IV access

Insert large-bore IV line for volume expansion

Insert CVP catheter for administration of drugs

Epinephrine and atropine can also be given through the ETT if you have no venous access

Draw ABGs from the femoral, brachial, or radial artery

Place arterial line if equipment and expertise available (cutdown may be necessary)

If aggressive management is warranted

A surgeon can open the chest and begin internal cardiac massage

Consider instituting CPB (can establish by percutaneous placement of femoral venous and arterial cannulae)

Consider pericardiocentesis or placement of a chest tube if there is a significant risk of pericardial tamponade or pneumothorax

If there is no response to the measures listed above

Seek expert advice early from cardiologist for arrhythmias unresponsive to conventional therapy

Consider use of high-dose α-adrenergic agonists in escalating doses

High-dose epinephrine IV, 5–10 mg, q5min

Phenylephrine IV, 1 mg

Norepinephrine IV, 1 mg

Complications

Death

Brain damage

Laceration of liver

Pneumothorax or hemothorax

Rib fracture

Suggested Readings

Textbook of Advanced Cardiac Life Support. American Heart Association, Dallas, 1987

Emergency Cardiac Care Committee and Subcommittees, American Heart Association: Guidelines for cardiopulmonary resuscitation and emergency cardiac care. JAMA 268:2171, 1992

Niemann JT: Cardiopulmonary resuscitation. N Engl J Med 327:1075, 1992

Schleien CL, Berkowitz ID, Traystman R et al: Controversial issues in cardiopulmonary resuscitation. Anesthesiology 71:133, 1989

Stiell IG, Hebert PC, Weitzman BN et al: High dose epinephrine in adult cardiac arrest. N Engl J Med 327:1045, 1992

3 DIFFICULT TRACHEAL INTUBATION

Definition

When difficulty is anticipated in placing the ETT in the trachea by standard techniques or when successful intubation of the trachea is not accomplished within the first two attempts by an experienced practitioner the intubation is considered difficult.

E
V 3
E
N
T

Etiology

Structural or mechanical obstruction to visualization of the larynx by direct laryngoscopy or to the passage of an ETT into the trachea

Typical Situations

Any patient with anatomy that makes direct laryngoscopy difficult
    Short "bull" neck
    Prominent maxillary incisors
    Limited range of neck or jaw movement
    Late stages of pregnancy
Congenital syndromes associated with difficulty in endotracheal intubation
Infections of the airway
Acquired anatomic abnormalities
    Intrinsic or extrinsic tumors of the airway
    Following radiation therapy to the head and/or neck
    Acromegaly
    Morbid obesity
    Patients with a history of sleep apnea
    Tracheal stenosis
    Significant neck swelling or hematoma compressing the airway

Prevention

Carefully assess airway anatomy
Use the classification schemes of Mallampati or Samsoon and Young
    Mallampati classification of visibility of oropharyngeal structures
        Class I: Visualize soft palate, uvula, tonsillar pillars, fauces
        Class II: Visualize soft palate, possibly uvula and fauces
        Class III: Visualize hard palate only
    Samsoon and Young modification of Mallampati classification
        Class I: Visualize soft palate, uvula, tonsillar pillars, fauces (same as Mallampati class I)
        Class II: Visualize soft palate, uvula, fauces
        Class III: Visualize soft palate, base of uvula only
        Class IV: Visualize hard palate only (same as Mallampati class III)

Manifestations

Expected Difficult Intubation
    An airway examination classified as Mallampati's class II or III or as Samsoon and Young's class III or IV
    Presence of other anatomic features that make the patient difficult to intubate
Unexpected Difficult Intubation
    Failure to intubate the trachea after two attempts by an experienced practitioner

Management

Expected Difficult Intubation

Err on the side of caution

> Review any available old anesthesia records of the patient's to see how the patient was managed during previous anesthetics
>
> Perform a careful airway assessment; obtain a second opinion about the airway if you are still unsure of how to proceed
>
> Consider alternatives to general anesthesia but remember that airway management will be difficult if a major complication or inadequate anesthesia occurs

Prepare contingency plans and obtain appropriate equipment

> Multiple laryngoscope blades
>
> Multiple ETT sizes
>
> Bougies, introducers, and light wand
>
> Emergency equipment for transtracheal jet ventilation connected to a source of O_2 and ready for use
>
> Fiberoptic laryngoscope
>
> A cricothyrotomy set and a person qualified to perform cricothyrotomy
>
> If cricothyrotomy would be difficult or impossible, consider CPB standby

Perform awake oral or nasal intubation

> This will be the safest option in most cases
>
> Awake intubation will be harder to perform if prior attempts at direct laryngoscopy have caused bleeding, secretions, or tissue edema
>
> Fiberoptic laryngoscopy
>
> Blind nasal intubation
>
> Retrograde intubation over a guidewire
>
> Light wand
>
> Awake direct laryngoscopy with topical anesthesia

For short cases consider general anesthesia with a volatile anesthetic via mask or nasal airway with spontaneous ventilation; however, **there is a risk of losing the airway**

> Do not attempt this without experienced help available; you will need to concentrate on the airway and will need to be able to delegate other tasks to someone else
>
> Use FiO_2 100%, monitor oxygenation and ventilation carefully
>
> Consider attempting direct laryngoscopy and intubation without using muscle relaxation once the patient is deeply anesthetized and the airway can be maintained. If there is an acceptable view of the glottis, consider using muscle relaxation to facilitate intubation
>
> If maintaining the airway is difficult, allow the patient to awaken
>
> If the airway cannot be maintained or if O_2 saturation falls, emergent airway management will be necessary
>
> > Attempt intubation <u>once</u>
> >
> > Move aggressively to transtracheal jet ventilation or cricothyrotomy

Unexpected Difficult Intubation

Call for help and emergency intubation equipment

Mask ventilate with 100% O_2, consider using cricoid pressure

> Assess adequacy of ventilation and oxygenation

EVENT 4

If mask ventilation is possible

Consider allowing spontaneous ventilation to return and the patient to awaken, and then converting to known difficult intubation

If a long-acting muscle relaxant has been administered, optimize attempts at intubation by using appropriate techniques, laryngoscope blades, and different anesthesiologists

If mask ventilation or intubation is impossible

Move early and aggressively to transtracheal jet ventilation. Do not wait for the O$_2$ saturation to fall precipitously

If transtracheal jet ventilation fails, move immediately to emergency cricothyrotomy or tracheostomy

After an unexpected difficult intubation, ensure that the patient is informed of the complications experienced and recommend that the patient obtain a Medic Alert bracelet (call 410-955-0631 in the United States) to inform future anesthetists about a potential problem

Complications

Damage to airway structures
Bleeding in the airway
Airway obstruction from loss of airway reflexes or laryngospasm
Hypoxemia
Esophageal intubation
Gastric distention
Regurgitation and aspiration of gastric contents
Damage to the cervical spine during attempts at intubation

Suggested Readings

Benumof JL: Management of the difficult adult airway. Anesthesiology 75:1087, 1991
Benumof JL, Scheller MS: The importance of transtracheal jet ventilation in the management of the difficult airway. Anesthesiology 71:769, 1989
Kross J, Zupan JT, Benumof JL: A contingency plan for tracheal intubation. Anesthesiology 72:577, 1990
Mallampati SR, Gatt SP, Gugino LD et al: A clinical sign to predict difficult tracheal intubation: a prospective study. Can Anaesth Soc J 32:429, 1985
Samsoon GL, Young JR: Difficult tracheal intubation. Anaesthesia 42:487, 1987

4 ESOPHAGEAL INTUBATION

Definition

Esophageal intubation is the placement of the ETT in the esophagus at the time of intubation or displacement of the ETT into the esophagus at a subsequent time.

Etiology

Difficulty in visualizing the larynx at the time of intubation
Difficulty in passing the ETT
Change in position of the ETT after correct placement

Typical Situations

After a difficult or "blind" intubation (see Event 3, *Difficult Tracheal Intubation*)
After intubation by an inexperienced laryngoscopist
After manipulation of the patient's head or neck

Prevention

Use proper intubation technique for optimal visualization of the larynx
Observe the ETT passing between the vocal cords
Secure the ETT carefully before allowing movement or positioning of the patient's head
Check the position of the ETT after each change of the patient's position or manipulation of the
     ETT
Visualize the carina during fiberoptic intubation

Manifestations

Abnormally low or absent expired CO_2 waveform after the first few breaths
Equivocal or absent thoracic breath sounds
Breath sounds or gurgling heard over the epigastrium
Abnormal lung compliance during hand or mechanical ventilation
Leakage around the ETT with a normal ETT cuff volume
In the awake patient, continued vocalization after the cuff of the ETT is inflated
Visualization of the ETT in the esophagus on direct laryngoscopy
Inability to palpate the cuff of the ETT in the sternal notch
Regurgitation of gastric contents up the ETT
LATE SIGNS
     Decreased O_2 saturation and cyanosis
     Bradycardia, PVCs, tachyarrhythmias, asystole
     Hypotension
     Ventricular fibrillation

Similar Events

Malfunction or disconnection of capnograph
Breath sounds difficult to hear
Complete or partial extubation
Endobronchial intubation (see Event 25, *Endobronchial Intubation*)
Severe bronchospasm (see Event 24, *Bronchospasm*)
Kinked ETT (see Event 5, *High Peak Inspiratory Pressure*)
Rupture of, or failure to inflate, the ETT cuff

Management

Development of hypoxemia within 10 minutes of intubation must be assumed to be due to esophageal intubation unless capnography demonstrates a normal CO_2 waveform or the ETT can be clearly visualized passing through the vocal cords (see Event 8, Hypoxemia).

Verify position of the ETT
> Check for a normal expired CO_2 waveform on the capnograph
> Listen for breath sounds in both axillae, and over the stomach
> Look for chest expansion
> Manually ventilate the patient, "feel" the compliance of the reservoir bag
> Perform direct laryngoscopy, visualize the position of the ETT relative to the vocal cords
> Get a second opinion if there are problems determining the position of the ETT

If esophageal intubation is confirmed or is still suspected
> Stop ventilating
> Leave the ETT in place with the cuff inflated
> Pass a suction catheter through the ETT and apply suction
> Secure the airway
>> Ventilate with 100% O_2 by mask with cricoid pressure, as needed to maintain the O_2 saturation above 90–95%
>>> Cricoid pressure may be ineffective with ETT in esophagus
>>> Mask seal may be difficult to achieve with an ETT and suction catheter in the mouth
>> Perform direct laryngoscopy and reintubate the trachea using a new ETT
>>> Regurgitation may occur as laryngoscopy is performed
>>> Laryngoscopy may be difficult with ETT in esophagus

Move aggressively to transtracheal jet ventilation or cricothyrotomy if the trachea cannot be intubated and oxygenation cannot be maintained (see Event 3, *Difficult Tracheal Intubation*)

> After securing the airway and confirming the position of the ETT, remove the ETT from the esophagus and pass a nasogastric tube to empty the stomach

Complications

Hypoxemia
Hypercarbia
Cardiac arrest
Airway, pharyngeal, or dental trauma from repeated laryngoscopy
Aspiration of gastric contents
Hypertension, tachycardia
Myocardial ischemia/infarction

Suggested Readings

Caplan RA, Posner K, Ward RJ, Cheney FW: Adverse events in anesthesia: a closed claims analysis. Anesthesiology 72:828, 1990
Sum-Ping ST, Mehta MP, Anderton JM: A comparative study of methods of detection of esophageal intubation. Anesth Analg 69:627, 1989

5 HIGH PEAK INSPIRATORY PRESSURE

Definition

An increase in the PIP of more than 5 cm H_2O during positive pressure ventilation or a PIP greater than 40 cm H_2O is considered high.

Etiology

Breathing circuit problem
    Ventilator/bag selector switch in the wrong position
    Stuck closed inspiratory, expiratory, or pop-off valve
    Accidental placement of a PEEP valve in the inspiratory limb of the breathing circuit
    Kinked or misconnected hose in the breathing circuit or scavenging system
    Failure of check valves or regulators in the anesthesia machine, allowing gas under high pressure into the breathing circuit
    Use of the O_2 flush when circuit is closed
    O_2 flush control stuck in the ON position
ETT problem
    Kink in the ETT
    Endobronchial, esophageal, or submucosal intubation
    Herniated ETT cuff obstructing the end of the ETT
    Foreign body, secretions, or mucus plugging the ETT
    Dissection of the interior surface of the ETT, leading to airway narrowing
Decreased pulmonary compliance
    Raised intra-abdominal pressure
    Pulmonary aspiration of gastric contents (see Event 23, *Aspiration of Gastric Contents*)
    Bronchospasm other than in association with pulmonary aspiration (see Event 24, *Bronchospasm*)
    Atelectasis
    Decreased chest wall or diaphragmatic compliance
    Pulmonary edema (see Event 17, *Pulmonary Edema*)
    Pneumothorax (see Event 28, *Pneumothorax*)
Drug-induced problem
    Narcotic-induced chest wall rigidity
    Inadequate muscle relaxation
    Malignant hyperthermia (see Event 38, *Malignant Hyperthermia*)

Typical Situations

During induction of anesthesia
Immediately after intubation
Light anesthesia
After change in patient or head position
Following manipulation of the ETT
After adding components to the breathing circuit
During or following surgery in or near the pleural cavities

Prevention

Check the breathing circuit and the ETT carefully before use
Place the ETT carefully
Use care when adding components to the breathing circuit
Plan anesthetic management to prevent bronchospasm, atelectasis, or buildup of secretions in
   patients at risk
Use a small dose of nondepolarizing muscle relaxant to pretreat patients prior to administration
   of opiates

Manifestations

High PIP
   If present, high-pressure alarm will sound
Decreased compliance of the reservoir bag during manual ventilation
Decreased minute ventilation
   Little or no excursion of the chest with inspiration
   Reduced expiratory return of gas on spirometer
   Reduced breath sounds
Abnormal sound of the ventilator during inspiration
Little or no end-tidal CO_2
Fall in O_2 saturation (see Event 8, *Hypoxemia*)
Profound hypotension not responsive to vasopressors or inotropes
Tachycardia

Similar Events

Faulty airway pressure gauge or airway pressure alarm

Management

Increase the FiO_2 to 100%
Verify the PIP
Switch to manual ventilation using the reservoir bag
   Assess the pulmonary/breathing circuit compliance
Disconnect the Y piece from the ETT and squeeze the reservoir bag
   If the airway pressure remains high, there is an obstruction in the breathing circuit
      Ventilate using a backup ventilation system (Jackson-Rees circuit, self-inflating
         bag, or mouth-to-ETT)
      Get help to replace or repair the obstruction in the circuit
   If the airway pressure falls, the problem is in the ETT or lungs, not in the breathing
      circuit
Auscultate both sides of the patient's chest
   Listen for symmetry of breath sounds, wheezes, or fine crackles (rales)
   If breath sounds are asymmetric
      Examine the ETT and consider endobronchial intubation (see Event 25,
         Endobronchial Intubation)

Check the blood pressure and heart rate, palpate the trachea, percuss the chest, and
consider pneumothorax (see Event 28, *Pneumothorax*)
If wheezes are present, consider bronchospasm (see Event 24, *Bronchospasm*)
If fine crackles are present bilaterally, consider pulmonary edema (see Event 17,
Pulmonary Edema)

Exclude ETT obstruction
Pass a suction catheter down the ETT and apply suction to clear any secretions
If it passes FREELY, the ETT is unlikely to be occluded
If the ETT is markedly obstructed
Deflate the ETT cuff and check again
Remove the ETT, retain it for later examination, mask-ventilate if necessary to
increase the O_2 saturation, then reintubate with a new ETT
If the patient was difficult to intubate, consider passing a fiberoptic laryngoscope
down the ETT to define the exact nature of the problem

Notify the surgical team of the problem and review any possible etiology with them
Check for other causes of decreased chest compliance
Malignant hyperthermia (see Event 38, *Malignant Hyperthermia*)
Inadequate depth of anesthesia or muscle relaxation
Administration of opiates
Unusual patient position or excessive surgical retraction
Abnormal anatomy of the patient (e.g., kyphoscoliosis)

Complications

Barotrauma
Hypotension, cardiovascular compromise due to raised intrathoracic pressure
Hypoxemia
Hypertension, tachycardia after resolution of high PIP, due to delayed action of vasopressors
and inotropes

Suggested Readings

Bashein G, MacEvoy B, Schreiber PJ: Anesthesia ventilators should have adjustable high-pressure alarms.
Anesthesiology 63:231, 1985
Biondi JW, Schulman DS, Soufer R et al: The effect of incremental positive end-expiratory pressure on
right ventricular hemodynamics and ejection fraction. Anesth Analg 67:144, 1988
Dorsch JA, Dorsch SE: Hazards of anesthesia machines and breathing systems. p. 289. In: Understanding
Anesthesia Equipment. 2nd Ed. Williams & Wilkins, Baltimore, 1984

6 HYPERTENSION

Definition

Hypertension is a rise in arterial blood pressure of more than 20% above baseline, or an
absolute value of arterial blood pressure above age-corrected limits.

Etiology

Pre-existing hypertension
    Essential hypertension
    Renovascular hypertension
    Pre-eclampsia
    Autonomic dysreflexia
Catecholamine release
    Laryngoscopy or intubation
    Surgical stimulation
    Emergence from anesthesia
    Acute withdrawal of antihypertensive medication
Hypoxemia
Hypercarbia
Administration of vasopressor medications
Raised ICP
Volume overload
Acute increase in afterload

Typical Situations

Anesthesia in patients with chronic hypertension
During intubation or on emergence from general anesthesia
Inadequate depth of anesthesia relative to surgical stimulus
In patients with pregnancy-induced hypertension (see Event 73, *Pre-eclampsia and Eclampsia*)
In patients who abuse drugs

Prevention

Treat preoperative hypertension adequately
    Continue preoperative administration of antihypertensive medications up to the time of
        surgery
    Postpone elective surgery if severe hypertension (diastolic pressure higher than 110 mm
        Hg) is present preoperatively
Consider the use of clonidine as oral premedication
Avoid ketamine for induction of anesthesia in known hypertensive patients
Anticipate times of high levels of surgical stimulation and prophylactically increase the depth
    of anesthesia
Avoid hypervolemia (e.g., TURP cases)
Carefully titrate vasoactive medications
Maintain oxygenation and ventilation at normal levels
Use blood pressure monitoring equipment properly
Treat severe pain, hypoxemia, or bladder distention in the postoperative period

Manifestations

Rise in or high arterial pressure (systolic, diastolic, or mean)
If hypertension is due to light anesthesia, the patient may exhibit

Tachypnea if breathing spontaneously
Tachycardia
Sweating
Tearing
Pupillary dilation
Movement
Heart rate may be <u>decreased</u> due to baroreceptor activity, especially if the etiology of hypertension is autonomic dysreflexia or raised intracranial pressure

Similar Events

Artifacts of blood pressure measurement system
   Motion artifact with NIBP device
   Inappropriately small NIBP cuff
   Faulty or inaccurately zeroed transducer
   Transducer at inappropriate height
   Resonance artifact

Management

Verify that hypertension is real
   If using a NIBP monitoring device
      Repeat measurement
      Check for artifact of NIBP system
      Consider moving blood pressure cuff to another site
      Measure cuff blood pressure manually
   If using an invasive system for measuring arterial blood pressure
      Check position and zero of arterial transducer, correlate with NIBP measurement
      Flush the arterial line
      Check calibration of transducer
      Check that there are no kinks in the arterial line tubing
Check drug administration
   If infusions of vasoactive drugs or IV anesthetics are being administered
      Check that infusion devices are set properly and are running at the desired rate
      Check the dosage calculations carefully
      Check the concentration of the medications being infused
      Check that the carrier IV line is running at an appropriate rate
   If administering a volatile anesthetic
      Check that the vaporizer is set correctly
      Check that all controls needed to activate the vaporizer are set correctly
      Check the level of liquid anesthetic in the vaporizer
      Check the inspired concentration of anesthetic by mass spectrometer or other analyzer
Ensure adequate oxygenation and ventilation
   Check ABGs if there is any question of hypoxemia or hypercarbia
Assess depth of anesthesia
   Assess clinical signs of anesthetic depth
   Look for a new surgical stimulus

Deepen anesthesia as necessary
>Increase concentration of volatile anesthetic
>Administer bolus of IV narcotic
>Administer bolus of IV anesthetic
>If using a continuous spinal or epidural technique, administer additional local anesthetic or narcotic via the catheter

For isolated hypertension not due to an identifiable cause
>Check for secondary manifestations of hypertension (tachycardia, ST-T wave changes [see Event 10, *ST Segment Changes*])
>If treatment is necessary, consider
>>ß blockade (use with caution in patients with COPD)
>>>Esmolol IV, 10–20 mg increments
>>>Propranolol IV, 0.25–0.5 mg increments
>>>Labetalol IV, 5 mg increments
>>Nitroprusside by IV infusion, 0.1–3 µg/kg/min
>>NTG by IV infusion, 0.1–2 µg/kg/min
>>α blockade
>>>Phentolamine IV, 0.5–1 mg (see Event 12, *Autonomic Dysreflexia*)
>>>Droperidol IV, 0.5–1.5 mg increments
>>Calcium channel blockade
>>>Verapamil IV, 2.5 mg increments
>>>Nifedipine SL, 10 mg

Review fluid management. If overhydration is likely, administer furosemide IV, 5–10 mg
Check for the presence of a distended bladder; place a urinary catheter if the bladder is distended
Raised ICP may require urgent therapy with mannitol IV, 0.5 g/kg; furosemide IV, 5–10 mg; or thiopental IV, 5–10 mg/kg over 30 minutes; or hyperventilation to arterial pCO_2 of 25 mm Hg, followed by rapid neurosurgical intervention
Look for signs of MH (see Event 38, *Malignant Hyperthermia*)

Complications

Myocardial ischemia/infarction
Arrhythmias
Congestive heart failure/pulmonary edema
Increased operative blood loss
Raised ICP
Disruption of vascular suture lines
Hypertensive encephalopathy or cerebral hemorrhage

Suggested Readings

Miller ED: Perioperative hypertension: an overview. p. 331. In: Annual Refresher Course Lectures. American Society of Anesthesiologists, Park Ridge, IL, 1991
Sprague DH, Just PW: High and low blood pressure—when to treat? Probl Anesth 1:273, 1987

7 HYPOTENSION

Definition

Hypotension is a fall in arterial blood pressure of more than 20% below baseline or an absolute value of systolic pressure below 90 mm Hg or of MAP below 60 mm Hg.

Etiology

Decreased preload
    Hypovolemia
    Vasodilation
    Surgical maneuvers restricting venous return
    Elevated intrathoracic pressure
    Patient position
    Pericardial tamponade
    Pulmonary embolism
Decreased contractility
    Inotropic depressant drugs
    Arrhythmias
    Cardiomyopathy or congestive heart failure
    Myocardial ischemia/infarction
    Hypoxemia
    Valvular heart disease
    Abrupt increase in afterload
Decreased SVR
    Vasodilation
    Side effects of drugs
    Sepsis
    Anaphylaxis
    Endocrine abnormalities (addisonian crisis, hypothyroidism, hypoglycemia, removal of pheochromocytoma)
    Abrupt change in mechanical afterload

Typical Situations

After anesthetic induction and before surgical incision
Pre-existing hypovolemia (e.g., trauma, chronic hypertension)
Spinal/epidural anesthesia
Surgery with major fluid shifts or near major vascular structures
History of cardiovascular disease
Position other than supine

Prevention

Carefully assess cardiovascular status preoperatively, checking for
    Increased heart rate or orthostatic hypotension
    CVP or jugular venous filling

Preoperative hematocrit

Skin turgor

Ensure adequate intravascular volume before induction of anesthesia

Correlate invasive blood pressure with NIBP early in case

Avoid high doses of anesthetic agents

Administer drugs slowly if hypotension is a known side effect

Use judicious doses of local anesthetics in single-shot regional techniques; carefully titrate local anesthetics in continuous regional techniques

Monitor surgical activities and track blood loss carefully

Manifestations

Fall in or low arterial pressure (systolic, diastolic, or mean)

Mental status changes (nausea, vomiting in conscious patient)

Arrhythmias

Weak or absent peripheral pulses

Inability of pulse oximeter or NIBP device to obtain a satisfactory reading

Decreased end-tidal CO_2 or decreased O_2 saturation

Decreased urine output

Diminished heart sounds

Similar Events

Artifact of blood pressure measurement system

Motion artifact with NIBP device

Incorrect size of NIBP cuff

Faulty blood pressure transducer

Transducer at inappropriate height

Spasm of radial artery or other lack of correlation between radial and central arterial pressure

Management

Ensure adequate oxygenation and ventilation

Check the O_2 saturation

Increase the FiO_2 if O_2 saturation is low or if hypotension is severe

Verify that patient is truly hypotensive

Palpate a peripheral pulse

IF the pulse is strong, consider artifact or transient

Repeat NIBP measurement

Measure blood pressure manually

Check the zero of the invasive blood pressure transducer

Check the arterial line for any open or loose stopcock or connector

Reduce or turn off any vasodilating drugs

Expand circulating blood volume

Lift the patient's legs above the level of the heart or put the patient into the Trendelenburg position

Administer fluids rapidly

If history of CHF, use multiple small boluses and re-evaluate frequently

8 E
V
E
N
T

Consider using colloids or blood for rapid volume expansion
Ensure sufficient large-bore IV access if continued volume replacement is necessary
Check with surgeons about venous compression and blood loss
Treat severe hypotension with IV bolus of vasopressor/inotrope
Use ephedrine, 5–50 mg, phenylephrine, 20–100 µg; or epinephrine, 10–100 µg
Repeat as necessary to maintain an acceptable blood pressure

Elucidate and correct the underlying cause
Hypovolemia is very common, but is NOT the only cause
Check urine output, hematocrit, and fluid balance
Check filling pressure if CVP or PA catheter is in place. If not, consider placing a CVP or PA catheter to assess filling pressure
Check cardiac output and SVR if PA catheter is in place. If not, consider placing a PA catheter if hypotension does not resolve with standard treatment or if other factors complicate patient management (e.g., pulmonary edema, oliguria)
Consider using infusions of inotropic or vasopressor drugs
Sustained use of vasopressors may be required in states of severe vasodilation (e.g., septic shock)
Consider placing an arterial line into the central arterial circulation (usually the femoral artery), especially if overall assessment is consistent with a failure of the radial artery pressure to correlate with central arterial pressure
Check ABGs for metabolic acidosis (see Event 39, *Metabolic Acidosis*)
Evaluate myocardial status
Check the ECG for signs of ischemia (see Event 10, *ST Segment Changes*)
Evaluate myocardial function with TEE, if available

Complications

CHF or pulmonary edema from excessive fluid administration
Hypertension from treatment of artifact or transient
Myocardial ischemia/infarction
Cerebral ischemia
Acute renal failure

Suggested Readings

Sprague DH, Just PW: High and low blood pressure—when to treat? Probl Anesth 1:273, 1987
Vincent JL: Fluids for resuscitation. Br J Anaesth 64:185, 1991

8 HYPOXEMIA

Definition

Hypoxemia is a fall in O_2 saturation of more than 5%, absolute value of O_2 saturation below 90%, or an absolute value of arterial pO_2 below 60 mm Hg.

Etiology

Low FiO_2
      Relative (inadequate for the patient's condition)
      Absolute (problems delivering O_2 to the breathing circuit)
Inadequate alveolar ventilation
V/Q mismatch
Anatomic shunt
Excessive metabolic O_2 demand
Low cardiac output

Typical Situations

Inadequate ventilation from any cause
      Failure to maintain the airway during general anesthesia
      Failure to ventilate adequately during general anesthesia
      Morbid obesity
Patients with increased A-a gradient
      Pre-existing lung disease
      Pulmonary edema
      Aspiration of gastric contents
      Atelectasis
      Pulmonary embolus
Patients at extremes of age are more likely to have anatomic features or disease states that compromise oxygenation

Prevention

Perform a careful check of the anesthesia machine, O_2 analyzer, and alarms before use
Maintain adequate ventilation, using appropriate clinical and electronic monitors
Monitor and adjust FiO_2 as necessary to maintain patient oxygenation
Keep lung volumes in high normal range with large tidal volumes during mechanical ventilation
Avoid spontaneous ventilation in patients with lung disease or when the patient is not in the supine position

Manifestations

Decreased or low O_2 saturation measured by pulse oximetry is the cardinal sign of hypoxemia
Pulse oximetry may not function properly in the presence of
      Hypothermia
      Poor peripheral circulation
      Artifacts due to electrocautery, motion, or ambient lighting
Cyanosis or dark blood in the surgical field
      Clinically detectable cyanosis corresponds to an arterial O_2 saturation of approximately 85% and requires 5 g of reduced hemoglobin. It may therefore be masked by anemia
Hypoxemia can be difficult to recognize clinically under anesthesia, as the circulatory and res-

piratory responses to hypoxemia are blunted by anesthetic agents. Late signs of hypoxemia include
  BRADYCARDIA
  Myocardial arrhythmias/ischemia
  Tachycardia
  Hypotension
  Cardiac arrest

Similar Events

Pulse oximeter artifact
Blood gas analysis of venous blood
Methemoglobinemia
Low cardiac output

Management

Assume that low O_2 saturation indicates hypoxemia until proven otherwise
  Development of hypoxemia within 10 minutes of intubation must be assumed to be due to esophageal intubation unless the ETT can be visualized passing through the cords or capnography demonstrates normal end-tidal CO_2
Increase FIO_2 to 100%
  Use high O_2 flow to equilibrate the breathing circuit rapidly
  Verify that FIO_2 approaches 100%
Check that ventilation is adequate
  Check end-tidal CO_2, if available (may not reflect adequacy of ventilation if V/Q mismatch is large)
  Switch to hand ventilation to assess pulmonary compliance
  Hand ventilate with large tidal volumes to expand collapsed lung segments
  Auscultate the breath sounds bilaterally, assess the adequacy and symmetry of chest movement
  Obtain ABGs. Ask blood gas laboratory to check for abnormal hemoglobin if clinically indicated
Check the position of the ETT
  Auscultation
  Direct visualization of ETT at mouth opening
  Direct visualization of ETT cuff below cords
  Fiberoptic bronchoscopy to visualize tracheal rings and the carina
  Adjust the position of the ETT if necessary (see Event 25, *Endobronchial Intubation*)
Verify function of the pulse oximeter
  Do not fixate on oximeter function. Monitor the patient carefully while ruling out artifacts and transients
  Correlate oximeter readings with activation of electrocautery
  Check the probe position
  Shield the probe from ambient light
  Assess adequacy of oximeter signal amplitude
  Change the site of the probe (from finger to ear)

If situation does not resolve, look for conditions that increase venous admixture
  Pulmonary aspiration of gastric contents
  Massive atelectasis/aspiration of foreign body
  Pulmonary emboli
  Bronchospasm
  Increased intracardiac shunting in congenital heart disease
  Check again to rule out pneumothorax, with a chest x-ray if necessary
Use aggressive pulmonary toilet
  Suction ETT
  Consider bronchoscopy
Consider the addition of PEEP to breathing circuit and maintain large tidal volumes (12–15 ml/kg)
Restore adequate circulating blood volume to maintain cardiac output and hemoglobin levels
Inform surgeons if difficulty in maintaining oxygenation persists
  Check for retractors causing difficulty with ventilation
  Check that patient in the prone position has not slipped off chest supports, placing pressure on the diaphragm; prepare to transfer the patient to the supine position emergently
  Terminate surgery as soon as possible
  Arrange for ICU transfer for postoperative care

Complications

Cardiac arrest (when hypoxemia precipitates cardiac arrest it is frequently associated with permanent neurologic injury regardless of the success of CPR)
Neurologic injury manifested as confusion, coma, delayed recovery from anesthesia
Arrhythmias
Hypotension
Bradycardia

Suggested Reading

Katz JA: Management of intra-operative ventilatory emergencies. p. 265. In Annual Refresher Course Lectures. American Society of Anesthesiologists, Park Ridge, IL, 1988

9 OPERATING ROOM FIRE

Definition

This event includes any fire in an operating room.

Etiology

An operating room fire requires three simultaneous elements
  Ignition source
  Fuel source
  Oxidizer

9 E
V
E
N
T

Typical Situations

Cases involving ignition sources
    Electrocautery
    Hot-wire cautery
    Fiberoptic light source
    Laser
Disregard for safe rules of operation of sources of ignition
Cases in which a high concentration of oxidizer (O_2 or N_2O) is present in or near the surgical site
Cases in which flammable solvents or ointments are used
Electrical faults, giving rise to sparks

Prevention

Use carefully and control devices that can act as ignition sources
Turn off ignition sources when not actively in use
Use low concentrations of O_2 (less than 30%) when an ignition source is present
Use nonflammable skin preparation solutions
Provide routine maintenance of operating room electrical equipment; remove electrical equipment from service if faults are detected
Avoid flammable anesthetic agents

Manifestations

Smoke
    Visible
    Smell
Visible charring of drapes or operating room table linens
Visible flames
Palpable heat
Sparks from electrical equipment or operating room lights
Explosion
Fire alarm

Similar Events

Fire elsewhere in the hospital

Management

Alert all personnel in the operating room immediately
Pat out or smother small fires on the surgical field
    A laser can burn a pinhole through the outer drape and ignite the inner drape
    Check under the patient drapes for smoldering fires in inner layers of drapes or blankets
    Turn off or unplug any electrical equipment involved
If the fire continues
    Call for help immediately
    Activate hospital fire alarm and notify fire department

Remove any burning material from the patient or from operating room personnel if possible

Extinguish the fire if it is safe for you to do so

Use Halon or CO_2 fire extinguisher

CO_2 extinguisher leaves a particulate residue

H_2O may extinguish the fire

H_2O may be ineffective if it beads up on water-repellent drapes

H_2O may spread the fire when the fuel source is a volatile liquid

Disconnect the circuit from the ETT or disconnect the hoses from the breathing circuit to prevent back propagation of fire into anesthesia machine

If the fire is not quickly controlled

Evacuate the patient, on the operating table if possible

Have auxiliary portable lighting available, as visibility may be very restricted

Notify staff in other operating rooms

After exiting, isolate the operating room to contain smoke or fire

Close the doors and any other openings into the operating room

Turn off piped gases, air conditioning, and ventilation to the affected operating room

Prepare to evacuate the entire operating room suite

Continue to fight the fire with extinguishers or fire hose if it is safe to do so

Evaluate and treat injuries to the patient or operating room personnel

Check for burns, bleeding, or other injuries

Maintain ventilation of the paralyzed patient

Replace damaged equipment, especially that needed for life support

Follow-up

Save suspect equipment or materials for investigation

Report all small fires through departmental quality assurance program regardless of outcome

Report significant fires or events with a negative outcome to the hospital risk manager

There may be a statutory responsibility to report a fire to local, state, or federal agencies

Complications

Burns
Smoke inhalation
Light anesthesia and awareness of the patient while disconnected from inhalation anesthetics

Suggested Reading

"The patient is on fire!" A surgical fires primer. Health Devices 21:19, 1992

10 ST SEGMENT CHANGES

Definition

This event includes elevation or depression of the ST segment of the ECG from the isoelectric level.

Etiology

Inadequate coronary perfusion for a given myocardial O_2 demand
Acute myocardial ischemia or infarction
Myocardial contusion
Acute pericarditis
Electrolyte abnormalities (hypo- or hyperkalemia, hypercalcemia)
Head injury or raised ICP
Early repolarization (normal variant)
Hypothermia (below 30˚C)
Defibrillation injury of myocardium

Typical Situations

In patients with pre-existing CAD
During any acute change in myocardial O_2 demand or delivery, secondary to
     Tachycardia, hypertension, or hypotension
     Hypoxemia or hemodilution
     Coronary spasm (Prinzmetal's angina)
After head or chest trauma
During vaginal delivery or cesarean section

Prevention

Carefully evaluate and prepare patients with CAD preoperatively
Carefully manage hemodynamics and hematocrit to optimize myocardial O_2 balance
Identify and evaluate pre-existing ST segment abnormalities preoperatively

Manifestations

Depression or elevation of ST segment from the isoelectric level
If the ST segment changes are due to myocardial ischemia, the awake patient may manifest
     Central chest pain radiating into the arms or throat
     Dyspnea
     Nausea and vomiting
     Altered level of consciousness or cognitive function
ST segment changes due to myocardial ischemia may be associated with
     The development of Q waves in the ECG
     Arrhythmias (PVCs, ventricular tachycardia, or fibrillation)
     Hypotension

Elevation of ventricular filling pressures
V wave on pulmonary artery wedge tracing

Similar Situations

Artifact of ECG
  Improper electrode position on the patient
  Alteration in position of heart relative to the electrodes due to changes in patient position
    or surgical manipulation
Abnormal cardiac conduction
Left ventricular hypertrophy
Drug effects
Ventricular pacing
Left ventricular aneurysm

Management

All ST changes should be considered ischemic in origin until proved otherwise.

Verify ST segment changes
  Evaluate electrode placement and ECG settings
  Evaluate multiple ECG leads
  Review previous ECGs or ST segment tracking data
Ensure adequate oxygenation and ventilation
  Check pulse oximeter
  Check capnograph if in use
  Check ABGs if there is any question of oxygenation or ventilation
Treat tachycardia and/or hypertension
  Tachycardia is the most important determinant of increased myocardial O_2 demand
  Increase the depth of anesthesia if appropriate
  β blockade
    Esmolol IV, 0.25–0.5 mg/kg bolus, 50–300 μg/kg/min infusion
    Labetolol IV, 5–10 mg bolus, repeat as necessary
    Propranolol IV, 0.25–1 mg bolus, repeat as necessary
    Use with caution if the patient is hypotensive or has severe COPD or asthma
  Treat hypertension
    NTG
      Sublingual (absorption uncertain, can cause hypotension)
      Transdermal paste, 1–2 in. applied to the chest wall (slow onset)
      IV infusion, 0.25–2 μg/kg/min (titrated to effect)
    Calcium channel blockade
      Nifedipine SL, 5–10 mg (absorption uncertain, can cause hypotension)
      Verapamil IV, 2.5 mg, repeat as necessary (avoid if β blockade present)
      Diltiazem IV, 2.5 mg increments, repeat as necessary
Treat hypotension and/or bradycardia
  Coronary perfusion pressure takes precedence over afterload reduction
  Optimize circulating fluid volume
    Use PA pressures as a guide, consider placement of a PA catheter if not in place

Support myocardial contractility as needed using inotropic agents

Use inotropes with caution since they may increase myocardial O_2 demand and worsen ischemia

Ephedrine IV, 5–10 mg increments

Dobutamine IV infusion, 2.5–10 µg/kg/min

Dopamine IV infusion, 2.5–10 µg/kg/min

Epinephrine IV infusion, 10–100 ng/kg/min

Avoid NTG or calcium channel blockade until hypotension or bradycardia are resolved

Consider combined use of phenylephrine and NTG infusions

Inform the surgeon

Discuss early termination of the surgical procedure

Discuss transfer to ICU for postoperative management

If no response to therapy, obtain cardiology consultation

If available, TEE can be used to assist diagnosis and to monitor the results of therapy. This technique requires considerable expertise in interpretation

Send blood samples to clinical laboratory

ABGs

Hemoglobin/hematocrit

Glucose

Electrolytes

CK, CK-MB isoenzyme (for comparison with subsequent measurements)

Treat underlying causes of ST segment changes other than myocardial ischemia

Complications

Myocardial infarction

Arrhythmias

Cardiac arrest

Complications of PA catheterization

Complications of TEE

Suggested Readings

Breslow MJ, Miller CF, Parker SD et al: Changes in T-wave morphology following anesthesia and surgery: a common recovery-room phenomenon. Anesthesiology 64:398, 1986

Dodds TM, Delphin E, Stone JB: Detection of perioperative myocardial ischemia using Holter monitoring with real-time ST segment analysis. Anesth Analg 67:890, 1988

Goldberger E, Wheat MW: Acute myocardial infarction. p. 145. In: Treatment of Cardiac Emergencies. 5th Ed. CV Mosby, St Louis, 1990

London MJ, Hollenberg M, Wong MG et al: Intraoperative myocardial ischemia: localization by continuous 12-lead electrocardiography. Anesthesiology 69:232, 1988

Chapter Four

Cardiovascular Events

11 ANAPHYLAXIS AND ANAPHYLACTOID REACTIONS

Definition

Anaphylaxis and anaphylactoid reactions are immediate hypersensitivity reactions involving a generalized response to a specific antigen:

Anaphylaxis involves antigen and IgE antibodies and requires previous sensitization to an antigen
Anaphylactoid reactions are mediated by histamine and may occur with the first exposure to an antigen
Complement activation follows both immunologic and nonimmunologic pathways mediated by histamine and other compounds

Etiology

Sensitization of the patient by prior exposure to an antigen, with production of antigen-specific Ig (IgE) antibodies (anaphylaxis)
Underlying physiologic events
    Degranulation of mast cells and basophils, with release of histamine, leukotrienes, and prostaglandins
    Activation of the complement system

Typical Situations

Approximately 500 deaths occur each year in the United States from anaphylaxis; penicillin allergy accounts for 75% of deaths.

After administration of substances that can trigger anaphylactic or anaphylactoid reactions
    Antibiotics
    Narcotics
    Protamine
    Aminoester local anesthetic agents
    Blood and blood products
    Iodinated contrast material
    Neuromuscular blocking agents
After repeated exposure of a patient to the same drugs at short intervals
In patients with a known allergy or sensitivity to a specific agent or with conditions making a reaction to an agent more likely
    Protamine reactions are more likely in patients with fish allergy or after treatment with protamine-zinc insulin
    Patients with a history of allergy to nondrug allergens have a higher risk of anaphylactic

or anaphylactoid reactions during anesthesia

Individuals with frequent exposure to latex products have a higher risk of a reaction to latex in the operating room

Patients who have undergone multiple surgical procedures

Patients who require intermittent bladder catheterization

Spinal cord injury

Chronic care patients

Health care workers

Prevention

Obtain a careful history of previous allergic reactions, atopy, or asthma

Administer a test dose followed by slow administration of antibiotics and other drugs known to precipitate allergic reactions

Avoid blood or blood product transfusion whenever possible

Check the identity of the patient and the blood products carefully prior to transfusion

If there is a history of latex allergy, establish a latex-free environment

Avoid contact with or manipulation of latex devices

Use nonlatex surgical gloves

Use syringe/stopcock methods or unidirectional valves for injecting medications

Do not instrument multiple-dose vials with natural rubber stoppers

Take the top of the vial completely off

Use the same medication from a glass ampule

Use glass syringes as an alternative to rubber-plunger plastic syringes

If a specific drug must be administered to a patient known to be at risk of an allergic reaction, administer prophylaxis

Corticosteroids

Dexamethasone IV, 20 mg, or methylprednisolone IV, 100 mg

H_1 antagonist

Diphenhydramine IV, 25–50 mg

Obtain a consultation from an allergist if a critical allergy must be defined

Manifestations

Anaphylaxis has the potential for sudden onset with catastrophic consequences.

Cardiac

Hypotension may be the only sign of anaphylaxis in the anesthetized patient

Cardiovascular collapse

Pulmonary hypertension

Arrhythmias, pulmonary edema

The awake patient may complain of dizziness or decreased level of consciousness

Respiratory

Bronchospasm

Increased PIP

Hypoxemia

Pulmonary edema

Stridor, laryngeal edema

The awake patient may complain of dyspnea and/or chest tightness

Cutaneous
> Rash, flush, or hives
> Pruritis
> Angioedema

Similar Events

Anesthetic overdose (see Event 62, *Volatile Anesthetic Overdose)*
Pulmonary edema (see Event 17, *Pulmonary Edema)*
Pericardial tamponade (see Event 16, *Pericardial Tamponade)*
Venous air embolism (see Event 20, *Venous Air or Gas Embolism)*
Vasovagal reaction
Septic shock
Stridor (see Event 29, *Postoperative Stridor)*
Pulmonary embolism (see Event 18, *Pulmonary Embolism)*
Aspiration of gastric contents (see Event 23, *Aspiration Of Gastric Contents)*
Pneumothorax (see Event 28, *Pneumothorax)*
Bronchospasm (see Event 24, *Bronchospasm)*
Skin manifestations of drug reactions not associated with anaphylaxis
Fat embolism
Hypotension from other causes (see Event 7, *Hypotension)*
Transfusion reaction (see Event 41, *Transfusion Reaction)*

Management

Stop administration of any possible antigen
> Retain blood products for analysis

Inform the surgeons
> Check to see whether they have injected or instilled a substance into a body cavity
> Prepare to terminate the surgical procedure if there is no response to treatment

Maintain the patient's airway and support oxygenation and ventilation
> Increase FiO$_2$ to 100%
> Intubate if necessary
> The airway and larynx can become very edematous

Decrease or stop administration of anesthetic agents if hypotension is present
> If bronchospasm is present and the patient is normotensive, volatile anesthetic agents
> may be administered to counteract bronchospasm

Expand the circulating fluid volume rapidly
> Immediate fluid needs may be <u>massive</u> (several liters of crystalloid)
> Insert a large-bore IV catheter

Administer epinephrine IV
> Epinephrine is the drug of choice for treatment of anaphylaxis
> For hypotension, 10–50 μg increments, repeat as necessary with escalating doses
> For cardiovascular collapse, use ACLS doses, 500–1000 μg boluses, repeat as necessary
> with escalating doses

Administer an H$_1$ antagonist
> H$_1$ blockers
>> Diphenhydramine IV, 50 mg

The use of H$_2$ antagonists is <u>not</u> recommended
In the absence of any other cause, consider latex allergy
> Remove all latex products in contact with the patient
>> Surgical gloves
>> Medications drawn up through a latex stopper
>> Urinary catheter

Administer corticosteroids
> Dexamethasone IV, 20 mg bolus
> Methylprednisolone IV, 100 mg bolus

Place invasive monitors as necessary for monitoring, infusion of vasoactive drugs, and blood sampling
> Arterial line
> CVP or PA catheter
> Urinary catheter

Complications

Inability to intubate, ventilate, or oxygenate
Cardiac arrest
Hypertension, tachycardia from vasopressors

Suggested Readings

Jantzen JH, Wangemann B, Wisser G: Adverse reactions to non-ionic iodinated contrast media do occur during general anesthesia. Anesthesiology 70:561, 1989

Holzman RS: Latex allergy: an emerging operating room problem. Anesth Analg 76:635, 1993

Kelly JS, Prielipp RC: Is cimetidine indicated in the treatment of acute anaphylactic shock? Anesth Analg 71:100, 1990

Levy JH: Anaphylactic Reactions in Anesthesia and Intensive Care. 2nd Ed. Butterworths, Boston, 1986

Stoelting RK: Allergy and Anesthesia. p. 146. In Review Course Lectures. International Anesthesia Research Society, Cleveland, 1991

Weiss ME, Adkinson NF Jr, Hirshman CA et al: Evaluation of allergic drug reactions in the perioperative period. Anesthesiology 71:483, 1989

12 AUTONOMIC DYSREFLEXIA

Definition

Autonomic dysreflexia is a massive unopposed reflex sympathetic discharge triggered by a physical stimulus below the level of a chronic spinal cord injury.

Etiology

Distention of the bladder or of a hollow viscus
Stimulation of the lower GI tract

Performance of a surgical procedure with inadequate anesthesia
Exposure to hot or cold temperature extremes
Tactile stimulation

Typical Situations

In patients with SCI after recovery from flaccid paralysis; may occur at any time but usually at
least 6 weeks after the injury
In patients whose level of SCI is above T8 (the higher the lesion, the higher the risk)
During performance of urologic procedures such as catheterization, cystoscopy, or cystomet-
rography
In patients with disorders of the lower GI tract
During procedures involving the rectum or colon
During recovery from spinal or general anesthesia
During labor and delivery

Prevention

Obtain a thorough history from patients with SCI. They are often aware of some of the stimuli
that will evoke this response in them
Check the baseline blood pressure for comparison with perioperative values
Provide adequate regional or general anesthesia for surgical procedures
Preoperative prophylaxis of patients at risk of autonomic dysreflexia
    Patients who are at high risk regardless of anesthetic technique
    Choices of prophylactic regimens include
        Phenoxybenzamine PO, 10 mg, 3 times daily to maximum of 60 mg/day
        Clonidine PO, 0.2–0.4 mg, preoperatively
        Nifedipine SL, 10 mg, immediately prior to surgery
        Trimethaphan IV, 1 mg/ml in D_5W, by infusion during surgery, titrated to main-
tain a normal blood pressure

Manifestations

Acute, paroxysmal onset of severe systolic and diastolic hypertension
    Normal blood pressure in most SCI patients is low
    Increased blood loss from surgical site
Additional signs of sympathetic hyperreactivity
    Reflex bradycardia (tachycardia and arrhythmias can also occur)
    Sweating, vasodilation, and flushing above the dermatomal level of the SCI
    Mydriasis, nasal obstruction, conjunctival congestion, eyelid retraction
    Muscle contraction below spinal cord lesion, including pallor, piloerection, and visceral
spasm
If the patient is awake
    Severe pounding headache, blurred vision, nasal congestion, dyspnea, nausea, or anxiety
    Increased spasticity

Similar Events

Light anesthesia
Epinephrine overdose
Pre-eclampsia/eclampsia in pregnant SCI patient (see Event 73, *Pre-eclampsia and Eclampsia*)
Intraoperative hypertension from other causes (see Event 6, *Hypertension*)
Pheochromocytoma
Migraine and cluster headaches

Management

Verify the blood pressure, check for additional signs and symptoms of sympathetic hyper-reactivity
Inform the surgeon and ask for the surgical stimulus to be stopped
If the patient is under general anesthesia
    Increase the depth of anesthesia with a volatile agent
    Place the patient in the reverse Trendelenburg position if possible
    Autonomic dysreflexia may occur during emergence from anesthesia
If the patient is awake
    Administer phentolamine IV, 1 mg
    If no response within 1 minute, administer double the previous dose
    Total dose required may exceed 40 mg
    If autonomic dysreflexia resolves, continue with surgery (autonomic dysreflexia may recur)
If autonomic dysreflexia does not resolve with treatment, abort surgery if possible
If emergent surgery must continue
    Place an additional peripheral or CVP line to administer potent vasodilators
    Insert an arterial line for direct measurement of blood pressure
    Institute pharmacologic therapy with a potent arteriolar vasodilator, titrating to response
        Nitroprusside, 0.25–1 µg/kg/min
        Trimethaphan infusion, 0.1–1 mg/min

Complications

Myocardial ischemia or infarction
Pulmonary edema
Hypertensive encephalopathy
Atrial and ventricular arrhythmias, heart block
Cardiac arrest
Seizures, coma, intracerebral or subarachnoid hemorrhage
Increased surgical blood loss
Hypotension secondary to therapy with vasodilators

Suggested Readings

Bendo AA, Giffin JP, Cottrell JE: Anesthetic and surgical management of acute and chronic spinal cord injury. p. 392. In Cottrell JE, Turndorff H (eds): Anesthesia and Neurosurgery. 2nd Ed. CV Mosby, St. Louis, 1986

Erickson RP: Autonomic hyperreflexia: pathophysiology and medical management. Arch Phys Med Rehabil 61:431, 1980

Schonwald G, Fish KJ, Perkash I: Cardiovascular complications during anesthesia in chronic spinal cord injured patients. Anesthesiology 55:550, 1981

Trop CS, Bennett CJ: Autonomic dysreflexia and its urological implications: a review. J Urol 146:1461, 1990

---

13 SINUS BRADYCARDIA

Definition

Sinus bradycardia is defined as a heart rate less than 60 bpm in an adult, in which the impulse formation begins in the sinus node.

Etiology

Decreased automaticity of sinus node
      Increased vagal tone
      Drug induced
      Hypoxemia
      Physiologic
           Congenital
           Physical conditioning
           Hypothermia
           Hypothyroidism
      Intrinsic disease of the sinus node
        ("sick sinus" syndrome)

Typical Situations

As an isolated finding during preoperative evaluation
Following administration of drugs that produce bradycardia
      Narcotics (especially fentanyl, sufentanil)
      Halothane
      ß-Adrenergic antagonists
      Calcium channel antagonists
      Anticholinesterases
      α_2-Agonists (clonidine, dexmedetomidine)
During periods of vagal stimulation
      Traction on the eye or the peritoneum
      Laryngoscopy and intubation
      Bladder catheterization
During hypertensive episodes as a baroreceptor reflex
During spinal or epidural anesthesia (not necessarily with high block)
Electroconvulsive therapy

Prevention

Premedicate patients at risk with an anticholinergic agent
     Atropine IM, 0.4 mg (adults)
     Glycopyrrolate IM, 0.2 mg (adults)
Treat bradycardia early
     During spinal or epidural anesthesia treat even asymptomatic patients
     Glycopyrrolate IV, 0.2–0.4 mg
     Atropine IV, 0.4–0.8 mg
Avoid traction on the peritoneum or the extraocular muscles
Avoid manipulation of or pressure on the carotid sinus

Manifestations

Bradycardia may be well tolerated, particularly if it develops slowly. Acute onset of bradycardia is more likely to be symptomatic.

Slow heart rate
     ECG
     Pulse oximeter
     Arterial line
     NIPB monitor
     Palpation of peripheral pulses
Hypotension
In the conscious patient
     Nausea, vomiting
     Mental status change
Junctional or idioventricular escape beats

Similar Events

Monitor artifact
     ECG lead disconnection or failure
     Failure of monitor to count QRS or pulse
Dropped beats (second-degree AV heart block, Mobitz type I and type II)
Third-degree AV block
Atrial fibrillation/flutter with poor perfusion

Management

Verify bradycardia and assess its hemodynamic significance
     Check redundant monitors of heart rate
     Check blood pressure
     Palpate a peripheral pulse
Ensure adequate oxygenation and ventilation
     Bradycardia is common in hypoxemic arrest
     Increase FiO_2 to 100%, turn off all volatile anesthetics

If the awake patient becomes obtunded or unconscious

Manage the airway

Call for help

If bradycardia is associated with severe symptoms (profound hypotension, loss of consciousness, seizures)

Epinephrine IV, 10 μg bolus, repeat with escalating doses as necessary

Early administration of epinephrine is <u>essential</u> if the patient is under spinal or epidural anesthesia

If bradycardia fails to resolve with epinephrine

Isoproterenol infusion IV, 1–3 μg/min

Pacemaker

Transcutaneous

Transvenous (effective, but logistically difficult in an emergency)

Commence CPR if necessary (see Event 2, *Cardiac Arrest*)

If bradycardia is associated with mild-to-moderate symptoms (modest decrease in blood pressure, nausea, vomiting, or mild alteration in sensorium)

Ephedrine IV, 5–10 mg increments

Atropine IV, 0.4 mg

Glycopyrrolate IV, 0.2 mg

Repeat as necessary

Scan the surgical field for operative causes

If in response to surgical stimulus, alert surgeon to stop the precipitating stimulus

If bradycardia is not associated with any obvious physiologic consequences

Monitor the patient closely

Treat asymptomatic patients under spinal or epidural anesthesia; sinus arrest, asystole, and cardiac arrest can occur without warning

Complications

Escape arrhythmias

Cardiac arrest

Complications of pacemakers

Tachyarrhythmias and hypertension secondary to drug treatment

Suggested Readings

Atlee JL: Recognition and management of specific dysrhythmias. p. 373. In: Perioperative Cardiac Dysrhythmias: Mechanisms, Recognition, Management. 2nd Ed. Year Book Medical Publishers, Chicago, 1990

Doyle DJ, Mark PWS: Reflex bradycardia during surgery. Can J Anaesth 37:219, 1990

Egan TD, Brock-Utne JG: Asystole after anesthesia induction with a fentanyl, propofol and succinylcholine sequence. Anesth Analg 73:818, 1991

Goldberger E, Wheat MW: The bradyarrhythmias and conduction disturbances. p. 68. In: Treatment of Cardiac Emergencies. 5th Ed. CV Mosby, St Louis, 1990

Gravlee GP, Ramsey FM, Roy RC et al: Rapid administration of a narcotic and neuromuscular blocker. Anesth Analg 67:39, 1988

Kelly JS, Royster RL: Noninvasive transcutaneous cardiac pacing. Anesth Analg 69:229, 1989

14 MYOCARDIAL INFARCTION

Definition

Myocardial infarction is myocardial cell death due to inadequate cellular perfusion. Transmural (Q wave) infarction involves the entire thickness of the myocardial wall; subendocardial (non-Q wave) infarction involves only the subendocardial portion of the myocardial wall.

Etiology

Acute occlusion of coronary artery
>A thrombus completely occludes the affected artery within 4 hours of the onset of symptoms in 80% of patients with acute transmural myocardial infarction
>Myocardial infarction is associated with coronary atherosclerosis in approximately 90% of cases

Inadequate coronary perfusion for a given myocardial O_2 demand
Acute dissecting aneurysm of the aorta

Typical Situations

In patients with pre-existing CAD
>Patients with angina pectoris
>Older patients
>Patients with peripheral vascular disease
>Patients with diabetes frequently have silent myocardial ischemia

During any acute change in myocardial O_2 demand or delivery, secondary to
>Tachycardia, hypertension, or hypotension
>Hypoxemia or hemodilution
>Coronary spasm (Prinzmetal's angina)

Patients with aortic or mitral stenosis
Patients with connective tissue disorders such as polyarteritis nodosa (adults) or Kawasaki's disease (children)
Following CABG surgery
Acute carbon monoxide poisoning

Prevention

Carefully evaluate and prepare patients with CAD preoperatively
>Verify the presence of CAD, evaluate myocardial function and reserve, and consider what therapy the patient requires before surgery

Avoid elective anesthesia and surgery in patients with unstable angina or with a history of myocardial infarction in the previous 6 months
Optimize hemodynamics and hematocrit during anesthesia

Manifestations

Myocardial infarction is distinguished from myocardial ischemia by
  Persistence and progression of ST segment and T wave changes
  Development of Q waves
  Evidence for myocardial cell necrosis (elevated cardiac isoenzymes)
The awake patient may manifest
  Central chest pain radiating into the arms or throat
  Dyspnea
  Nausea and vomiting
  Altered level of consciousness or cognitive function
ECG abnormalities
  ST segment depression or elevation
  Hyperacute T waves, tall prominent T waves
  Q waves
  Arrhythmias (PVCs, ventricular tachycardia, or fibrillation)
  Conduction abnormalities (AV block, bundle branch block)
Hemodynamic abnormalities
  Hypotension
  Elevation of ventricular filling pressures
  V wave on pulmonary artery wedge tracing
  Tachycardia
  Bradycardia

Similar Events

Myocardial ischemia (see Event 10, *ST Segment Changes*)
Pulmonary embolism (see Event 18, *Pulmonary Embolism*)
Acute dissecting aneurysm of the aorta not involving the coronary arteries
Esophageal spasm, costochondritis, acute cholecystitis, acute peptic ulcer/perforation, or acute
  pancreatitis
Primary pulmonary pathology
Nonischemic abnormalities of ST segment or T wave (see Event 10, *ST Segment Changes*)
Artifact of ECG
  Improper electrode position on the patient
  The position of the heart relative to the electrodes may be altered owing to changes in
    patient position or surgical manipulation

Management

Verify manifestations of ongoing myocardial ischemia
  Assess clinical signs and symptoms
  Evaluate electrode placement and ECG settings
  Evaluate multiple ECG leads
  Obtain a 12-lead ECG as soon as feasible, review previous ECGs
  Evaluate hemodynamic status

Inform the surgeon

Terminate surgery as soon as possible

Request ICU bed for postoperative care

Treat ventricular arrhythmias (see Event 15, *Nonlethal Ventricular Arrhythmias*)

Lidocaine IV, 1.0–1.5 mg/kg bolus, then infusion of 1–4 mg/min

Procainamide IV, 500 mg loading dose over 10–20 minutes, then infusion of 2–6 mg/min

Monitor blood pressure carefully

Place an arterial line

Treat tachycardia and/or hypertension

Tachycardia is the most important determinant of increased myocardial O_2 demand

Increase the depth of anesthesia if appropriate

β Blockade

Esmolol IV, 0.25–0.5 mg/kg bolus, 50–300 μg/kg/min infusion

Labetolol IV, 5–10 mg bolus, repeat as necessary

Propranolol IV, 0.25–1 mg bolus, repeat as necessary

Use with caution if the patient is hypotensive or has severe COPD or asthma

NTG

Sublingual (absorption uncertain, can cause hypotension)

Transdermal paste, 1–2 in. applied to the chest wall (slow onset)

IV infusion, 0.25–2 μg/kg/min (titrated to effect)

Calcium channel blockade

Nifedipine SL, 5–10 mg (absorption uncertain, can cause hypotension)

Verapamil IV, 2.5 mg, repeat as necessary (avoid if ß blockade present)

Diltiazem IV, 2.5 mg increments, repeat as necessary

If hypotension develops

Coronary perfusion pressure takes precedence over attempts at afterload reduction

Maintain blood pressure with phenylephrine IV, 0.25–1 μg/kg/min by infusion

Optimize circulating fluid volume

Use PA pressures as a guide, consider placement of a PA catheter if not already in place

Support myocardial contractility as needed using inotropic agents

Use inotropes with caution since they may increase myocardial O_2 demand and worsen ischemia

Dobutamine IV infusion, 5–10 μg/kg/min

Dopamine IV infusion, 5–10 μg/kg/min

Epinephrine IV infusion, 10–100 ng/kg/min

Avoid NTG or calcium channel blockade until hypotension or bradycardia are resolved

Consider combined use of phenylephrine and NTG infusions

If cardiac arrest occurs

Begin ACLS (see Event 2, *Cardiac Arrest*)

Ensure adequate oxygenation and ventilation—monitor with pulse oximeter and capnograph

Treat pain and anxiety in the awake patient by careful titration of sedatives and narcotics

Send blood samples to clinical laboratory for

ABGs

Hemoglobin/hematocrit

Electrolytes

CK, CK-MB isoenzyme (for comparison with subsequent measurements)
Obtain cardiology consultation to determine postoperative management of patient
    Assessment for cardiac catheterization
    Circulatory support with a circulatory assist device (IABP)
    PTCA or CABG surgery
    Thrombolytic therapy

Complications

CHF
Arrhythmias
Cardiac arrest
Thromboembolic complications (see Event 18, *Pulmonary Embolism*)
Papillary muscle dysfunction or rupture
Rupture of the interventricular septum or the ventricular wall

Suggested Readings

Goldberger E, Wheat MW: Acute myocardial infarction. p. 145. In: Treatment of Cardiac Emergencies. 5th
    Ed. CV Mosby, St. Louis, 1990
Goldberger E, Wheat MW: Complications of acute myocardial infarction. p. 175. In: Treatment of Cardiac
    Emergencies. 5th Ed. CV Mosby, St. Louis, 1990

---

15 NONLETHAL VENTRICULAR ARRHYTHMIAS

Definition

Nonlethal ventricular (wide QRS complex) arrhythmias are those not requiring ACLS, although they may eventually lead to ventricular fibrillation.

Etiology

PVCs
Abnormal automaticity of ventricular myocardium
Re-entry
Drug toxicity
R on T phenomenon (a PVC or a pacemaker spike occurring at the apex of the T wave, initiating ventricular tachycardia)

Typical Situations

PVCs are seen frequently in normal persons and can be provoked by tea, coffee, alcohol, tobacco, or emotional excitement

Patients with myocardial ischemia or infarction
Hypoxemia and/or hypercarbia
Potassium and/or acid-base disturbance
Patients with mitral valve prolapse
Inappropriate depth of anesthesia for level of surgical stimulus
Mechanical stimulation of the heart
    Handling of the heart during cardiothoracic surgery
    Passage of a PA catheter through the right ventricle
Acute hypertension and/or tachycardia
Acute hypotension and/or bradycardia
Drugs
    Halothane plus topical, SC, or IV catecholamine; seen less frequently when other volatile
      anesthetic agents are administered
    Digitalis toxicity
    Tricyclic antidepressant toxicity
    Aminophylline toxicity
    Antiarrhythmic drugs (quinidine, procainamide, disopyramide)
    Antihistamines (astemizole, terfenadine)
Hypothermia (core temperature less than 32°C)

Prevention

Recognize and treat preoperative ventricular arrhythmias
Correct perioperative electrolyte abnormalities
Identify patients taking drugs known to cause ventricular arrhythmias
Use less than 1 µg/kg of epinephrine for infiltration or regional nerve block when the patient is
    receiving halothane

Manifestations

Wide QRS complex on ECG not preceded by a P wave
PVCs
    May not produce ejection of blood into the aorta or a palpable pulse if the coupling inter-
      val to prior beat is short
    There is usually a compensatory pause between the PVC and the next normal beat
Ventricular tachycardia
    A succession of five or more PVCs
    Some ventricular tachycardias support adequate circulation and do not degenerate into
      lethal arrhythmias
Torsade de pointes
    Paroxysms of ventricular tachycardia in which the QRS axis changes direction continu-
      ously, with a periodicity of 5–20 beats

Similar Events

ECG artifact
Supraventricular rhythm with aberrant conduction
AV re-entrant rhythms

Bundle branch blocks, especially in the presence of tachycardia
Escape rhythms originating in the bundle branches or ventricle

Management

Ensure adequate oxygenation and ventilation
Check the hemodynamic significance of the rhythm
    Palpate the peripheral pulses
    Check the blood pressure
    Examine the arterial waveform (if present)
If the arrhythmia causes significant hemodynamic impairment
    If halothane is being administered, switch to another volatile or IV anesthetic agent
    Administer lidocaine IV, 1–1.5 mg/kg bolus
    Consider electric countershock (200–300 J) if hemodynamic impairment is severe
Diagnose the arrhythmia
    Print rhythm strip if recorder available
    Check multiple ECG leads if type of arrhythmia is uncertain
If ventricular tachycardia is present
    Repeat lidocaine IV bolus 15 minutes after initial dose
    Administer lidocaine infusion at 1–4 mg/min
    Consider electric countershock
    If ventricular tachycardia is due to digitalis toxicity
        Do not cardiovert
        Administer lidocaine IV, 1–1.5 mg/kg bolus, infusion 1–4 mg/min
        Administer potassium chloride IV until the serum K^+ is above 5.5 mEq/L
        Administer phenytoin IV, 50 mg/min to a total dose of 250 mg
If torsade de pointes is present
    Administer $MgSO_4$ IV, 1–2 g bolus, followed by an infusion at 1 mg/min
    Consider electric countershock (200–300 J), but torsades de pointes is often refractory
    Correct electrolyte abnormalities
    Obtain a STAT consultation from a cardiologist
If PVCs only are present and there is tachycardia and hypertension
    The rhythm may be due to light anesthesia
        Deepen anesthesia with a bolus of IV anesthetic agent
        Increase the inspired concentration of volatile agent unless the agent is halothane
Evaluate the patient for evidence of myocardial ischemia
    Assess ST segments and T waves (see Event 10, *ST Segment Changes*)
    Consider using TEE to evaluate regional wall motion

Other antiarrhythmic drugs can be used if the arrhythmia is refractory to the above measures
    Procainamide IV, 25–50 mg/min up to a total dose of 500 mg, followed by an infusion of
        2–6 mg/min
    Bretylium IV bolus, 5–10 mg/kg over 8 minutes followed by an infusion of 1–2 mg/min
Address additional underlying etiologies
    Check the patient's body temperature
        If the patient is hypothermic, take active measures to restore body temperature
            (see Event 37, *Hypothermia*)

If the patient is hyperthermic, exclude MH (see Event 38, *Malignant Hyperthermia*)
Send samples to the clinical laboratory for measurement of
  Electrolytes (Na^+, K^+, and Mg^{2+})
  ABGs

Complications

Progression of nonlethal arrhythmia to cardiac arrest
Cerebral hypoperfusion
Drug side effects
  Hyperkalemia or cardiac arrest from rapid K^+ administration
  Lidocaine toxicity
  Lidocaine can ablate a ventricular escape rhythm, producing asystole
  Hypertension followed by hypotension from bretylium
  Widening of QRS, hypotension from procainamide
  Hypotension, respiratory depression, AV block, or ventricular fibrillation from phenytoin

Suggested Readings

Atlee JL: Recognition and management of specific dysrhythmias. p. 373. In: Perioperative Cardiac Dysrhythmias. 2nd Ed. Year Book Medical Publishers, Chicago, 1990
Atlee JL, Bosnjak ZJ: Mechanisms for cardiac dysrhythmias during anesthesia. Anesthesiology 72:347, 1990
Goldberger E, Wheat MW: Ventricular tachyarrhythmias. p. 112. In: Treatment of Cardiac Emergencies. 5th Ed. CV Mosby, St. Louis, 1990

16 PERICARDIAL TAMPONADE

Definition

Pericardial tamponade is the accumulation of blood or fluid in the closed pericardial space, limiting ventricular filling and resulting in hemodynamic compromise.

Etiology

Bleeding after cardiac surgery
Coagulopathy
Perforation of the heart
Rheumatologic or autoimmune diseases
Pericardial malignancy or tumor metastasis
Pericardial infection, typically as a complication of sepsis
Chronic renal failure
Radiation-induced pericardial effusion

Typical Situations

After cardiothoracic surgery
> Clots may cause tamponade even in the presence of an open pericardium and patent mediastinal drains

After placement of an intracardiac monitoring line or pacemaker lead
> Erosion by a CVP catheter in the right atrial position is especially common

Perforation of a coronary artery or the myocardium during cardiac catheterization, PTCA, or cardiac biopsy

Following blunt trauma or a penetrating injury to the chest
> Tamponade after trauma may be delayed and insidious in onset

After myocardial infarction
> Myocardial wall rupture
> Bleeding of the pericardium itself in patients receiving anticoagulant or thrombolytic therapy

In patients with chronic renal failure requiring hemodialysis

Patients with malignancies, especially after receiving radiation therapy to the mediastinum
> Pericardial effusion occurs in 30% of patients receiving more than 4000 rads of irradiation to the mediastinum for lymphoma; 40% of these patients will require extensive surgical pericardectomy

Prevention

Achieve adequate surgical and medical hemostasis during and after cardiothoracic surgery

Treat coagulopathy as necessary, with therapy guided by laboratory assessment of coagulation

Place intracardiac monitoring lines and pacemaker leads carefully
> CVP catheter tip should not lie in the right atrium
> Obtain a chest x-ray following surgery to confirm the position of the CVP catheter tip

Control underlying medical problems that predispose the patient to pericardial effusion

Perform pericardiocentesis of large but asymptomatic pericardial effusion prior to surgery

Manifestations

The pericardium has a low compliance, and the rate of fluid accumulation will determine the rapidity of onset of symptoms. If the fluid accumulation is rapid, 150–200 ml of blood can critically compromise myocardial function. If it accumulates slowly, symptoms may not occur with fluid volumes of 1 L or more.

Hypotension (see Event 7, *Hypotension*)

Decreased cardiac output

Narrow pulse pressure, exaggeration of pulsus paradoxus
> Normal limit of pulsus paradoxus is a decrease in systolic blood pressure on inspiration of less than 10 mm Hg

Equalization of all cardiac diastolic filling pressures at a relatively high value

Following cardiac surgery
> Pericardial tamponade should always be considered in the differential diagnosis of the patient with low cardiac output
> Increased drainage from the mediastinal chest tube
>> May be followed by decreased drainage if clots obstruct the mediastinal drain

Pericardial fluid visible on the echocardiogram
Diminished heart tones and precordial cardiac pulsations
Pericardial rub
Low-amplitude ECG with ST changes (see Event 10, *ST Segment Changes*)
Increased size of the cardiac silhouette on chest x-ray

Similar Events

CHF
Constrictive pericarditis
Exacerbation of asthma
Hypovolemia
Acute aortic dissection

Management

If Pericardial Tamponade Is Suspected and the Patient Is <u>*Symptomatic*</u>
Ensure adequate oxygenation and ventilation
    Administer supplemental O_2
Expand the circulating fluid volume
    Place a large-bore IV for rapid IV infusion
Place invasive monitoring lines
    CVP line for monitoring and drug administration
    PA line for monitoring cardiac filling pressures and cardiac output
Provide inotropic support
    Dobutamine, 5–10 µg/kg/min
    Dopamine, 5–10 µg/kg/min
    Epinephrine, 50–100 ng/kg/min
If the patient has had recent cardiothoracic surgery
    If the patient's hemodynamic status is severely compromised, have an appropriately
        trained surgeon open the chest immediately to relieve the pericardial tamponade
    If the patient is stable, transport the patient to the operating room for this procedure
If the patient has NOT had recent cardiothoracic surgery
    Perform pericardiocentesis by the subxiphoid route
        May remove enough fluid to temporarily improve the patient's condition prior to
            emergency surgery
        A negative tap does not exclude the presence of large blood clots compressing the
            heart

If Pericardial Tamponade Is Suspected and the Patient Is <u>*Stable*</u>
Review the patient's history and drug administration record
Check coagulation status of the patient
    PT and PTT
    Platelet count
    Bleeding time
Monitor the patient carefully using invasive techniques
Obtain chest x-ray and cardiac ultrasound for diagnosis
Obtain consultation from a cardiologist or cardiothoracic surgeon

Anesthetic Management of the Patient with Pericardial Tamponade
Best described as <u>fast</u>, <u>full</u>, and <u>tight</u>

> Maintain heart rate in the range of 90–140 bpm
> Correct hypovolemia and optimize filling pressures to compensate for the vasodilation that frequently occurs with induction of anesthesia
> Induce anesthesia with ketamine IV, 0.25–1 mg/kg
> Use succinylcholine IV, 1–2 mg/kg, for muscle relaxation for rapid intubation
> Provide additional IV anesthesia as tolerated with ketamine, 10–20 mg; fentanyl , 25–50 µg; midazolam, 0.25–0.5 mg
> Maintain vasoconstriction and myocardial contractility by avoiding volatile anesthetic agents and IV agents known to be myocardial depressants

Complications

Cardiac arrest
Acute cardiac failure
Laceration of heart or lungs during pericardiocentesis
Myocardial ischemia or infarction
Infection

Suggested Readings

Goldberger E, Wheat MW: Acute pericardial tamponade. p. 237. In: Treatment of Cardiac Emergencies. 5th Ed. CV Mosby, St Louis, 1990

Nicholls BJ, Cullen BF: Anesthesia for trauma. J Clin Anesth 1:115, 1988

Palatianos GM, Thurer RJ, Pompeo MQ, Kaiser GA: Clinical experience with subxiphoid drainage of pericardial effusions. Ann Thorac Surg 48:381, 1989

---

17 PULMONARY EDEMA

Definition

Pulmonary edema is accumulation of fluid in the alveoli of the lung.

Etiology

High pulmonary capillary hydrostatic pressure
Low pulmonary capillary oncotic pressure
"Leaky" pulmonary capillary membranes
Inadequate lymphatic clearance of normal alveolar fluid

Typical Situations

Fluid overload
> With massive fluid resuscitation
> With fluid absorption (e.g., during TURP surgery)

In patients with chronic CHF
In patients with renal failure and decreased ability to excrete excess fluid
Acute myocardial dysfunction
Acute myocardial ischemia or infarction
Acute valvular dysfunction
ARDS (increased pulmonary capillary permeability) secondary to
Hypotension
Gram-negative sepsis or DIC
Smoke inhalation injury
Pulmonary aspiration of acid gastric contents
Obstetric causes (e.g., pregnancy-induced hypertension, intrauterine fetal death)
Certain immunologic disorders
Neurogenic (after major head trauma)
Postobstruction or re-expansion pulmonary edema
Following opiate reversal with naloxone

Prevention

Monitor fluid replacement carefully
Use invasive hemodynamic monitoring in patients at risk of pulmonary edema or CHF
Monitor for signs of possible fluid absorption during TURP
Treat the underlying problem in ARDS

Manifestations

In the awake patient
Dyspnea, "air hunger," and restlessness, even with normal O_2 saturation and end-tidal CO_2
Hypoxemia and hypercarbia will develop later
In the mechanically ventilated patient
Increased PIP secondary to decreased pulmonary compliance
Reduction of tidal volume if the lung compliance is outside the performance envelope of the ventilator
Frothy sanguineous pulmonary edema fluid in the ETT or under the face mask
Elevated cardiac filling pressures
Jugular venous distention
Increased CVP or PA pressure
Fine crackles (rales) in the lung fields on auscultation
Hypotension and arrhythmias if pulmonary edema is secondary to myocardial ischemia
Hypertension and tachycardia if pulmonary edema is secondary to hypervolemia
Abnormalities on the chest x-ray
Increased pulmonary vascularity
Cardiomegaly
Perivascular cuffing
Kerly B lines
Interstitial infiltrate
"White-out" of lung fields

17

Similar Events

Bronchospasm (see Event 24, *Bronchospasm*)
Endobronchial intubation (see Event 25, *Endobronchial Intubation*)
Kinked or obstructed ETT (see Event 5, *High Peak Inspiratory Pressure*)
Pneumothorax (see Event 28, *Pneumothorax*)
Residual neuromuscular blockade

Management

Assess respiratory effort and adequacy of ventilation
> If respiratory effort is inadequate, consider residual neuromuscular blockade or pneumothorax as possible etiologies
> Intubate the patient that is not already intubated if pulmonary edema persists in the presence of severe hypoxemia or hypercarbia or if loss of consciousness develops

Administer supplemental O_2
> Administer O_2 with a high flow using a nonrebreathing face mask
> Assist ventilation if necessary with CPAP
> For the intubated and ventilated patient increase the FIO_2 and consider adding PEEP to the circuit to ensure maximal oxygenation

Reduce the cardiac preload
> Sit the awake patient upright or put the anesthetized patient in the reverse Trendelenburg position if not contraindicated by the surgical procedure or hypotension
> Administer furosemide IV, 10–20 mg bolus (use an increased dose if the patient is already on diuretic therapy)
>> Consider placing a urinary catheter
> Administer morphine IV, 2 mg increments, with caution, watching for respiratory depression
> If the etiology is myocardial ischemia, commence an infusion of NTG IV, 0.25–1 µg/kg/min unless the patient is hypotensive

Obtain ABGs, chest x-ray, and a 12-lead ECG

Optimize myocardial contractility
> Discontinue myocardial depressant drugs
> Place invasive hemodynamic monitors
> Consider inotropic support
>> Dopamine, 3–10 µg/kg/min; or dobutamine, 5–10 µg/kg/min
>> Amrinone IV, 0.75–1.5 mg/kg loading dose (over 30 minutes), infusion of 5–15 µg/kg/min; or milrinone IV, 50 µg/kg loading dose (over 10 minutes), infusion of 0.375–0.75 µg/kg/min
> If bronchospasm is also present, consider aminophylline IV, 5 mg/kg by slow IV infusion over 15 minutes (may also promote diuresis)

Call for help
> Devote primary attention to monitoring the patient and establishing a diagnosis. Assign assistants the tasks of setting up lines

Terminate the surgical procedure as quickly as possible; make arrangements to transfer the patient to the ICU for continuation of care

Obtain an urgent cardiology consultation

Use TEE as a diagnostic tool if the equipment and an operator are available

Complications

Hypovolemia and hypotension from overaggressive diuresis or reduction of preload

Hypokalemia

Hypoxemia

Suggested Readings

Allen SJ: Pathophysiology of pulmonary edema: implications for clinical management. p. 222. In: Annual Refresher Course Lectures. American Society of Anesthesiologists, Park Ridge, IL, 1988

Matsumiya N, Dohi S, Kimura T, Naito H: Re-expansion pulmonary edema after mediastinal tumor removal. Anesth Analg 73:646, 1991

18 PULMONARY EMBOLISM

Definition

A pulmonary embolism is a partial or complete obstruction of the pulmonary arterial circulation by substances originating elsewhere in the cardiovascular system.

Etiology

Substances that can cause a pulmonary embolism

Blood clot

Fat

Amniotic fluid (See Event 68, *Amniotic Fluid Embolism*)

Air (see Event 20, *Venous Air or Gas Embolism*)

Typical Situations

There is a high risk of development of deep vein thrombosis in patients who

Have recently had surgery

Have a history of previous deep vein thrombosis or venous insufficiency of the lower extremities

Are postpartum or are immobilized for long periods of time

Have had a recent fracture or leg injury

Have a malignancy (especially metastatic disease)

Have a history of CHF or myocardial infarction

Have undergone splenectomy with rebound thrombocytosis

Are elderly

Are obese

Fat embolism is typically seen in patients who have undergone
  Major trauma or a fracture of a long bone
  Surgical high pressure injection or reaming into the marrow cavity of long bones

Prevention

Prophylaxis for patients at risk of deep vein thrombosis
    Graduated compression stockings
        When used alone, these devices do not protect the high-risk patient
    Intermittent pneumatic compression boots
    Heparin SC, 5000 units, 1–2 hours before surgery and continuing until the patient is ambulatory
Insert an IVC filter in patients at high risk of pulmonary embolism from deep vein thrombosis, when nonpharmacologic methods are inadequate, and when anticoagulants are contraindicated

Manifestations

A massive pulmonary embolism may manifest either as a cardiac arrest in EMD or asystole, or as acute hemodynamic compensation that rapidly progresses to a cardiac arrest.

If the patient is conscious
    The classic signs of pulmonary embolism are dyspnea, pleuritic chest pain, and hemoptysis (see Event 26, *Massive Hemoptysis*)
    The chest x-ray is usually normal, but there may be a change in vessel diameter, vessel "cutoff," increased radiolucency in areas of hypoperfusion, atelectasis, and/or a pleural effusion
    Fine crackles (rales), wheezes, or a pleural rub may be heard on auscultation of the chest
    Hypoxemia or increase of the A–a gradient
In the patient who is under general anesthesia
    Tachypnea if the patient is not paralyzed
    Hypotension and tachycardia
    Hypoxemia, increase of A–a gradient, or cyanosis, even with an FIO_2 of 100%
    Decreased end-tidal CO_2
    Increased PA pressures
        Acute right heart failure may occur
    ECG changes
        Right heart strain, ST-T wave changes, bradycardia, EMD, or asystole
In fat embolism
    Widespread petechiae may be visible
    DIC and thrombocytopenia are common, with ecchymoses and overt bleeding from incisions, IV sites, and mucous membranes
    Fat globules may be seen in the urine, sputum, or retinal vessels
In amniotic fluid embolism
    Squames may be seen on microscopic examination of the sputum

Similar Events

Hypoxemia from other causes (see Event 8, *Hypoxemia*)

Hypotension from other causes (see Event 7, *Hypotension*)
Increased dead space from other causes
Pulmonary hypertension from other causes
Right ventricular failure

Management

The diagnosis of pulmonary embolism is difficult to make in the patient under general anesthesia.

Ensure adequate oxygenation and ventilation
Administer supplementary O_2
For the nonintubated patient
Use a rebreathing face mask with an FIO_2 of 100%
Consider endotracheal intubation, mechanical ventilation, and PEEP
For the intubated patient
Increase FIO_2 to 100%
Consider use of PEEP
Check ABGs
End-tidal CO_2 measurements will not reliably indicate the adequacy of ventilation

Support the circulation
Expand the circulating fluid volume
Administer inotropic drugs
Ephedrine IV, 5–20 mg, repeat as necessary
Epinephrine IV, 10–50 μg, repeat as necessary
Dopamine, dobutamine, or epinephrine infusion (see Event 7, *Hypotension*)
Place invasive monitors for diagnosis and management of right ventricular failure or low cardiac output
If there is pulmonary hypertension with right ventricular failure consider using an infusion of NTG (0.25–1 μg/kg/min) as a pulmonary vasodilator
Use with great caution because of systemic vasodilation and hypotension

If there has been an acute cardiovascular collapse and pulmonary embolism is known to be present or is extremely likely
Consider emergency percutaneous CPB
Consider emergency pulmonary embolectomy
Establish the diagnosis
Rule out other causes of hypoxemia, dead space, or hemodynamic compromise
Obtain a V/Q scan or a pulmonary angiogram
An angiogram is the definitive diagnostic test but is more difficult to perform
If pulmonary thromboembolism of a blood clot is confirmed, anticoagulation will prevent further embolization
Anticoagulation therapy may be contraindicated if there is an underlying bleeding site or if surgical hemostasis is not satisfactory
Heparin IV, 5000 unit bolus, followed by a heparin infusion of 1000 units/hr, adjusted to maintain the aPTT at least twice normal
Thrombolytic therapy remains controversial and is contraindicated in the early postoperative period
Insert an IVC filter in patients with recurrent pulmonary embolism who have received adequate

gulation or in patients in whom anticoagulation is contraindicated
tion of or clipping of the IVC at laparotomy may be necessary when percutaneous
sertion of the filter is impossible

ʻons

ırction

nplications of anticoagulation therapy

adings

of a

F: Pulmonary thromboembolism: disease recognition and patient management.
·146, 1990
1ous thrombosis and anaesthesia. Br J Anaesth 66:4, 1991
Vallavicenzia JL: Deep venous thrombosis and pulmonary embolism. Surg Clin
1991

t rate

ı embolism: detection by pulse oximetry. Anesthesiology 68:951, 1988

ıction,

ıaveling
ex; nor-

PRAVENTRICULAR ARRHYTHMIAS

P waves

different
vandering

hmia is an abnormal cardiac rhythm arising from a supraventricular

de

icular rate
y is usual-

ıse is irreg-

entricular tissue (tachyarrhythmias)

ade and ret-
hycardia" if
plex or seen

tricular tissue (AV nodal rhythm)

tients with normal hearts

lcohol

on
liac surgery
her cardiac disorders with accessory conduction pathways

Hypoxemia, hypercarbia, acidosis, alkalosis
Pyrexia
Electrolyte imbalance, hypermetabolic states
Hyperthyroidism
Acute or chronic pulmonary disease
Valvular heart disease
Pericarditis, myocarditis

Prevention

Identify and treat patients with supraventricular arrhythmias preoperatively

Manifestations

If there is a rapid ventricular response, it may be difficult to determine the exact focus *tachyarrhythmia.*

Sinoatrial node
   Sinus tachycardia: evenly spaced P and QRS waves, 1:1 AV conduction, hea
      greater than 100 bpm
   Sinus arrhythmia: impulses arise from SA node at a varying rate, 1:1 AV cond
      normal QRS morphology, variation in rate is typically linked to ventilation

Atrial
   Premature atrial beats: usually benign normal variant
   Nonsinus atrial rhythm: impulses arise from atrial tissue other than SA node, t
      both antegrade and retrograde; P waves inverted or buried in the QRS comp
      mal QRS morphology
   Wandering atrial pacemaker: impulses arise from different points in the atria;
      vary in shape; PR interval varies
   Multifocal atrial tachycardia: impulses originate irregularly and rapidly from
      points in the atria; P waves vary in shape; PR/RR intervals vary; similar to
      atrial pacemaker but at a higher heart rate
   Atrial flutter: re-entrant rhythm in the atria at a rate of 220–300 bpm; ventr
      depends on degree of AV block, typically 2:1, 3:1, or 4:1; QRS morpholog
      ly normal
   Atrial fibrillation: impulses originate randomly in the atria; ventricular respor
      ularly irregular and depends on degree of AV block; QRS is usually norma

AV node ("junction")
   Junctional rhythm: impulses arise from the AV node and conduct both antegr
      rograde at a rate of 40–55 bpm (can be "accelerated idioventricular tad
      heart rate is greater than 55 bpm); P wave may be buried in the QRS con
      immediately after QRS; QRS morphology is usually normal

Similar Events

ECG artifact
Artificial pacing of right atrium
Light anesthesia

Management

Ensure adequate oxygenation and ventilation
Check the blood pressure
> If hypotension is severe
>> Administer vasopressor (see Event 7, *Hypotension*)
>> Consider immediate cardioversion

Diagnose the arrhythmia
> Palpate the peripheral pulses
> Use ECG hard copy if available
> Check multiple ECG leads to get the best atrial waveform
> Esophageal or intracardiac ECG leads may be helpful if available
> The diagnosis of a tachyarrhythmia may be easier if the ventricular response rate can be slowed, which can be achieved with
>> Vagal maneuvers
>> Adenosine IV, 3–6 mg bolus
>> Edrophonium IV, 5–10 mg bolus
>> Phenylephrine IV, 25–50 µg bolus

Treat the underlying rhythm and/or slow the ventricular response
> Atrial flutter
>> Esmolol IV, 10 mg increments, will increase the degree of AV block and slow the ventricular response rate
>> Digoxin IV, 0.25 mg q6h, will usually convert flutter to fibrillation, which may then revert spontaneously to sinus rhythm
>> If digoxin fails, add quinidine PO, 200 mg
>> Atrial pacing at a rate 20% faster than the native atrial rate: pace for at least 30 seconds, then gradually slow the pacemaker rate
>> Cardioversion 10–25 J, increase energy if necessary
> Atrial fibrillation
>> Digoxin IV, 0.5–1 mg
>> Verapamil IV, 2.5–5 mg, repeat as necessary q5min to maximum of 20 mg
>> Esmolol IV, 5–10 mg, repeat q5min as necessary; IV infusion at 50–200 µg/kg/min
>> Cardioversion 100–200 J
> AV node re-entry tachycardia
>> Verapamil IV, 2.5–5 mg, repeat as necessary q5min to maximum of 20 mg
>> Adenosine IV, 3–6 mg bolus
> Paroxysmal re-entrant tachyarrhythmias (including Wolff-Parkinson-White syndrome and other accessory tracts)
>> Adenosine IV, 3–6 mg bolus
>> Verapamil IV, 2.5–5 mg, repeat as necessary q5min to maximum of 20 mg
> AV nodal rhythm ("junctional rhythm")
>> No treatment may be necessary if the patient is hemodynamically stable
>> Atropine IV, 0.4–0.8 mg bolus
>> Ephedrine IV, 5–10 mg bolus
>> Pacemaker (transcutaneous, transesophageal, atrial, ventricular)

Avoid using calcium channel blockade and β blockade together (profound bradycardia)
It can be difficult to distinguish between ventricular tachycardia and supraventricular tach-

yarrhythmias with aberrant conduction. If in doubt treat as ventricular tachycardia with cardioversion

Complications

Myocardial ischemia/infarction (in patients at risk)
Adverse drug reactions
Complications of cardioversion
> Heart block
> Conversion to a more lethal rhythm
> Myocardial damage from repeated cardioversions (unusual)
Complications of pacing
> Induction of arrhythmias
> Cardiac perforation

Suggested Readings

Emergency Cardiac Care Committee and Subcommittees, American Heart Association: Guidelines for cardiopulmonary resuscitation and emergency cardiac care. JAMA 268:2171, 1992
Goldberger E, Wheat MW: Supraventricular tachyarrhythmias. p. 86. In: Treatment of Cardiac Emergencies. 5th Ed. CV Mosby, St. Louis, 1990
Rooke A: Diagnosis and treatment of common intraoperative dysrhythmias. p. 113. In: Annual Refresher Course Lectures. American Society of Anesthesiologists, Park Ridge, IL, 1990

20 VENOUS AIR OR GAS EMBOLISM

Definition

A venous air or gas embolism occurs by embolization of air or other gas to the right side of the heart or to the pulmonary vessels.

Etiology

Entrainment of ambient air into an open flowing vein or dural sinus
Infusion of air or other gas under pressure into a vein

Typical Situations

Surgical procedures in which the operative site is above the level of the heart
Surgical procedures requiring insufflation of gas
Invasive procedures that connect the low-pressure venous circulation to the atmosphere during spontaneous ventilation with negative intrathoracic pressure
Any invasive procedure in which the patient is connected to a high-pressure gas source

Prevention

Avoid positioning the patient such that the surgical field is above the level of the heart

Mechanically ventilate the patient when the surgical field must be above the level of the heart
When there is a risk of gas embolism, maintain a high venous pressure by using IV fluids and/or PEEP
Avoid administering N_2O to patients at risk of gas embolism
Remove all air from plastic IV solution bags prior to pressurized infusion

Manifestations

Manifestations depend on the size of the patient, the volume of air embolized, the rate at which embolization occurs, and the monitors used.

Ultrasound monitoring
    Bubbles of gas in the heart on a TEE, if present
    Change in the sound of a precordial Doppler
        A very sensitive technique for detection of venous air emboli; volumes as low as 0.25 ml can be detected
        The transducer must be positioned over the right heart structures (right or left parasternal area)
        Correct positioning of the transducer may be tested with a small IV bolus of room temperature fluid administered through a CVP catheter
Decrease in the end-tidal CO_2 concentration
    An abrupt fall in the end-tidal CO_2 concentration (greater than 2 mm Hg) due to transient arteriolar-capillary obstruction
    Any event that reduces pulmonary blood flow acutely will cause a similar decrease (see Event 18, *Pulmonary Embolism*)
Increase in the end-tidal N_2 concentration
    Detection of an increased N_2 concentration in the end-tidal gases and not in the inspired gases is pathognomonic of an <u>air</u> embolism
    The change in expired end-tidal N_2 concentration will be at most 2–3%
A loud, coarse, continuous "mill wheel" murmur on auscultation (esophageal stethoscope)
Gas in blood aspirated from CVP catheter (more than 20 ml indicates a large air embolus)
Hypotension (a greater than 15 mm Hg fall indicates a large air embolus)
Bradycardia
Rise in PA pressures unless the right ventricular outflow tract is obstructed with gas

Similar Events

Brain stem retraction and ischemia
Non-air pulmonary embolism (see Event 18, *Pulmonary Embolism*)
Other cause of hypotension (see Event 7, *Hypotension*)
Artifact on Doppler ultrasound device due to electrocautery, rapid fluid infusion, or movement of the precordial probe
Entrainment of air into a respiratory gas analyzer

Management

Notify the surgeon immediately of a possible gas embolization
    The surgeon should check possible entry sites in the wound
    The nurses should check surgical insufflation equipment
    Stop all pressurized gas sources

Confirm the diagnosis

>Listen carefully to the precordial Doppler signal

>Check the end-tidal CO_2

>Check the end-tidal N_2, if available

>Check the blood pressure

>Listen for mill wheel murmur

>Check PA pressures, if available

>Check for gas in blood aspirated from the CVP catheter, if present

If gas embolism is confirmed

>The surgeons should flood the surgical field with saline or pack the wound with saline-soaked sponges

>Discontinue N_2O, administer 100% O_2

>Provide Valsalva maneuver by manual ventilation to prevent further air from entering the heart and to reveal the vascular entry site to the surgeon

>Infuse IV fluid rapidly

>Reposition the patient, if feasible

>>First, tilt the operating table to lower the surgical site below the heart level

>>If necessary, place patient in left side-down position

>Consider applying 5 cm H_2O PEEP

>Use vasopressors and inotropes as needed to support the circulation

If hemodynamic compromise is severe

>Perform CPR if cardiac arrest occurs (see Event 2, *Cardiac Arrest*)

>Direct aspiration of air from the heart or great vessels via a thoracotomy may be necessary

>Internal cardiac massage may be required

Complications

Complications of severe hypotension

>Myocardial ischemia

>Cerebral hypoperfusion

Paradoxical gas embolism to the arterial circulation

>Patent foramen ovale or other right-to-left shunt

>Massive venous gas embolism crossing the pulmonary capillaries to the arterial circulation

Pulmonary edema

Contamination of the wound from repositioning

Complications of thoracotomy and CPR if performed

Suggested Readings

Cucchiara RF: Is the sitting position justifiable for the neurosurgical patient? p. 331. In: Annual Refresher Course Lectures. American Society of Anesthesiologists, Park Ridge, IL, 1986

Cucchiara RF, Nugent M, Seward JB: Air embolism in upright neurosurgical patients: detection and localization by 2-D echocardiography. Anesthesiology 60:353, 1984

Losasso TJ, Muzzi DA, Dietz NM, Cucchiara RF: Fifty per cent nitrous oxide does not increase the risk of venous air embolism in neurosurgical patients operated upon in the sitting position. Anesthesiology 77:21, 1992

Matjasko J, Petrozza P, Mackenzie CF: Sensitivity of end-tidal nitrogen in venous air embolism; detection in dogs. Anesthesiology 63:418, 1985

Michenfelder JD: Air embolism. p. 268. In Orkin F, Cooperman L (eds): Complications in Anesthesiology. JB Lippincott, Philadelphia, 1983

Chapter Five

Pulmonary Events

21 AIRWAY BURN

Definition

Airway burn occurs when there is thermal or chemical injury to the mucosa of the airway between the mouth and the alveoli.

Etiology

Ignition of the ETT during laser surgery
Inhalation of hot gases
> Inspired gases too hot
> Direct exposure to fire
> Exposure to smoke or toxic gases

Typical Situations

Laser surgery in the pharynx, the larynx, or the tracheobronchial tree
Malfunction of inspired gas heater or humidifier
> Faulty heater or thermostat
> Use of O_2 flush with servocontrol heater or humidifier
Patients with acute burns

Prevention

Protect the ETT during laser surgery in the airway by using appropriate protocols
> Use protected or "laser-proof" ETT
> Fill the ETT cuff with colored water or saline
> Maintain a low FIO_2 (less than 30%), avoid N_2O
> If higher FIO_2 is required to maintain an acceptable O_2 saturation, advise surgeon, consider aborting laser surgery
> Have a clamp available to occlude the ETT in case of ETT fire
Monitor the temperature of inspired gases when using a heater/humidifier
> Keep inspired gas temperature below 40°C
Protect patient from exposure to operating room fire or smoke

Manifestations

Immediate manifestations
> Laser-ignited ETT fire
>> Visible ignition or burning of the ETT
>> Smell of burning, smoke, flames in the surgical field
>> Fire may propagate into the breathing circuit
> Overheated gases
>> Breathing circuit tubing feels hot to the touch
>> High temperature alarm sounds on the heater/humidifier
>> Unexpected increase in patient's core temperature

Later manifestations
> Airway edema or airway rupture (see Event 22, *Airway Rupture* and Event 28, *Pneumothorax*)
> Decreased arterial pO_2 and O_2 saturation (see Event 8, *Hypoxemia*)
> Decreased pulmonary compliance
> Pulmonary edema (see Event 17, *Pulmonary Edema*)
> Bronchospasm (see Event 24, *Bronchospasm*)
> ARDS

Similar Events

Pulmonary edema from other causes (see Event 17, *Pulmonary Edema*)
ARDS from other causes
Pneumonia
Bronchospasm (see Event 24, *Bronchospasm*)
Partial airway obstruction

Management

For Laser-Induced ETT Fire
Stop the flow of O_2 to the ETT
> Clamp the ETT immediately
> Disconnect the patient from the breathing circuit

If a significant fire has occurred
> Remove the damaged ETT immediately
> However, if the O_2 saturation is already low and the ETT is intact, the patient can be ventilated through the damaged ETT; however, particulate matter may embolize distally into the tracheobronchial tree
> Mask-ventilate by hand with 100% O_2

Reintubate the patient as soon as possible
> Rapid development of airway edema may make later reintubation difficult
> If reintubation is not possible, proceed to either transtracheal jet ventilation, tracheostomy, or cricothyrotomy
> Provide supportive care and mechanical ventilation
> Add PEEP as necessary to maintain oxygenation
> Consider administering high-dose steroids (e.g., methylprednisolone IV, 0.1–1 g)

Call for an immediate consultation by an otolaryngologist or a thoracic surgeon to evalu-

ate the extent of the airway burn
>Fiberoptic bronchoscopy when the patient is stable

Impound any device thought to be defective for inspection by a biomedical engineer

For Overheated Gases

Remove heater/humidifier from the breathing circuit

Evaluate and treat the patient
>Increase the FIO_2 as necessary to maintain oxygenation
>Provide supportive care as described above
>Consider administering high-dose steroids as described above

Call for an immediate consultation by an otolaryngologist or a thoracic surgeon to evaluate the extent of the airway burn
>Fiberoptic bronchoscopy when the patient is stable

Impound any device thought to be defective for inspection by a biomedical engineer

Complications

Permanent pulmonary injury
>Pulmonary fibrosis
>Restrictive pulmonary disease

Hypoxemia/hypercarbia
Inability to reintubate
Pneumothorax
Pneumonia

Suggested Readings

Hayes DM, Gaba DM, Goode RL: Incendiary characteristics of a new laser resistant endotracheal tube. Otolaryngol Head Neck Surg 95:37, 1986

Sosis M: Anesthesia for laser surgery. Int Anesthesiol Clin 28:119, 1990

Wolf GL, Simpson JI: Flammability of endotracheal tubes in O_2 and N_2O enriched atmosphere. Anesthesiology 67:236, 1987

---

22 AIRWAY RUPTURE

Definition

Airway rupture includes traumatic perforation or disruption of any part of the airway.

Etiology

Mechanical or thermal energy rupturing airway walls
Hyperextension of the neck, combined with a direct blow to the unprotected trachea

Penetrating injury of the chest

Erosion of the tracheobronchial wall by an ETT cuff

Typical Situations

Following thoracic injury

Blunt trauma possibly associated with thoracic compression and in presence of a closed glottis

Frequently no external evidence of injury is present

Penetrating injury of the chest

During or following thoracic surgery

During laser surgery to the airway

Associated with the use of a double lumen ETT, especially with a high-pressure endobronchial cuff

With nasal intubation or instrumentation

Intubation of the airway with any rigid object

During bronchoscopy

During placement of a metal ETT for laser surgery

Prevention

Avoid excessive force during instrumentation of the airway

Do not allow the stylet to protrude beyond the tip of the ETT during intubation

Avoid overinflation of the ETT cuff or the endobronchial cuff of a double lumen ETT

Repeatedly check the occlusion pressure of the ETT cuff

Maintain full relaxation of the patient during endoscopy or laser surgery of the airway

Manifestations

Lacerations or partial rupture of the airway may easily be missed until some other event or a late complication (such as bronchial stenosis) demonstrates its presence.

Rupture of nasopharynx

Inability to pass ETT easily

ETT not visible in the pharynx on direct laryngoscopy

Blood or bloody secretions from nasopharynx or ETT

Inability to ventilate through nasotracheal ETT passed blindly

Nasopharyngeal swelling and visible hematoma

Rupture of tracheobronchial tree

Respiratory distress

Dyspnea

Hypoxemia

Cyanosis

Hemoptysis

Subcutaneous emphysema

Pneumothorax

Chest x-ray may be diagnostic

Laryngeal or tracheal injuries are frequently associated with visible cervical, mediastinal, and subcutaneous air, <u>without</u> accompanying pneumothorax

Bronchial injury is associated with pneumomediastinum, with pneumothorax, and possibly with overlying rib fractures. Rarely, chest x-ray may show "fallen lung sign," in which the transected bronchus allows the lung to fall <u>away</u> from the mediastinum, not toward the mediastinum as in a pneumothorax

Air leak from the site of a penetrating injury of the chest

Persistent air leak after placement of a chest tube is suggestive of bronchial rupture

Difficulty in establishing ventilation after intubation

High PIP

Decreased breath sounds

Similar Events

Other causes of airway obstruction

Pneumothorax (see Event 28, *Pneumothorax*)

Management

Nasopharyngeal Rupture

Intubate the trachea by direct laryngoscopy <u>before</u> removing misplaced ETT

If the ETT is removed first severe hemorrhage may occur

Obtain a consultation from an ENT surgeon, immediately if hemorrhage is severe

Tracheobronchial Tree Rupture

Suspect airway rupture in major trauma cases with subcutaneous or mediastinal air, a pneumothorax, or other major abdominal, cervical, or thoracic injuries

Ensure adequate oxygenation and ventilation

Administer supplemental O_2

If respiratory failure is impending

Intubate the trachea via direct laryngoscopy

Ventilate with 100% FIO_2, observe carefully for tension pneumothorax

Assess the site of airway rupture

Perform fiberoptic bronchoscopy in all cases of major thoracic trauma

Will require an experienced bronchoscopist

Should be performed awake with topical anesthesia if feasible

Will allow the diagnosis and exact site of airway rupture to be confirmed

May allow aspirated material or secretions to be removed

If tracheal rupture is recognized

Advance the ETT beyond the site of rupture if possible

Double lumen ETT may be required to maintain oxygenation

If bronchial rupture is diagnosed

Intubate the unaffected side under fiberoptic guidance

Double lumen ETT may be necessary

Placement of a bronchial blocker may be useful, particularly if pulmonary hemorrhage is found during bronchoscopy

Resuscitate the patient as necessary

Diagnose and manage other injuries

Exclude the presence of a pneumothorax

If nonemergent intubation is required for bronchoscopy or surgery

Treat as a known difficult intubation (see Event 3, *Difficult Tracheal Intubation*)

Fiberoptic intubation with topical anesthesia is the method of choice

Sedate the patient with low doses of narcotic or benzodiazepine

>Fentanyl IV, 50 μg, repeated as necessary

>Midazolam IV, 0.5 mg, repeated as necessary

Administer 100% O_2 and, if necessary, manually ventilate with gentle breaths, avoiding high PIP

Surgical correction of the ruptured airway is the definitive management

In patients with cervical injury, consider performing fiberoptic bronchoscopy as the ETT is removed to identify tracheal injuries

Complications

Retropharyngeal abscess

Airway obstruction

Hypoxemia

Cardiac arrest

Mediastinitis

Pneumonia distal to bronchial rupture

Tracheal or bronchial stenosis

Suggested Readings

Baxter A: Using a conventional ventilator in the presence of a bronchopleural fistula. Anesthesiology 64:835, 1986

Emery RE: Laser perforation of a main stem bronchus. Anesthesiology 64:120, 1986

Hannallah M, Gomes M: Bronchial rupture associated with the use of a double-lumen tube in a small adult. Anesthesiology 71:457, 1989

Roxburgh JC: Rupture of the tracheobronchial tree. Thorax 42:681, 1987

Sacco JJ, Halliday DW: Submucosal epiglottic emphysema complicating bronchial rupture. Anesthesiology 66:555, 1987

Spencer JA, Rogers CE, Westaby S: Clinico-radiological correlates in rupture of the major airways. Clin Radiol 43:371, 1991

---

23 ASPIRATION OF GASTRIC CONTENTS

Definition

Aspiration of gastric contents is defined as inhalation of gastric contents into the tracheobronchial tree.

Etiology

Passive regurgitation or active vomiting of gastric contents in patients who are unable to protect their airway

Typical Situations

Any patient with impaired laryngeal reflexes
  Anatomic abnormalities in and around the larynx
  Altered level of consciousness
  Anesthesia of the larynx or pharynx
Patients with muscle weakness or paralysis
Patients with an incompetent gastroesophageal junction
  Hiatus hernia
  Previous esophageal surgery
Patients with a "full stomach" or raised intra-abdominal pressure
Patients with large amounts of gas in the stomach
  Prolonged positive pressure mask ventilation
  Difficult tracheal intubation
Ineffective cricoid pressure either by an inexperienced assistant or in a patient with unusual anatomy
  Failure to maintain cricoid pressure until the correct placement of the ETT has been confirmed
Patients who are acutely intoxicated with alcohol have a lower gastric pH and may be obtunded

Prevention

In patients at risk of aspiration of gastric contents
  Avoid general anesthesia if possible
  Delay nonemergent surgery as long as possible (up to 6 hours) to allow the stomach to empty and to allow time for medications that assist gastric emptying and reduce gastric acidity to be effective
  Avoid depression of laryngeal reflexes by excess sedation or regional or topical anesthesia
  Administer nonparticulate antacids immediately prior to induction of anesthesia
    Sodium citrate PO, 30 ml
  Administer H_2 antagonists at least 30 minutes prior to the induction of anesthesia
    Cimetidine PO or IV, 300 mg
    Ranitidine PO, 150 mg, or IV, 50 mg
  Administer metoclopramide IV, 10 mg, to stimulate gastric emptying
If general anesthesia is necessary
  Assess the patient's airway carefully <u>prior</u> to inducing general anesthesia
  Apply nasogastric suctioning prior to induction of general anesthesia
    If a nasogastric tube is left in place, it may produce incompetence of the gastroesophageal sphincter
    Particulate matter may occlude the nasogastric tube, giving a false sense of security
  Use effective cricoid pressure by a trained and experienced assistant
    Maintain cricoid pressure until the ETT position is ensured (see Event 4, *Esophageal Intubation*)
  Intubate the trachea and inflate the ETT cuff as rapidly as possible
  Apply nasogastric suctioning prior to extubation
  Extubate the patient only after recovery of protective laryngeal reflexes
Consider awake intubation
  Topical anesthesia of the larynx before securing the airway may ablate protective

reflexes at a time that regurgitation or vomiting is likely to occur

Fiberoptic intubation can be performed in the upright position, making regurgitation less likely

Cough reflexes may be preserved by using specific nerve blocks and topical anesthesia of the oropharynx alone, without transtracheal injection of local anesthesia

Consider tracheostomy under local anesthesia if fiberoptic intubation is impossible and a difficult intubation is anticipated

Manifestations

Gastric contents visualized in the oropharynx

Severe hypoxemia

Increased PIP

Bronchospasm

Copious tracheal secretions

Coughing, laryngospasm, rales, or chest retraction

Dyspnea, apnea, or hyperpnea

Chest x-ray findings

Unremarkable in 15–20% of cases of aspiration

Pneumonic infiltrates and atelectasis

Similar Events

Hypoxemia from other causes (see Event 8, *Hypoxemia*)

Obstruction of the ETT

Bronchospasm from other causes (see Event 24, *Bronchospasm*)

Pulmonary edema (see Event 17, *Pulmonary Edema*)

ARDS

Pulmonary embolism (see Event 18, *Pulmonary Embolism*)

Pneumonia

Other causes of high PIP (see Event 5, *High Peak Inspiratory Pressure*)

Management

If gastric contents and/or pulmonary aspiration are recognized at the time of intubation

Perform immediate tracheal suctioning prior to positive pressure ventilation

If the ETT is in the trachea, place the patient head down, with right lateral tilt

Pass a suction catheter down the ETT

Do not make prolonged efforts at suctioning the trachea, especially if the patient's O_2 saturation is falling

Maintain oxygenation

Positive pressure ventilation with 100% FIO_2

PEEP

If particulate aspiration has occurred, perform bronchoscopy

Lavage plus suctioning may be necessary to remove particulate material

Obtain a sample of the pulmonary aspirate for pH, Gram stain, and culture

Cancel elective surgery. Emergency surgery should be restricted to the minimum procedure consistent with patient safety

Provide supportive care
> Fluid management with crystalloid rather than colloid
> Administer H_2 blockers for stress ulcer prophylaxis
>> Cimetidine IV, 300 mg q6h
>> Ranitidine IV, 50 mg q6h
> Intermittent pulmonary toilet is advisable because uninjured pulmonary cilia will continue to sweep particles and edema fluid to the bronchi
>> Lavage via the ETT is usually not indicated

Consider the administration of antibiotics
> Choice of antibiotic should be based on the results of a Gram stain of the pulmonary aspirate
> Prophylaxis is indicated for known aspiration of feculent material

Steroids have not been shown to be of benefit during the period of acute hypoxemia and may impair the long-term healing process of the lung

Bronchodilators may be helpful in relieving large airway closure in less damaged areas of the lung

Consider extracorporeal membrane oxygenator support if oxygenation cannot be maintained

Consider lung transplant

Complications

Pneumonia, ARDS, sepsis
Barotrauma secondary to high PIP

Suggested Readings

Cheek TG, Gutshe BB: Pulmonary aspiration of gastric contents. p. 407. In Shnider SM, Levinson G (eds): Anesthesia for Obstetrics. 3rd Ed. Williams & Wilkins, Baltimore, 1993

Gibbs CP, Modell JH: Management of aspiration pneumonitis. p. 1293. In Miller RD (ed): Anesthesia. 3rd Ed. Churchill Livingstone, New York, 1990

Palmer SK: Aspiration pneumonia: prevention and management. p. 263. In: Annual Refresher Course Lectures, American Society of Anesthesiologists, Park Ridge, IL, 1988

24 BRONCHOSPASM

Definition

Bronchospasm is a reversible narrowing of the medium and small airways due to smooth muscle contraction.

Etiology

Bronchial asthma
COPD with a reversible component of airway narrowing

Airway irritation
Medications

Typical Situations

Patients with known asthma, COPD, or recent upper respiratory tract infection
Mechanical irritation of the airway
      Placement of oral airway
      Intubation
      Endobronchial intubation
Chemical irritation of the airway
      Pungent anesthetic gases
      Soda lime dust
      Smoke inhalation
Administration of drugs that can precipitate bronchospasm
      Histamine release
      β-Antagonists
      Anticholinesterases
Aspiration of gastric contents (see Event 23, *Aspiration of Gastric Contents*)
Pulmonary embolism (see Event 18, *Pulmonary Embolism*)

Prevention

Avoid anesthesia and elective surgery when the patient is at risk of bronchospasm
      Acute upper respiratory tract infections
      Exacerbation of asthma or COPD
Optimize therapy with bronchodilators and/or systemic steroids prior to anesthesia in patients
    with known asthma or COPD
If it is necessary to proceed with surgery in a patient at risk of bronchospasm
      Regional anesthesia may be a viable alternative to eliminate stimulation of the trachea by
          the ETT
      Consider using ketamine for anesthetic induction instead of thiobarbiturates
Achieve an adequate depth of anesthesia prior to intubation
      Lidocaine IV, 1.5 mg/kg, 1–3 minutes prior to intubation
      Deepen anesthesia with volatile anesthetic agent prior to intubation
      Halothane may be preferable to other agents because it is less pungent

Manifestations

Increased PIP
Audible wheezing, usually during expiration
      No wheezing will be audible if bronchospasm is severe and there is little or no gas flow
Decreased pulmonary compliance
Decreased arterial pO_2 and O_2 saturation
Decreased tidal volume
Hypercarbia
      End-tidal CO_2 may be absent if bronchospasm is severe and there is little or no gas flow

Similar Events

Aspiration of gastric contents (see Event 23, *Aspiration Of Gastric Contents*)
Kinked or obstructed ETT (see Event 5, *High Peak Inspiratory Pressure*)
Pneumothorax (see Event 28, *Pneumothorax)*
Amniotic fluid embolism (see Event 68, *Amniotic Fluid Embolism*)
Pulmonary edema (see Event 17, *Pulmonary Edema*)
Pulmonary embolism (see Event 18, *Pulmonary Embolism)*
Endobronchial intubation (see Event 25, *Endobronchial Intubation)*
Anaphylaxis/anaphylactoid reactions (see Event 11, *Anaphylaxis and Anaphylactoid Reactions*)
Air trapping

Management

Ensure adequate oxygenation and ventilation
Increase FIO_2 to 100% if O_2 saturation is compromised
Ventilate the patient by hand
Provides important information regarding pulmonary compliance
May reduce the mean and peak airway pressures
If hand ventilation will be an ongoing requirement, call for help
Verify that the problem is truly bronchospasm
Auscultate the chest
Check the position, placement, and patency of ETT
Pass a suction catheter down the ETT
If in doubt about the ETT, consider removing it and replacing it with a new ETT
For mild bronchospasm
Remove any airway irritant
Increase anesthetic depth with a volatile anesthetic agent if the patient is not hypotensive
Administer β agonist to the lungs by metered-dose inhaler, repeat in 10 minutes if there
is no response and no tachycardia
A large dose of any aerosolized medication may be required when administered
via the ETT
Metaproterenol: initial dose, 4–8 metered puffs
Albuterol: initial dose, 4–8 metered puffs
Ipratropium bromide: initial dose, 4–8 metered puffs
For moderate to severe bronchospasm
Institute measures as in mild bronchospasm
Consider the possibility of silent aspiration of gastric contents
Suction through the ETT and collect aspirate for analysis of pH
If bronchospasm does not resolve
Administer nebulized <u>undiluted</u> β agonist (nebulized saline may be irritating to lungs,
especially during severe bronchospasm)
Institute IV bronchodilator therapy
Aminophylline: loading dose, 5 mg/kg; maintenance infusion, 0.5–0.9 mg/kg/hr
Isoproterenol IV infusion, 1–3 µg/min titrated to the pulse rate, blood pressure,
and bronchodilation response
Epinephrine IV: 0.1 µg/kg bolus; infusion, 10–25 ng/kg/min, titrated to the pulse
rate, blood pressure, and bronchodilation response

Administer corticosteroids

    Methylprednisolone IV, 100 mg bolus

Obtain a high-performance ventilator (such as an ICU ventilator)

    Pulmonary compliance/resistance may exceed the performance envelope of the anesthesia machine ventilator

Stop the surgical procedure as soon as possible

Transfer patient to ICU for postoperative management if resolution incomplete

Complications

Hypoxemia

Hypercarbia

Cardiac arrest

Hypotension

Arrhythmias

Barotrauma

Suggested Readings

Bishop MJ: Bronchospasm: managing and avoiding a potential anesthetic disaster. p. 272. In: Annual Refresher Course Lectures, American Society of Anesthesiologists, Park Ridge, IL, 1990

Crogan SJ, Bishop MJ: Delivery efficiency of metered dose aerosols given via endotracheal tubes. Anesthesiology 70:1008, 1989

Hirschman CA: Airway reactivity in humans: anesthetic implications. Anesthesiology 58:170, 1983

25 ENDOBRONCHIAL INTUBATION

Definition

Endobronchial intubation is the unintentional placement of the ETT in a mainstem or segmental bronchus, resulting in excessive ventilation of one lung or lung segment and hypoventilation of the other(s).

Etiology

ETT advanced too far during initial placement

Manipulation of the head or ETT after tracheal intubation

Aberrant tracheal/bronchial anatomy

Typical Situations

Inadequate assessment of the insertion depth of the ETT during initial placement

    Inexperienced anesthetist

Difficult intubation
ETT placed through a tracheostomy
Placement of uncut ETT
During certain types of surgery
Neurosurgery
The head is frequently placed in a flexed or extended position; flexion can advance the ETT by up to 3 cm
Head or neck surgery, especially when the airway is shared with the surgeon
Thoracic surgery
Double lumen ETT
Surgical manipulation of trachea and bronchi
When the patient is placed in the steep Trendelenburg or lithotomy position
Pediatric patients in whom the distance between the larynx and the carina is short

Prevention

Cut excess length from the ETT before insertion
Advance the ETT so that the cuff is just beyond the vocal cords
Carefully note the markings on the ETT at the teeth or gums after insertion
Secure the ETT firmly to the patient
Maintain security of the ETT when positioning the patient
Recheck the position of the ETT and auscultate the breath sounds after positioning the patient

Manifestations

Endobronchial intubation most commonly involves the ETT in the right mainstem bronchus.

Increased PIP
Decreased breath sounds on the nonventilated side
Asymmetric chest movement with ventilation
Changes in oxygenation
O_2 saturation may remain at or near 100% , especially if the $FiO2$ is 100%
Atelectasis will occur in the nonventilated lung, increasing the shunt fraction
Decrease in arterial pO_2, O_2 saturation, and increased A-a gradient
Changes in end-tidal CO_2
End-tidal CO_2 may increase, decrease, or remain unchanged depending on the V/Q characteristics of the ventilated lung
Increased time lag in the patient's response to changes in the concentration of volatile anesthetics because of the increase in shunt fraction
Tidal volume may decrease if the pulmonary compliance exceeds the ventilator's performance envelope
Fiberoptic bronchoscopy
The carina is not visualized distal to the tip of the ETT
The division between segmental bronchi may resemble the carina
The tip of the ETT may be visualized at or below the level of the carina on a chest x-ray

Similar Events

Kinked or obstructed ETT (see Event 5, *High Peak Inspiratory Pressure*)

Pneumothorax (see Event 28, *Pneumothorax*)
Pulmonary embolism (see Event 18, *Pulmonary Embolism*)
Bronchospasm (see Event 24, *Bronchospasm*)
Lobar or segmental atelectasis or collapse

Management

Maintain oxygenation and ventilation
If the O_2 saturation is less than 95%, increase the FIO_2 to 100%
Auscultate both sides of chest for asymmetry of breath sounds
Auscultate in the axilla to reduce the breath sounds transmitted across the midline and heard on the opposite side
If the orifice of the right upper lobe bronchus is occluded by a right mainstem intubation, this difference may be difficult to hear
Inspect the ETT
Check that the insertion depth of the ETT is appropriate
Palpate the intraoral part of the ETT for kinks
If the ETT is visible in the surgical field, ask the surgeon to check the depth of insertion of the ETT or for kinks in the ETT
If endobronchial intubation is diagnosed
Deflate the cuff and pull back the ETT cautiously
Be prepared to reintubate the trachea
Auscultate the chest for symmetric breath sounds
Check the PIP

If uncertain about the placement of the ETT, perform fiberoptic laryngoscopy or obtain a chest x-ray
Ensure the patency of the ETT
Pass a suction catheter down the ETT to rule out obstruction

Complications

Hypoxemia
Hypercarbia
Atelectasis
Pneumonia of the atelectatic lung or segment
Barotrauma to the hyperventilated lung

Suggested Readings

Gammage GW: Airway. p. 151. In Gravenstein N (ed): Manual of Complications During Anesthesia. JB Lippincott, New York, 1990
Gilbert D, Benumof JL: Biphasic carbon dioxide elimination waveform with right mainstem bronchial intubation. Anesth Analg 69:829, 1989
Owen RL, Cheney FW: Endobronchial intubation: a preventable complication. Anesthesiology 67:255, 1987
Riley RH, Marcy JH: Unsuspected endobronchial intubation—detection by continuous mass spectrometry. Anesthesiology 63:203, 1985

26 MASSIVE HEMOPTYSIS

Definition

Expectoration of more than 600 ml of blood in 24 hours constitutes massive hemoptysis.

Etiology

Pulmonary infection
Pulmonary neoplasm
Cardiovascular disease
Coagulopathy

Typical Situations

Thoracic trauma or surgery
Pulmonary infection
      Tuberculosis
      Aspergilloma
      Lung abscess
Pulmonary neoplasm
      Bronchogenic or metastatic carcinoma
      Endobronchial polyp
Rupture of a PA by the balloon of a PA catheter
Pulmonary infarction
Mitral stenosis and/or pulmonary hypertension
Atheromatous or mycotic aneurysms of the thoracic aorta, or previous repair of an aneurysm of
    the thoracic aorta
Coagulopathy

Prevention

Prepare for the possibility of massive hemoptysis during thoracic or intrabronchial procedures
Avoid overinflation and persistent wedging of PA catheter

Manifestations

Hemoptysis in the awake patient
Blood in the ETT of the anesthetized patient
      Blood does not clear with suctioning
Hypoxemia
Hypercarbia
Hypotension
Bronchospasm

Similar Events

Hemorrhage from oral cavity or nasopharynx
Hematemesis
Fulminant pulmonary edema (see Event 17, *Pulmonary Edema*)

Management

Death is usually due to <u>asphyxiation</u>, not blood loss.

Intubate the patient if there is respiratory distress
    Intubation will be difficult
    Wear a face mask and protect your eyes
    Attempt awake intubation via direct laryngoscopy
        Use topical anesthesia, although it is not very effective
        Have at least <u>two</u> suction units available, as bleeding can be massive
        A rigid bronchoscope may be necessary to establish the airway
    Once the patient is intubated
        Suction the ETT
        If hypotension is not present, carefully sedate the patient to help reduce the rate of hemorrhage
            Morphine IV, 1–2 mg q5min
            Midazolam IV, 0.5–1 mg q5min

Ventilate with 100% FIO_2
    Monitor oxygenation via pulse oximetry or repeated ABGs
    Avoid high airway pressures if possible to avoid air embolism

If the ETT fills with blood and ventilation is impossible
    Push the single lumen ETT into the trachea as far as possible to perform deliberate endobronchial intubation
        The ETT <u>may</u> be guided down the left mainstem bronchus by turning the patient's head during intubation (right ear to right shoulder)
        If the right mainstem bronchus is intubated, the upper lobe bronchus will be obstructed
    If the ETT goes down the <u>bleeding</u> bronchus
        Maintaining oxygenation and ventilation takes precedence over stopping the bleeding
            Attempt to reposition the ETT into the nonbleeding bronchus
            Try to ventilate alongside the endobronchial ETT by inserting an addtional small ETT through the glottis
            Consider placing a Fogarty catheter down the ETT and occluding the bronchus, then withdrawing the ETT into the trachea
    If the ETT goes down the <u>nonbleeding</u> side
        Suction the ETT to remove residual blood
        Ventilate the patient with 100% O_2
        If oxygenation continues to be a problem, prepare to insert a double lumen ETT

Consider separate ventilation of the lungs using a double lumen ETT
    Do <u>not</u> remove the ETT without leaving a guide in the trachea. Hemoptysis may make subsequent visualization of glottis impossible
    Place a bougie or stiff guide down the single lumen ETT, making sure the guide is longer than the double lumen ETT that you plan to pass over the guide
    Remove the single lumen ETT and reintubate the trachea with the double lumen ETT
        Using direct laryngoscopy, pass the double lumen ETT over the guide into the larynx
        The double lumen ETT can be passed blindly over the guide into the larynx

Prepare for and administer massive transfusion if necessary
>Insert several large-bore IV catheters
>Place an arterial line and a CVP catheter early in the course of treatment

Obtain emergent consultation from a thoracic surgeon and an interventional radiologist
>Determine the site of bleeding and assess the need for emergency thoracotomy
>Chest x-ray or surgeon's report may identify the likely site of bleeding
>Bronchoscopy is the most appropriate first step in the evaluation but may be very diffi-cult if the bleeding has not stopped
>Arteriography or bronchography are indicated if the bleeding is not catastrophic

Take measures to stop the bleeding
>Embolization of bronchial, pulmonary, and/or intercostal arteries under fluoroscopic guidance
>Iced saline lavage or application of topical vasoconstrictors through a bronchoscope
>Tamponade of the bleeding site or occlusion of the bronchus leading to the bleeding site with a Fogarty balloon catheter
>Correct any coagulopathy

Emergency thoracotomy
>Should be reserved for those patients with adequate lung function in whom the site of hemorrhage can be identified and who continue to suffer massive hemoptysis

For induction of anesthesia in the nonintubated patient whose hemoptysis has been controlled
>Treat patients as if they have a "full stomach"
>>Use rapid sequence induction and cricoid pressure
>Intubation may be difficult with large amounts of blood in the oropharynx, making the larynx difficult to visualize
>Awake intubation is controversial
>>Anesthetizing the larynx with local anesthetic may make aspiration more likely
>>Laryngoscopy may provoke vomiting in the awake patient
>Use a double lumen ETT if possible, to protect the nonbleeding lung from aspiration
>Anticipate the need for postoperative ventilation

Complications

Massive hemoptysis usually complicates severe underlying lung disease. Mortality is related to the rate of blood loss (600 ml or more in less than 4 hours is associated with a 70% mortality rate).

Aspiration pneumonitis secondary to blood in the lungs
Hypoxemia
Hypotension
Cardiac arrest

Suggested Readings

Benumof JL, Alfery DD: Anesthesia for thoracic surgery. p. 1517. In Miller RD (ed): Anesthesia. 3rd Ed. Churchill Livingstone, New York, 1990

Jones DK, Davies RJ: Massive hemoptysis. Br Med J 300:889, 1990

MacIntosh EL, Parrott JCW, Unruh HW: Fistulas between the aorta and tracheobronchial tree. Ann Thorac Surg 51:515, 1991

Thompson AB, Teschler H, Rennard SI: Pathogenesis, evaluation and therapy for massive hemoptysis. Clin Chest Med 13:69, 1992

27 HYPERCARBIA

Definition

Abnormally high levels of CO_2 in the blood or end-tidal gas is called hypercarbia.

Etiology

Inadequate alveolar ventilation relative to CO_2 production
Compensatory mechanism for metabolic alkalosis

Typical Situations

Increased CO_2 production
       Shivering
       Pyrexia, sepsis
       Parenteral nutrition with high glucose loads
       Malignant hyperthermia
Decreased CO_2 elimination
       Depression of the respiratory center by drugs or cerebral disease
       Airway obstruction
       Mechanical failure of ETT, breathing circuit, or ventilator
       Neuromuscular disorders or residual effects of muscle relaxants
       Pain-induced decrease in tidal volume following thoracic or upper abdominal surgery
       Altered lung mechanics
       Cardiopulmonary arrest

Prevention

Use appropriate ventilator settings during mechanical ventilation
       10–15 ml/kg tidal volume
       6–10 breaths/min (adults)
Avoid excessive doses or combinations of respiratory depressant drugs
Set alarms on ventilator and capnograph to warn of hypoventilation
Monitor end-tidal CO_2 levels
Clinically monitor the ventilation of patients breathing spontaneously
       Especially important postoperatively for patients who have received spinal opiates

Manifestations

Increased end-tidal CO_2
Clinical signs of hypercarbia (may be masked by general anesthesia)
       Sympathoadrenal stimulation triggered by the CNS
              Hypertension
              Tachycardia
              PVCs
       Tachypnea in spontaneously ventilating patient

Semiparalyzed patient may try to overbreathe the ventilator

Peripheral vasodilation

Inability to fully reverse muscle relaxants

Failure to awaken secondary to the anesthetic effect of increased arterial CO_2 (see Event 45, *Postoperative Alteration in Mental Status*)

Similar Events

Physiologic increase in arterial pCO_2 to 45–47 mm Hg during sleep

Capnograph artifact

Management

Temporary and mild hypercarbia (arterial pCO_2 of 45–50 mm Hg) during anesthesia is common (particularly if the patient is ventilating spontaneously) and is unlikely to harm the patient.

Ensure adequate oxygenation

If the O_2 saturation is low or decreasing, increase the FIO_2

Ensure adequate ventilation

If the patient is ventilating spontaneously

Establish a patent airway, with mechanical aids if necessary

Reduce the depth of anesthesia

Intubate the trachea and begin mechanical ventilation if hypercarbia or hypoxemia cannot be reversed

If the patient is being ventilated mechanically

Increase the minute ventilation

Check for a malfunction in the ventilator or a major leak in the anesthesia breathing circuit (see Event 6, *Ventilator Failure* and Event 57, *Major Leak in the Anesthesia Breathing Circuit*)

Leak in breathing circuit

Ventilator malfunction

Check the inspired CO_2 level; the presence of more than 1–2 mm Hg inspired CO_2 indicates rebreathing of CO_2 due to

Incompetent valve in breathing circuit (see Event 50, *Circle System Valve Stuck Open*)

Exhausted soda lime in CO_2 absorber

Increase the fresh gas flow to convert the circle system to a semiopen system

The inspired CO_2 level should drop markedly

Administration of exogenous CO_2

Obtain an ABG analysis to confirm hypercarbia

Look for causes of increased CO_2 production

Sepsis

Pyrexia

MH (CO_2 production will increase dramatically)

For hypercarbia occurring after emergence from anesthesia

Maintain controlled ventilation until adequate spontaneous ventilation can be sustained

If the ETT is still in place, do not remove it

If the trachea has been extubated, maintain the patency of the airway, and reintubate the trachea if necessary

Ensure adequate reversal of neuromuscular blockade (see Event 46, *Postoperative Failure To Breathe*)

 Evaluate the response to electrical stimulation of nerves

  Train-of-four

  Tetanus

  Double burst stimulation

 Check the patient's ability to sustain head lift for more than 5 seconds

 Check the patient's maximum inspiratory force

  Greater than 25 cm H_2O will sustain ventilation but protective airway reflexes may not be intact

 If reversal of neuromuscular blockade is incomplete

  Administer additional anticholinesterase to a maximum of 70 μg/kg of neostigmine

  Maintain mechanical ventilation until reversal of neuromuscular blockade is ensured

Reverse respiratory depressant drugs

 Antagonize narcotic effect with naloxone IV, 40 μg increments

 Antagonize benzodiazepine effect with flumazenil IV, 1 mg increments

Check for syringe or ampule swaps (see Event 60, *Syringe or Ampule Swap*)

Complications

Hypertension and tachycardia

Pulmonary hypertension, right heart failure

Hypoxemia

Arrhythmias

Cardiac arrest

Suggested Readings

Benumof JL: Respiratory physiology and respiratory function during anesthesia. p. 505. In Miller RD (ed): Anesthesia. 3rd Ed. Churchill Livingstone, New York, 1990

Gravenstein JS, Paulus DA, Hayes TJ: Capnography in Clinical Practice. Butterworths, Boston, 1989

28 PNEUMOTHORAX

Definition

Pneumothorax is the presence of gas in the pleural space.

Etiology

Connection from the atmosphere to the pleural space

Rupture of an alveolus or bronchus into the pleural cavity

Typical Situations

Following CVP line placement, regional block of nerves, or surgery in close proximity to the
pleural cavity
Subclavian approach to CVP line placement
Intercostal nerve blocks, supraclavicular brachial plexus or stellate ganglion block
Nephrectomy, splenectomy, percutaneous liver biopsy
Spontaneous pneumothorax in patients with bullous disease of the lungs
Barotrauma from ventilation of the lungs with a high PIP
Excessive tidal volume
Expiratory obstruction of the breathing circuit
Ball valve effects in trachea due to tumor or endobronchial cuff of double lumen ETT
Chest trauma
Rib fractures
Injury may be **recent** or **remote**
Following diagnostic procedures
Laryngoscopy, bronchoscopy, or esophagoscopy
Pleurocentesis
Percutaneous lung biopsy
During laparoscopy (due to CO_2 insufflation)
Use of high-speed pneumatic drills in oral/dental surgery

Prevention

Identify patients at risk of pneumothorax
Avoid N_2O if there is a significant risk of pneumothorax
Consider prophylactic chest tube placement if the risk of pneumothorax is high
Increase vigilance during surgery on or near the pleural space
Place CVP lines carefully
Avoid the subclavian approach immediately before general anesthesia or if the patient is
being mechanically ventilated
If the subclavian approach must be used, obtain a chest x-ray to rule out pneumothorax
before proceeding with surgery
Initial chest x-ray may not show a pneumothorax if air accumulates slowly
Use care when using a double lumen ETT
Reduce the risk of cuff herniation by not overinflating the endobronchial cuff
Verify correct placement of the bronchial cuff by auscultation and fiberoptic bron-
choscopy after changes in the patient's position

Manifestations

Pneumothorax is difficult to diagnose during general anesthesia.

In the awake patient
Cough, tachypnea, and dyspnea
Hypoxemia, cyanosis
Tachycardia
Chest pain
In the anesthetized patient

Hypoxemia

Hypercarbia

Increased PIP and decreased pulmonary compliance

Hypotension, tachycardia

Asymmetric breath sounds, hyperresonant percussion over the affected hemithorax

Subcutaneous emphysema of the oropharynx, face, or neck (especially during oral/dental surgery)

Tracheal deviation from the midline

Neck veins may appear distended

Bulging hemidiaphragm may be visible during abdominal surgery

Characteristic chest x-ray picture

Loss of lung markings, visible edge of the partially collapsed lung

Deviation of the mediastinum away from the pneumothorax

Similar Events

Obstructed ETT (see Event 5, *High Peak Inspiratory Pressure*)

Endobronchial intubation (see Event 25, *Endobronchial Intubation*)

Bronchospasm (see Event 24, *Bronchospasm)*

Aspiration of gastric contents (see Event 23, *Aspiration Of Gastric Contents*)

Expiratory valve or pop-off valve stuck in the closed position (see Event 48, *Circle System Expiratory Valve Stuck Closed* and Event 58, *Pop-Off Valve Failure*)

Pulmonary edema (see Event 17, *Pulmonary Edema*)

Management

Turn off N_2O, increase FiO_2 to 100%

Confirm the diagnosis of pneumothorax

Auscultate both sides of the chest as pneumothoraces may be bilateral

Percuss the chest if possible

Look and feel for tracheal deviation

Rule out endobronchial intubation, obstructed ETT, and valves stuck closed

Notify the surgeon

If significant hypotension is present without another probable etiology, treat for possible tension pneumothorax (may be lifesaving)

Support the circulation

Expand the circulating fluid volume

Administer vasopressors or inotropic drugs

Drugs may not reach the heart if a tension pneumothorax compromises venous return

Insert a large-bore IV catheter into the pleural space of the side with decreased breath sounds or hyperresonant percussion

Insert just cephalad to rib body to avoid the neurovascular bundle

Insert either in the second intercostal space, midclavicular line or in the fourth intercostal space, midaxillary line

If tension pneumothorax is relieved, a "hiss" may be heard

Hemodynamic improvement may occur after catheter insertion

Evacuation of air with a small IV catheter may be diagnostic but may not completely relieve a tension pneumothorax

A chest tube <u>must</u> be inserted following placement of an IV catheter, whether positive for air or not

Consider the possibility of bilateral pneumothoraces

If a bronchopleural fistula is noted after placement of chest tube

Increase fresh gas flow into the anesthesia circuit

Increase minute ventilation to maintain normocarbia

Consider placing a double lumen ETT for split lung ventilation

Consider high-frequency jet ventilation if available

Complications

Hypoxemia
Hypotension
Arrhythmias
Cardiac arrest
Venous or arterial gas embolism

Suggested Readings

Denlinger JK: Pneumothorax. p. 173. In Orkin FK, Cooperman LH (eds): Complications in Anesthesia. JB Lippincott, Philadelphia, 1983

Kneeshaw JD: Tension pneumothorax—wrong tube? Br J Anaesth 64:222, 1991

Laishley RS, Aps C: Tension pneumothorax and pulse oximetry. Br J Anaesth 66:250, 1991

Samuel J, Schwartz S: Tension pneumothorax during dental anesthesia. Anesth Analg 67:1187, 1988

29 POSTOPERATIVE STRIDOR

Definition

Stridor is a harsh, high-pitched inspiratory sound caused by airway obstruction.

Etiology

Laryngospasm (persistent coaptation of the vocal cords)
Laryngeal edema
Paralysis of one or both vocal cords
Obstruction or compression of the airway by a mass

Typical Situations

Laryngospasm
Extubation during emergence from anesthesia

Secretions in or near the larynx

Recent upper respiratory infection

Laryngeal edema

Laryngeal surgery or instrumentation

Major fluid resuscitation, especially with prolonged use of the Trendelenburg position

Hematoma or swelling secondary to lymphatic obstruction following neck surgery

In parturients, following prolonged second stage of labor

Paralysis of vocal cord

Following cervical or thoracic surgery, or pathology of recurrent laryngeal nerve

Inadequate reversal of muscle relaxants

Mass, secretions, blood, or fluid in the upper airway

Following airway surgery (e.g., tonsillectomy)

Secretions in heavy smoker

Pre-existing airway pathology

Retained surgical pack

Vocal cord polyp or laryngeal tumor

Prevention

Administer steroids prior to extubation to minimize airway edema following trauma, instrumentation, or surgery of the airway

Do not extubate the patient if there is facial edema following surgery

Ensure full reversal of neuromuscular blockade

Suction secretions from the upper airway before extubation and as necessary afterward

Remove all foreign bodies from the airway at the end of surgery

Extubate the trachea when the patient is awake or when anesthesia is deep enough to ablate airway reflexes

Maintain the patency of the airway as necessary after extubation

Manifestations

Noisy, high-pitched inspiratory sound

Reduced inspiratory volume

Retraction of the chest or neck during inspiration accompanied by use of the accessory muscles of respiration

Restlessness and dyspnea that are aggravated by increasing respiratory efforts or attempts to cough up secretions

Hypoxemia and cyanosis

Increasing end-tidal CO_2 and arterial pCO_2

Similar Events

Airway obstruction from other causes

Bronchospasm (see Event 24, *Bronchospasm*)

Epiglottitis [see Event 76, *Epiglottitis (Supraglottitis)*]

Intrathoracic airway obstruction

Anxiety reaction

Management

Place the patient on 100% O$_2$ by face mask
Assist ventilation with CPAP
> Encourage the patient to take slow, steady breaths

Apply mechanical airway support maneuvers
> Jaw thrust
> Oral or nasal airway

Suction the oropharynx to remove secretions
If there is any question about the adequacy of reversal of neuromuscular blockade, administer additional anticholinesterase to the patient
If stridor does not resolve and respiratory distress continues
> Call for help
> Prepare for emergency reintubation
> Have an assistant prepare for transtracheal jet ventilation and/or cricothyrotomy
> Administer a small dose of succinylcholine IV, 0.3 mg/kg, or IM, 0.6 mg/kg, and continue mask ventilation

If hypoxemia occurs and cannot be corrected, move aggressively
> Reintubate the trachea
> If tracheal intubation is difficult, begin transtracheal jet ventilation and/or cricothyrotomy

Treatment of specific underlying situations
> Following neck surgery
>> Call for the surgeon immediately
>> Remove any dressings from the wound
>> If a hematoma is found, cut the wound sutures
>>> Will require surgical exploration of the wound for hemostasis and reclosure
>> Reintubate the trachea if there is no immediate improvement in the patient's airway
>>> Intubation may be difficult because of larynx/airway edema
>>> Perform intubation under optimum conditions in the operating room if the patient is stable

> Following airway surgery
>> Call for the surgeon immediately
>> Administer steroids
>>> Dexamethasone IV, 8–20 mg
>> Consider inhalation therapy with racemic epinephrine
>>> Call for respiratory therapist
>> Consider the possibility of retained gauze, throat packs, or other foreign body in the airway
>> Prepare for direct examination of the airway and/or reintubation

Complications

Hypoxemia
Inability to reintubate
Airway trauma due to difficult intubation
Aspiration of gastric contents

Pulmonary edema due to excessive negative intrathoracic pressure
Contamination of surgical wounds opened to relieve pressure in the neck
Cardiac arrest

30 UNPLANNED EXTUBATION

Definition

An uplanned extubation is any unplanned dislodgement or removal of the endotracheal tube from the trachea.

Etiology

Mechanical traction on the ETT
Endotracheal tube inadequately secured

Typical Situations

When the patient's position is changed
    Moving the operating table relative to the anesthesia machine
    Moving the patient from one bed or table to another
During manipulation of the head and neck
When manipulating the anesthesia breathing circuit hoses or surgical drapes
When attempting to reposition an ETT
During placement of a nasogastric tube

Prevention

Use a Rae ETT where appropriate
Secure the ETT in place following intubation
    Prepare the skin with benzoin solution
    Tape the ETT to the skin securely
    Note the markings of the ETT at the gums or teeth
Avoid attaching the ETT to the operating table
Ensure that the ETT is in proper position prior to surgical draping
Hold the ETT securely in place and observe as the patient's position is changed
Disconnect the anesthesia breathing circuit from the ETT when moving the patient to avoid
    traction on the ETT
    Make sure that the circuit is reconnected to the ETT and that the ventilator is activated
        after completing patient movement
Hold the ETT in place during procedures such as fiberoptic bronchoscopy or direct laryn-
    goscopy
If the patient is in the lateral or prone position, be prepared to move the patient into the supine
    position should reintubation become necessary

Manifestations

An apparent major leak in the anesthesia breathing circuit
> The ventilator bellows or reservoir bag collapses
> A leak may develop slowly, as the extubation may not be complete
> The smell of volatile anesthetic may be apparent
> Sounds of a gas leak may be heard
> An excessive amount of air in the ETT cuff may be required to achieve a seal

No breath sounds or abnormal breath sounds heard through the esophageal or precordial stethoscope
Decreased or zero PIP
Decreased or zero expiratory gas flow measured by a spirometer in the anesthesia breathing circuit
Little or no expired CO_2
The ETT may be visualized outside the trachea
If the patient is breathing spontaneously
> Little or no movement of the reservoir bag

Gastric distention may occur if the ETT is in the pharynx or esophagus
Late signs of hypoventilation
> Hypoxemia
> Hypercarbia

Similar Events

ETT cuff rupture
Disconnection or other major leak in the anesthesia breathing circuit or anesthesia machine (see Event 57, *Major Leak in the Anesthesia Breathing Circuit*)
Loss of O_2 pipeline supply (see Event 56, *Loss of Pipeline Oxygen*)

Management

Confirm the diagnosis
> Switch to manual ventilation, feel the compliance of the lungs and anesthesia breathing circuit during ventilation
> Palpate the pilot balloon of the ETT to check the pressure in the ETT cuff

Compensate for the leak in the anesthesia breathing circuit
> Increase the FIO_2 to 100%
> Increase the fresh gas flow into the breathing circuit if a leak is present

Inform the surgeon
> If necessary, clear your access to the airway
> If the airway is in or near the surgical field, halt the surgery and cover the wound with a sterile drape

Perform a direct laryngoscopy to determine the position of the ETT
> Reposition or replace the ETT into the trachea

If repositioning or reintubation is not easily accomplished
> **Immediately** mask ventilate the patient with 100% FIO_2 if the O_2 saturation is less than 95%
> Attempt reintubation when the patient is maximally oxygenated

If oxygenation cannot be maintained, move aggressively to transtracheal jet ventilation or cricothyrotomy

If the patient is in the prone or lateral position

Call for help

If the patient's O_2 saturation is lower than 95% or there is no CO_2 waveform on the capnograph

If the patient is in the lateral position, attempt reintubation

Otherwise, move emergently to turn the patient supine for mask ventilation and reintubation

If the patient's O_2 saturation is higher than 95% and there is a CO_2 waveform on the capnograph

Continue to ventilate manually with small tidal volumes and low airway pressures

If experienced assistance is available, consider fiberoptic endoscopy to confirm the diagnosis and to reposition the ETT

If the patient was difficult to intubate at the beginning of the case

Call for help

Maintain mask ventilation with 100% FIO_2

Assemble the equipment needed for a difficult intubation (see Event 3, *Difficult Tracheal Intubation*)

Consider the alternatives if the patient cannot be reintubated

Transtracheal jet ventilation

Cricothyrotomy or tracheostomy

Terminate surgery and awaken the patient

Complications

Aspiration of gastric contents

Esophageal intubation

Contamination of the surgical wound

Disconnection or accidental removal of monitoring lines or sensor monitors during repositioning of the patient

Hypoxemia

Cardiac arrest

Chapter Six
Metabolic Events

31 ADDISONIAN CRISIS

Definition

Addisonian crisis is a relative or absolute deficiency of adrenal corticosteroid hormones resulting in hemodynamic or other compromise.

Etiology

Primary adrenal insufficiency
Secondary adrenal insufficiency
Failure of hormone synthesis
    Etomidate inhibits the synthesis of adrenal corticosteroids, but there are no reports of its precipitating addisonian crisis

Typical Situations

Patients with primary or secondary adrenal insufficiency
Abrupt termination of steroid therapy
Patients with a recent history of steroid therapy who are stressed by major surgery or perioperative infections

Prevention

Administer preoperative corticosteroids to any patient who has received adrenal suppressive doses of corticosteroids (more than 5 mg/day of prednisone or equivalent) within the year prior to surgery
    Hydrocortisone IV, 100 mg prior to induction of anesthesia, followed by 200–300 mg/day in divided doses
Identify patients with primary or secondary adrenal insufficiency
Have a high index of suspicion for adrenal insufficiency in patients with significant systemic diseases that are often treated with corticosteroids

Manifestations

Onset may be delayed to the postoperative period and may be very acute.

Hypotension
Shock
Nausea and vomiting

Similar Events

Septic shock
Hypotension secondary to other etiologies (see Event 7, *Hypotension*)

Management

If hypotension or cardiovascular collapse occurs in the patient at risk of adrenal insufficiency
  Rapidly expand circulating fluid volume (crystalloid and/or colloid)
  Administer hydrocortisone IV, 100 mg bolus, repeat q6h
  Hemodynamic support with vasopressors, inotropes as necessary
  Identify and treat underlying causes of adrenal insufficiency if possible
Ensure that other more likely etiologies of hypotension and shock are not responsible for hypotension
  Hypovolemia
  Anesthetic or drug overdose
  Primary cardiovascular impairment
  High intrathoracic pressure

Complications

Cardiac arrest
Complications of steroid therapy

Suggested Readings

Graf G, Rosenbaum S: Anesthesia and the endocrine system. p. 1237. In Barash P, Cullen BF, Stoelting RK (eds): Clinical Anesthesia. 2nd Ed. JB Lippincott, New York, 1992
Hertzberg LB, Shulman MS: Acute adrenal insufficiency in a patient with appendicitis during anesthesia. Anesthesiology 62:517, 1985
Williams GH, Dluhy RG: Diseases of the adrenal cortex. p. 1713. In Wilson JD, Braunwald E, Isselbacher KJ et al (eds): Harrison's Principles of Internal Medicine. 12th Ed. McGraw-Hill, New York, 1991

32 DIABETIC KETOACIDOSIS

Definition

Diabetic ketoacidosis is a metabolic acidosis associated with high levels of ketoacids (acetoacetate and β-hydroxybutyrate) in the blood and urine of the diabetic patient.

32

Etiology

An absolute or relative deficiency of insulin causing mobilization and oxidation of fatty acids, with resulting production of ketoacids

Typical Situations

In patients with type I (insulin-dependent) diabetes
When an appropriate insulin dose has been administered but the patient's insulin requirements are increased due to
>Trauma
>Intercurrent infection
>Excessive fluid losses or inadequate fluid intake
>Increased catabolic stress
When there has been an absolute deficiency of insulin
>The appropriate dose has not been administered
>The absorption of SC or IM insulin has been delayed by poor peripheral perfusion

Prevention

Prevention of DKA, rather than prevention of hyperglycemia, is the primary aim of surgical care of the diabetic patient.

Identify insulin-dependent patients preoperatively and optimize therapy
>The appropriate perioperative insulin regimen must be based on prior insulin requirements, the patient's history, the timing of surgery, and frequent measurements of blood and urine glucose
>>Most insulin-dependent patients should receive some insulin on the day of surgery
>Maintain euglycemia or mild hyperglycemia during anesthesia and surgery
>>Typically the blood glucose will be 100–250 mg/dl
Treat infections early and aggressively with antibiotics
Treat fluid losses or dehydration aggressively with fluid replacement

Manifestations

The conscious patient may complain of nausea, vomiting, or abdominal pain
Hypovolemia
>Hypotension
>Postural hypotension
>Tachycardia
Metabolic acidosis, increased anion gap (see Event 39, *Metabolic Acidosis*)
Hyperventilation secondary to acidosis
Altered sensorium, coma
Polyuria or oliguria depending on the patient's underlying fluid volume status

Similar Events

Other forms of metabolic acidosis (see Event 39, *Metabolic Acidosis*)
Hyperosmolar nonketotic coma

Hypovolemia from other causes (see Event 7, *Hypotension*)
Abdominal pain from other causes
Hyperglycemia from other causes

Management

Confirm the diagnosis
> Obtain blood and urine samples for
>> ABGs
>> Serum glucose
>>> Laboratory results for glucose and ketoacids may differ from values measured by fingerstick and Dextrostix
>> Serum ketoacids
>> Serum electrolytes (including PO_4^{3-}, Mg^{2+})
>> Hematocrit
>> Creatinine and BUN
>> Urine ketoacids

Ensure adequate oxygenation and ventilation
> Intubate the trachea if the patient is obtunded or if respiratory distress is present

Expand the circulating fluid volume
> The minimum initial fluid requirement (in adults) is typically 1–2 L of crystalloid
> Additional fluid administration should be based on the patient's response
>> If the patient has CAD, CHF, or renal failure, place an arterial line and a PA catheter for monitoring and to guide fluid management

Begin insulin therapy
> Administer regular insulin IV, 10 units
> Initiate an IV infusion of regular insulin at 5–10 units/hr

Administer sodium bicarbonate <u>only</u> for profound acidosis (pH below 7.1–7.2) (see Event 39, *Metabolic Acidosis*)

Repeat measurements of serum glucose, electrolytes, and ABGs q1–2h until the values normalize
> When blood glucose reaches 250–300 mg/dl
>> Consider adding glucose to IV solutions
>> Reduce rate of insulin therapy
> Replace K^+ deficit once urine output is ensured (see Event 35, *Hypokalemia*)
>> Most patients with DKA have a large total body K^+ deficit

Replace PO_4^{3-}, Mg^{2+} as indicated by laboratory measurements
Treat underlying precipitants of DKA
Obtain a consultation from an internist or endocrinologist to assist in the patient's postoperative management

Complications

Hypotension
Hypoglycemia
Hypokalemia
Hyperkalemia
Pulmonary edema
Thrombotic events

Suggested Readings

Foster DW: Diabetes mellitus p. 1739. In Wilson JD, Braunwald E, Isselbacher KJ et al (eds): Harrison's Principles of Internal Medicine. 12th Ed. McGraw-Hill, New York , 1991

Hirsch IB, McGill JB, Cryer PE, White PF: Perioperative management of surgical patients with diabetes mellitus. Anesthesiology 74:346, 1991

Milaskiewicz RM, Hall GM: Diabetes and anaesthesia: the past decade. Br J Anaesth 68:198, 1992

33 HYPERKALEMIA

Definition

Hyperkalemia is a serum K^+ level of greater than 5.5 mEq/L.

Etiology

Excessive intake
      Excessive parenteral or oral K^+ supplement
      Massive blood transfusion
      Administration of hyperkalemic cardioplegia solution
Inadequate excretion of K^+
      Renal failure
      Adrenal insufficiency
      K^+-sparing diuretics
      Administration of ACE inhibitors (indirectly reduce the secretion of aldosterone)
Shift of K^+ from the tissues to the plasma
      Extensive tissue damage (muscle crushing injury, hemolysis, internal bleeding)
      Administration of succinylcholine
      Respiratory or metabolic acidosis
      Acute release of K^+ into the plasma from transplanted organs with a high K^+ content
      Hyperkalemic periodic paralysis
      Malignant hyperthermia

Typical Situations

Major trauma
Release of aortic cross-clamp
During IV K^+ replacement
Patients with renal failure, with or without ongoing renal dialysis
Burn victims

Prevention

Use appropriate protocols for patients at risk of hyperkalemia
      Avoid succinylcholine
      Measure serum K^+ concentration frequently
      Use continuous ECG monitoring
Administer K^+ supplements carefully, with replacement only to physiologic levels
Avoid acidosis
Preoperatively dialyze patients with renal failure who have significant hyperkalemia

Manifestations

Serum K^+ higher than 5.5 mEq/L
ECG abnormalities and arrhythmias
      Do not appear until the serum K^+ rises above 6.5–7.0 mEq/L
      Tall, peaked T waves
      Prolonged PR interval, loss of P waves, or atrial asystole
      Complete heart block
      Prolonged QRS complex
      Sine wave-type ventricular arrhythmia
      Ventricular fibrillation or asystole
If serum K^+ rises rapidly, the first detectable manifestation may be ventricular fibrillation or
    asystole
Skeletal muscle weakness

Similar Events

Sample handling error
      Poor venipuncture technique with hemolysis of sample
      In vitro hemolysis in the laboratory
Pseudohyperkalemia
      Thrombocytosis
      Leukocytosis
Transient rise following use of succinylcholine

Management

If ECG changes after induction of anesthesia suggest hyperkalemia
      Immediately hyperventilate the patient
      Administer 10% calcium gluconate IV, 10–30 ml

Whenever Hyperkalemia Is Suspected
Stop administration of any K^+-containing solutions
      IV K^+ replacement
      LR IV solution (contains 4.0 mEq/L)
Confirm diagnosis by STAT measurement of serum K^+
      Measure serum K^+ frequently in patients at risk of hyperkalemia

Moderate or severe hyperkalemia

> Check ECG for changes of hyperkalemia
> Increase the blood pH
>> Draw blood for an ABG measurement
>> Administer sodium bicarbonate IV, 50–150 mEq
>> Treat underlying metabolic acidosis, if present
> Administer dextrose 50% IV, 50 g, and regular insulin IV, 12 units
> Administer calcium gluconate 10% IV, 10–30 ml
> Force a diuresis
>> Increase fluid administration
>> Administer loop diuretics IV (e.g., furosemide, 5–20 mg)
> Obtain emergency consultation from a nephrologist or internist to institute emergency peritoneal dialysis or hemodialysis

Mild hyperkalemia (serum K⁺ less than 6.0 mEq/L)

> Administer cation exchange resins by rectal or oral routes

Complications

Complications of therapy
> Hyperosmolality
> Hypoglycemia
> Hypokalemia
> Dialysis-related problems (vascular access, heparin-related)

Complications of hyperkalemia
> Arrhythmias
> Ventricular fibrillation

Suggested Readings

Levinsky NG: Fluids and electrolytes. p. 278. In Wilson JD, Braunwald E, Isselbacher KJ et al (eds): Harrison's Principles of Internal Medicine. 12th Ed. McGraw-Hill, New York, 1991
Tetzlaff JE, O'Hara JF, Walsh MT: Potassium and anaesthesia. Can J Anaesth 40:227, 1993
Vaughan RS: Potassium in the perioperative period. Br J Anaesth 67:194, 1991

34 HYPOGLYCEMIA

Definition

A blood glucose level of less than 70 mg/dl constitutes hypoglyemia.

Etiology

Underproduction of glucose
Overutilization of glucose
Inability to utilize intracellular glucose

Typical Situations

Patients with inadequate glucose intake
      Chronic starvation
      Presurgery fasting
      Discontinuation of hyperalimentation
Patients with metabolic diseases
      Hormone deficiencies
      Enzyme deficiency in the glycogenic pathway
      Acquired liver disease
Patients taking drugs that alter glucose metabolism
      Oral hypoglycemic agents
      Alcohol
      Propranolol
      Salicylates
Patients with excessive circulating insulin
      Administration of insulin
      Insulinoma
      Newborn infants of diabetic mothers
"Dumping syndrome" following upper GI surgery

Prevention

Identify and treat patients at risk of hypoglycemia preoperatively
      Optimize the patient's metabolic status prior to surgery
      Measure serum glucose frequently
Establish a preoperative infusion of a glucose-containing solution in diabetic patients who are
    receiving insulin
      Reduce the patient's daily insulin dose the day of surgery
Do not administer oral hypoglycemic agents the morning of surgery
Continue hyperalimentation in the perioperative period or replace it with a 10% dextrose solution

Manifestations

All manifestations of hypoglycemia can be masked by general anesthesia or β blockade.

CNS manifestations
      In the awake patient
            Altered mental status
            Headache, lethargy
            Seizures
      In the anesthetized patient
            Failure to awaken from general anesthesia
            Seizures
Sympathetic nervous system stimulation
      Hypertension

Sweating
Tachycardia
Cardiovascular collapse is a late sign of hypoglycemia

Similar Events

Light anesthesia
Hypoxemia
TURP syndrome (see Event 36, *Hyponatremia and Hypo-osmolality*)
Seizures from other causes (see Event 47, *Seizures*)
Failure to awaken from general anesthesia due to other causes (see Event 45, *Postoperative Alteration in Mental Status*)

Management

Confirm the diagnosis
> Obtain blood for STAT glucose analysis

Treat suspected or known hypoglycemia
> Therapy for hypoglycemia carries little risk, whereas failure to treat hypoglycemia may be catastrophic
> Administer dextrose 50% IV, 1 ml/kg bolus, while waiting for clinical laboratory results
> Start a dextrose 5% IV infusion at 1–2 ml/kg/hr

Stop or reduce administration of insulin or other drugs that lower blood glucose levels
Monitor serum glucose frequently

Correct underlying metabolic problems
If there is no response to 50% dextrose IV, consider other etiologies for CNS manifestations

Complications

CNS injury
Cardiac arrest
Hyperglycemia and hyperosmolality from excessive glucose administration

Suggested Readings

Foster DW, Rubenstein AH: Hypoglycemia. p. 1759. In Wilson JD, Braunwald E, Isselbacher KJ et al (eds): Harrison's Principles of Internal Medicine. 12th Ed. McGraw-Hill, New York , 1991
Roizen MF: Anesthetic implications of concurrent diseases. p. 793. In Miller RD (ed): Anesthesia. 3rd Ed. Churchill Livingstone, New York, 1990
Strunin L: How long should patients fast before surgery? Time for new guidelines. Br J Anaesth 70:1, 1993
Tonneson AS: Crystalloids and colloids. p. 1439. In Miller RD (ed): Anesthesia. 3rd Ed. Churchill Livingstone, New York, 1990

35 HYPOKALEMIA

Definition

A plasma K^+ concentration of less than 3.0 mEq/L constitutes hypokalemia.

Etiology

GI deficiency or loss
    Deficient dietary intake
    Nasogastric suction
    GI loss due to diarrhea or vomiting
Renal loss
    Diuretic therapy
    Excess mineralocorticoid or glucocorticoid effect
    Renal tubular diseases
    Mg^{2+} depletion
Cellular shifts
    Metabolic or respiratory alkalosis
    Insulin effect
    Hypokalemic periodic paralysis
    Hyperaldosteronism
    β_2-Adrenergic agonists and α-adrenergic antagonists enhance K^+ entry into the cell

Typical Situations

Acute hypokalemia presents the greater hazard to the patient's safety; chronic hypokalemia is less significant.

Patients with diarrhea, vomiting, or preparation for large bowel surgery
Patients receiving diuretics, particularly loop diuretics
Following cardiac surgery
After treatment of hyperkalemia
Hyperventilation

Prevention

Replacement of K^+ for patients receiving K^+-wasting diuretics
IV replacement of fluids and electrolytes during cathartic preparation for bowel surgery
Monitor serum K^+ and replace as necessary during and after CPB
Avoid conditions that reduce serum K^+ acutely
    Hyperventilation
    Metabolic alkalosis
    β_2-Adrenergic stimulation

Manifestations

Serum potassium less than 3.0 mEq/L

Cardiac
    ECG abnormalities
        Do not usually occur until serum K^+ is less than 3.5 mEq/L
        T-wave flattening or inversion
        Increased U-wave amplitude
        ST segment depression
        Tachycardia, PVCs
        Digitalis toxicity may worsen significantly if combined with hypokalemia
    AV arrhythmias
    Cardiac conduction defects
    Cardiac arrest
Neuromuscular
    Increased sensitivity to neuromuscular blocking drugs
    Skeletal muscle weakness causing
        Respiratory failure
        Paralysis
    Decreased activity of the GI system, with paralytic ileus
Renal
    Polyuria
    Metabolic alkalosis
Endocrine
    Hyperglycemia

Similar Events

Laboratory error
Myocardial arrhythmias from other causes
Inadequate reversal of nondepolarizing muscle relaxants
Other causes of ST-T wave abnormalities (see Event 10, *ST Segment Changes*)

Management

If serum K^+ is higher than 2.6 mEq/L, there are no ECG changes, and the patient is not receiving digitalis acute K^+ replacement is not necessary and elective surgery can proceed.

Postpone elective surgery and use oral K^+ replacement if
    Serum K^+ is less than 2.6 mEq/L
    Hypokalemia is acute
    Arrhythmias are present
    Patient has other complicating signs or symptoms
    Patient is taking digoxin
For urgent or emergent surgery, if serum K^+ is less than 2.6 mEq/L or if the patient is symptomatic
    Replace K^+ by the IV route to achieve a serum K^+ of at least 3.5 mEq/L before induction of anesthesia
        Administer through a CVP line if possible
        Infuse no faster than 1 mEq/min, except for treatment of life-threatening ventricular arrhythmias in a patient known to be hypokalemic
        Monitor the ECG during the infusion (see Event 33, *Hyperkalemia*)

Watch out for "runaway" IV
Prevent K^+ from accumulating in the IV tubing or blood-warming devices
Measure serum K^+ hourly during rapid administration of K^+

In the hypokalemic patient
Be sure that muscle relaxants are fully reversed and that the patient has recovered appropriate neuromuscular function before the trachea is extubated
Measure ABGs if neuromuscular function is slow to recover following surgery

Complications

Difficulty reversing nondepolarizing muscle relaxants
Hyperkalemia, myocardial arrhythmias, or cardiac arrest from excessive rate of K^+ replacement
Pain or thrombophlebitis at IV site from use of noncentral line for K^+ replacement

Suggested Readings

Hirsch IA, Tomlinson DL, Slogoff S et al: The overstated risk of preoperative hypokalemia. Anesth Analg 67:131, 1988
Levinsky NG: Fluids and electrolytes. p. 278. In Wilson JD, Braunwald E, Isselbacher KJ et al (eds): Harrison's Principles of Internal Medicine. 12th Ed. McGraw-Hill, New York , 1991
Vaughan RS: Potassium in the perioperative period. Br J Anaesth 67:194, 1991
Vitez TS, Soper LE, Wong KC, Soper P: Chronic hypokalemia and intraoperative dysrhythmias. Anesthesiology 63:130, 1985

36 HYPONATREMIA AND HYPO-OSMOLALITY

Definition

Hyponatremia/hypo-osmolity is defined as abnormally low serum Na^+ (less than 130 mEq/L) and/or abnormally low serum osmolality (less than 270 mOsm/L).

Etiology

Hemodilution
Decreased renal free water clearance
Pseudohyponatremia (low serum Na^+ with normal or elevated osmolality)

Typical Situations

Cystoscopic surgery
Absorption of hypotonic irrigation fluid into the prostatic venous channels
Hyperglycinemia secondary to the use of glycine-containing irrigation fluid

This is usually pseudohyponatremia since the serum osmolality may be near normal
Infusion of hypotonic IV fluids, especially D_5W
Impaired mechanisms of renal free water excretion
 Chronic renal failure
 Administration of drugs
  Oxytocin
  NSAIDs
  Thiazide diuretics
 Decreased renal blood flow associated with major surgery
 SIADH
Psychogenic polydipsia
Patients with metabolic abnormalities causing pseudohyponatremia
 Hyperglycemia
 Hyperproteinemia
 Hyperlipidemia

Prevention

During TURP surgery
 Avoid sterile water as the irrigation agent
 Minimize resection time
 Achieve adequate hemostasis of venous sinuses
 Avoid high irrigation pressures
Avoid fluid replacement with hypotonic solutions
Check electrolyte levels frequently for patients who
 Have chronic renal failure
 Are undergoing major surgery
 Are receiving drugs that can cause hyponatremia
 Have metabolic abnormalities

Manifestations

Osmotically induced cerebral edema associated with rapid decreases in serum Na^+ concentration
 In the awake patient
  Restlessness, disorientation
  Visual disturbances
  Nausea, vomiting
  Altered mental status
 In any patient
  Preseizure irritability
  Seizures
Symptoms of circulating fluid volume overload
 Tachycardia or bradycardia
 Hypertension
 Increased CVP
 Decreased O_2 saturation
 Dyspnea

Pulmonary or laryngeal edema
Intravascular hemolysis

Similar Events

Anxiety during regional anesthesia
Hypoxemia from other causes (see Event 8, *Hypoxemia*)
Altered mental status due to
> Sedative drugs
> Organic brain syndrome
Myocardial ischemia, infarction

Management

These management guidelines are oriented to the common situation of hyponatremia occurring during TURP surgery.

Inform the surgeon of the problem
> Suggest replacing sterile water irrigation fluid with the glycine-containing irrigation solution, which has a nearly normal osmolality
> Advise the surgeon to discontinue prostatic resection, achieve hemostasis, and terminate the procedure as soon as possible

Ensure adequate oxygenation and ventilation
> Administer supplemental O_2 as necessary
> If pulmonary or laryngeal edema develops, call for help
>> Laryngeal edema can make airway management and intubation extremely difficult

Send blood to the clinical laboratory for STAT serum Na^+ <u>and</u> serum osmolality
> If serum Na^+ is low but osmolality is normal or near normal, pseudohyponatremia is present
>> Glycine may be an unmeasured osmolar compound
>> Hyperglycinemia may cause symptoms similar to those of true hyponatremia

Reduce the pressure of fluids irrigating the bladder

If there are signs of circulating fluid volume overload
> Slow IV fluid administration or blood transfusion to a minimum
> Administer furosemide IV, 5–20 mg bolus

Treat hyponatremia if the patient is symptomatic or if there is true hyponatremia with a serum Na^+ less than 120 mEq/L
> Administer furosemide IV, 5–20 mg bolus, if the patient is not hypotensive
> Switch IV fluids to NS for slow restoration of normal Na^+ concentration
> Do not use hypertonic saline unless the patient is markedly symptomatic or has very low Na^+ **and** low osmolality
>> Hypertonic saline may produce significant hypervolemia and neurologic injury

Monitor CVP or PCWP if clinically indicated
> If pulmonary edema is present
> If the patient has a history of CAD or CHF
> If there are ST-T wave changes on the ECG

Complications

Hyperosmolality secondary to use of hypertonic saline

37
E
V
E
N
T

Cerebral edema

Central pontine myelinolysis or diffuse cerebral demyelination secondary to too rapid restoration of serum Na$^+$

Suggested Readings

Mazze RI: Anesthesia and the renal and genitourinary systems. p. 1791. In Miller RD (ed): Anesthesia. 3rd Ed. Churchill Livingstone, New York, 1990

Rose BD: Hypoosmolal states—hyponatremia. p. 601. In Clinical Physiology of Acid-Base and Electrolyte Disorders. 3rd Ed. McGraw-Hill, New York, 1989

Swales JD: Management of hyponatremia. Br J Anaesth 67:146, 1991

37 HYPOTHERMIA

Definition

Hypothermia is defined as a core body temperature below 35°C during the perioperative period.

Etiology

Pre-existing hypothermia
Depression of metabolic heat production by anesthesia
Increased heat loss to the environment
    Radiation
    Conduction
    Convection

Typical Situations

Cool operating room
Significant portions of the patient's body exposed to the air
Use of cold or room temperature fluids
    Skin preparation solutions
    Irrigation fluids
    IV fluids or blood
Ventilation of the lungs with cool, dry gas through an ETT
When the abdominal or thoracic cavity is open
    Large amount of evaporative losses (a special case of conduction)
During pediatric surgery (high ratio of body surface area to weight)
Direct contact between the patient and the operating table
Long cases
Trauma cases
Following exposure to the elements or near drowning

Prevention

Increase operating room temperature to at least 21°C
Provide a local warm environment for the patient by use of a forced-air warming device
Cover exposed areas of the patient whenever possible
> Particularly the head, which is 18% of body surface area

Warm all IV fluids, blood products, and irrigation fluids
Use passive or active breathing circuit humidification
Minimize exposure of viscera to the air
Use reflective blankets to minimize both convective and radiative losses
Use warming lights for infants and neonates during preparation for anesthesia and surgery

Manifestations

Body temperature is lower than normal
Shivering in the unparalyzed or awake patient
Cutaneous vasoconstriction, piloerection
Decreased level of consciousness, reduced anesthetic requirement
If hypothermia is severe (body temperature less than 30°C)
> Decreased myocardial contractility
> Increased ventricular irritability
> Ventricular fibrillation (usually at 25–30°C)
> Increased blood viscosity
> Abnormal blood coagulation

Similar Events

Temperature measurement artifact
Local abnormalities in temperature reading
> Esophagus cooled by topical pericardial cooling during CPB

Management

If hypothermia is severe (below 30°C), especially after near drowning
> Consider CPB for rewarming
> Monitor for and treat myocardial irritability and arrhythmias
> Otherwise apply treatment as for major hypothermia (below)

For major intraoperative hypothermia (below 35°C)
> Maintain neuromuscular blockade
> Maintain normocarbia by adjusting mechanical ventilation
> Warm the patient using
>> Radiant heaters
>> Heated and humidified inspired gases
>> Warm IV fluids
>> Forced-air warming system
>> Increased temperature of the operating room or ICU room
>> Warming blanket

Complications

Severe shivering
        Shivering can increase O_2 consumption by up to 800%
        Cardiac output must increase to meet tissue demands
        Myocardial ischemia
        Arrhythmias
Hypotension from rapid vasodilation during rewarming
Slow metabolism of drugs
Slow awakening from anesthesia

Suggested Readings

Lennon RL, Hosking MP, Conover MA, Perkins WJ: Evaluation of a forced-air system for warming hypothermic postoperative patients. Anesth Analg 70:424, 1990
Sessler DI: Temperature monitoring. p. 1227. In Miller RD (ed): Anesthesia. 3rd Ed. Churchill Livingstone, New York, 1990
Sessler DI, Rubinstein EH, Maoyeri A: Physiologic responses to mid perianesthetic hypothermia in humans. Anesthesiology 75:594, 1991
Sladen, RN: Temperature regulation in the operating room. p. 146. In: Review Course Lectures. International Anesthesia Research Society, Cleveland, 1993
Zoll RH: Temperature monitoring. p. 264. In Ehrenwerth J, Eisenkraft JB (eds): Anesthesia Equipment. Mosby-Year Book, St Louis, 1993

38 MALIGNANT HYPERTHERMIA

Definition

Malignant hyperthermia is a lethal disorder of skeletal muscle metabolism triggered by volatile anesthetics or muscle relaxants.

Etiology

MH is an inherited disorder (autosomal dominant with partial penetrance)
Certain drugs can trigger MH in susceptible patients
        Succinylcholine
        Volatile anesthetic agents
Exercise or stress alone can trigger MH in susceptible individuals

Typical Situations

In patient with a history (or a family history) of a prior episode of MH
In patient with masseter spasm on administration of succinylcholine (see Event 81, *Masseter Muscle Spasm*)

More common in pediatric patients

In association with certain congenital abnormalities (strabismus, musculoskeletal deformities, central core disease)

Prevention

Obtain an anesthetic history for the patient and the patient's family

Avoid administering triggering agents

Use an appropriate anesthetic protocol for known susceptible individuals or if the history is suggestive of MH susceptibility

Manifestations

Manifestations may occur in the operating room, in the PACU, or after discharge from the PACU.

Unexplained tachycardia, cardiovascular instability, and arrhythmias

Increased CO_2 production resulting in

Increased arterial pCO_2 and end-tidal CO_2

Tachypnea in spontaneously ventilating patient, overbreathing of ventilator in nonparalyzed patient receiving mechanical ventilation

Rapid exhaustion of CO_2 absorbent, increased heat production in soda lime container

Muscle rigidity (see Event 81, *Masseter Muscle Spasm*)

Hyperthermia

A late manifestation

Core temperature may increase by up to 1°C q5min, and reach a value as high as 45°C

Cyanosis, reduced O_2 saturation

Abnormal laboratory values

Metabolic acidosis (lactic acid)

Hyperkalemia

Markedly elevated blood CK

Myoglobinuria secondary to rhabdomyolysis

Sweating

Similar Events

Monitor artifact (temperature, end-tidal CO_2)

Light anesthesia

Fever secondary to

Infection

Hyperthyroidism

Pheochromocytoma

Infected IV fluids or blood products

Inadvertent overheating of the patient by warming devices

Injury to the hypothalamic thermoregulatory center

Drug reactions causing tachycardia or hyperthermia (neuroleptic malignant syndrome, MAO inhibitors, cocaine, atropine, scopolamine)

Elevated end-tidal CO_2 for other reasons (see Event 27, *Hypercarbia*)

Management

If MH Is Suspected
Confirm the diagnosis of MH
> Check the ECG (heart rate, arrhythmias)
> Check O_2 saturation
> Check end-tidal CO_2 and its response to hyperventilation
> Check temperature, place a temperature probe if necessary, feel temperature of skin and CO_2 absorber
> Draw an ABG sample to look for combined respiratory and metabolic acidosis
> **If uncertain of diagnosis, err on the side of caution by treating MH**

If the Diagnosis of MH Is Made
Declare an MH emergency
> Notify the surgeons and nurses, terminate the surgical procedure as soon as feasible
> Call for help
> Call for the MH kit

Turn off volatile anesthetic agents and N_2O, administer 100% O_2
> Use an O_2 tank and self-inflating bag to ventilate the patient
> If there is no self-inflating bag, use very high flow O_2 and ventilate using the reservoir bag and a new anesthesia breathing circuit
> Assign one person to hyperventilate the patient

Assign one or more individuals to mix dantrolene. Dantrolene is lifesaving and takes precedence over other supportive measures
> Dantrolene comes as a lyophilized powder; each vial contains 20 mg dantrolene and 3 g mannitol
> Each vial must be reconstituted with **60 ml sterile water**
> Multiple vials will be needed for an older child or an adult

Administer dantrolene IV, 2.5 mg/kg
> Administer further doses of dantrolene as necessary, titrated to the heart rate, muscle rigidity, and temperature, to a maximum of 10 mg/kg

Initiate cooling if temperature is elevated
> Place core temperature probes (esophageal, nasal, bladder)
> Surface cooling with ice and or water
> Administer cold IV solutions
> Gastric or rectal lavage with cold solution
> Consider cold peritoneal lavage or cooling via CPB
> STOP COOLING WHEN CORE TEMPERATURE REACHES 38°C

Administer HCO_3^- 1–2 mEq/kg initially, then as indicated by ABG data
Correct hyperkalemia (see Event 33, *Hyperkalemia*)
> Fluid infusion
> Furosemide IV, 5–20 mg
> IV glucose and insulin

Treat myocardial arrhythmias
> Correcting metabolic abnormalities will usually correct the arrhythmias
> Procainamide IV, 3 mg/kg, to maximum 15 mg/kg is the agent of choice
> Lidocaine IV, 1–1.5 mg/kg, is safe to use

Place a urinary catheter

If there is decreased urine output or if there is evidence of myoglobinuria, force a diuresis

Mannitol IV, 0.5–1 g/kg (including the 3 g mannitol per vial of dantrolene)

Furosemide IV, 5–20 mg

Increase IV fluid infusion rate

Send blood samples to clinical laboratory for

CK

Serum K^+

PT, PTT, platelet count

Measure mixed venous blood gases if CVP catheter is in place

MH will be associated with

Marked venous desaturation (normal mixed venous O_2, 70–80%)

Elevated mixed venous pCO_2 (normal 46 mm Hg)

If uncertain at any time of how to proceed

Consult the MH Hotline (209-634-4917), ask for "Index Zero"

Transfer patient to ICU when stable

Watch carefully for signs of recurrent MH

Repeat dantrolene, 4 mg/kg/day, in divided doses for 48 hours, discontinue if no recurrence of symptoms

Convert to oral dantrolene when patient is extubated and stable

Refer patient for a medical history bracelet and counseling (in the United States contact the Malignant Hyperthermia Association of the United States at 203-655-3007)

Complications

Hypothermia from excessive cooling

Side effects of dantrolene therapy

Muscle weakness

Double vision

Dizziness

Nausea

Diarrhea

DIC

Renal failure from myoglobinuria

Interactions between dantrolene and other drugs (especially calcium channel blockers, which may produce hypotension and hyperkalemia when given concurrently)

Suggested Readings

Gronert GA, Schulman SR, Mott J: Malignant hyperthermia. p. 935. In Miller RD (ed): Anesthesia. 3rd Ed. Churchill Livingstone, New York, 1990

Kaplan RF: Malignant hyperthermia. p. 226. In: Annual Refresher Course Lectures, American Society of Anesthesiologists, Park Ridge, IL, 1992

39 METABOLIC ACIDOSIS

Definition

Metabolic acidosis is defined by abnormally high levels of circulating acid in the blood, producing a blood pH of less than 7.35 and an HCO_3^- concentration of less than 21 mEq/L.

Etiology

Elevated blood levels of metabolic acids (<u>increased</u> anion gap)
     Anion gap = $[Na^+] - ([Cl^-] + [HCO_3^-])$
     Normal range 9–13
Abnormally low blood levels of bicarbonate (<u>normal</u> anion gap)

Typical Situations

Inadequate perfusion of peripheral tissues resulting in lactic acidosis
     Increased lactic acid production by ischemic or hypoxic tissues accompanied by decreased hepatic utilization of lactic acid
     Shock or profound hypotension (see Event 7, *Hypotension*)
          Hypovolemic
          Cardiogenic
          Septic
     Severe hypoxemia (see Event 8, *Hypoxemia*)
     Cardiac arrest (see Event 2, *Cardiac Arrest*)
     Release of arterial tourniquet or cross-clamp (transient acidosis)
Increased production of metabolic acids
     Diabetic ketoacidosis (see Event 32, *Diabetic Ketoacidosis*)
     Ingestion of
          Aspirin (produces organic acids)
          Methanol or ethylene glycol (produce formic acid and glycolic acid/oxalic acid, respectively)
          Cyanide from IV administration or ingestion of sodium nitroprusside (produces lactic acid)
     Chronic renal failure (accumulation of urea and other by-products of protein metabolism)
     MH (see Event 38, *Malignant Hyperthermia*)
Loss of circulating HCO_3^-
     Diarrhea
     Pancreatic fistula
     Renal tubular acidosis
     Early stages of acute renal failure
Large-volume fluid resuscitation with NS
     Hyperchloremia, low blood level of HCO_3^-

Prevention

Maintain cardiac output and tissue perfusion
Maintain urine output
Avoid excessive use of NS for fluid resuscitation
Monitor electrolyte levels frequently during cases requiring large volumes of IV fluid

Manifestations

Hyperventilation
> In spontaneously ventilating patient
> Overbreathing of ventilator in nonparalyzed ventilated patient

Decreased pH on ABG determination
Arrhythmias
Decreased myocardial contractility and cardiac output
Vasodilation and hypotension
Decreased cardiovascular response to endogenous and exogenous catecholamines

Similar Events

Hyperventilation due to other causes
Laboratory artifact
Respiratory acidosis (see Event 27, *Hypercarbia*)

Management

Confirm acidosis
> Obtain an ABG analysis

Ensure adequate oxygenation and ventilation
> Hyperventilate to an arterial pCO_2 of 28–30 mm Hg to compensate for metabolic acidosis
> > PCO_2 less than 25 mm Hg will produce marked cerebral vasoconstriction
> Increase FiO_2 to 100% if acidosis is severe

Administer $NaHCO_3$ only to patients who have severe metabolic acidosis not associated with tissue hypoxia (pH less than 7.1–7.2)
> Administer HCO_3^- only as needed to maintain the pH above 7.1–7.2
> Administration of large amounts of HCO_3^- during cardiac arrest can result in severe hypernatremia, hyperosmolality, increased lactic acidosis, and decreased survival
> Administration of HCO_3^- does not increase the pH of the blood when CO_2 excretion is impaired

Ensure adequate cardiac output, perfusion pressure, and tissue O_2 delivery
> Expand the circulating fluid volume
> > Consider placing a PA catheter to guide fluid management and to measure the cardiac output
> Administer vasopressors as necessary to maintain an adequate blood pressure (see Event 7, *Hypotension*)
> Optimize O_2 transport
> > Treat anemia

Maximize arterial pO_2
Consider monitoring mixed venous O_2 saturation

Establish the cause of the acidosis
    Review the clinical course and management to date
    Check serum electrolyte levels
        Calculate the anion gap
        Monitor K^+ carefully
    Send blood to clinical laboratory to measure blood levels of lactic acid and/or ketoacids
    Send blood or urine for a toxicology screen
        Institute appropriate therapy for toxic ingestion
    If the patient has received sodium nitroprusside and there is no other cause for metabolic
        acidosis, treat for possible cyanide toxicity
        Send blood to laboratory to measure blood levels of cyanide
        Administer sodium nitrite IV, 4–6 mg/kg, over 3 minutes, followed by sodium
           thiosulfate IV, 150–200 mg/kg, over 10 minutes

Complications

Cardiac arrest
Tetany due to too rapid alkalization of blood
Hypernatremia, hypertension, fluid overload due to fluid resuscitation

Suggested Readings

Arieff AI: Indications for use of bicarbonate in patients with metabolic acidosis. Br J Anaesth 67:165, 1991

Hindman BJ: Sodium bicarbonate in the treatment of sub-types of acute lactic acidosis: physiologic considerations. Anesthesiology 72:1064, 1990

Levinsky NG: Acidosis and alkalosis. p. 289. In Wilson JD, Braunwald E, Isselbacher KJ et al (eds): Harrison's Principles of Internal Medicine. 12th Ed. McGraw-Hill, New York , 1991

40 OLIGURIA

Definition

Oliguria is defined as urine production at a rate below 0.5 ml/kg/hr.

Etiology

Decreased renal perfusion
Increased secretion of vasopressin
Primary renal failure
Obstruction or diversion of urine outflow

Typical Situations

During surgical procedures involving large amounts of blood loss or fluid shifts
>   Inadequate fluid replacement

When vasopressin production is stimulated by anesthesia or surgery
>   Surgical stress
>   Administration of narcotics or other drugs
>   Positive pressure ventilation or application of PEEP

When aortic or renal artery flow is impaired by
>   Cross-clamping of the aorta (above <u>or</u> below the renal arteries)
>   Renal artery stenosis

Patients with CHF or myocardial dysfunction
Patients with renal failure
Surgery on or near the bladder or ureters
Patients who have undergone preparation for surgery on the large bowel
Patients presenting with trauma or shock

Prevention

Identify patients with diseases that make them at high risk of oliguria
>   Postpone elective surgery until the underlying diseases can be treated appropriately
>   Monitor urine output and the cardiovascular system more carefully if surgery is necessary

Maintain normal circulating fluid volume and cardiac output during anesthesia and surgery
>   Insensible losses and fluid shifts to the "third space" are often underestimated

Manifestations

Urine output below 0.5 ml/kg/min
Empty bladder (if visible or palpable)

Similar Events

Failure to drain urine from the bladder
>   Obstructed urinary catheter or collecting tubing
>   Urine pooling at dome of bladder (e.g., Trendelenburg position)
>   Disconnection of some part of the urine collecting system from the urinary catheter to the urimeter

Obstruction or laceration of one or both ureters

Management

If urine output stops <u>acutely</u>
>   Look for acute surgical events such as the placement of an aortic cross-clamp or pressure on the bladder or ureters from surgical retraction
>   Rule out a mechanical obstruction to urine drainage
>>   Ensure that the urinary catheter is still in place
>>>   If the urinary catheter has a temperature probe and its indicated temperature is significantly lower than temperatures measured at other sites, the urinary catheter may be outside of the patient

Track the course of the urine collecting system from the patient to the urimeter
Check for a kink or a disconnection of the tubing
Irrigate the urinary catheter
Ask the surgeon to feel the fullness of the bladder and to check for ureteric obstruction if these are in the surgical field
Evaluate the patient for evidence of hypovolemia or decreased cardiac output
Check for
Hypotension or tachycardia
Low CVP or PA pressure
Review blood loss and fluid administration
Consider covert blood loss, insensible losses, and shifts of fluid to the third space
Consider expanding the circulating fluid volume as a therapeutic trial
Administer crystalloid (NS or LR) in 250–500 ml increments
Administer colloid (hetastarch or 5% albumin) in 100–250 ml increments
If a PA catheter is present, expand fluid volume to achieve a PCWP of 15–20 mm Hg
Check hemoglobin and hematocrit; transfuse PRBCs if there is significant anemia
In cases in which risk factors for acute renal failure are present
Review the patient's history to evaluate for acute precipitants of renal failure
Shock or hypotension
Crush syndrome (myoglobinuria)
Transfusion reaction (hemoglobinuria)
Place a PA catheter to ensure that circulating fluid volume and cardiac output are appropriate (see above)
If cardiac output is low after fluid volume is optimized, administer inotropic support
Dopamine, 3–10 µg/kg/min
Dobutamine, 3–10 µg/kg/min
Epinephrine, 3–100 ng/kg/min
If cardiac output is normal or elevated
Consider low-dose dopamine, 2–3 µg/kg/min
After optimizing cardiac output consider diuretic therapy to increase urine output
Furosemide IV, 5–10 mg bolus; 10–50 mg if the patient is already receiving diuretic therapy
Mannitol IV, 25 g bolus

If the case is otherwise routine, the patient is previously healthy, and there have been no episodes of hypotension, sepsis, or other predisposing factors of acute renal failure
Ensure the integrity of the urinary collecting system and the absence of hypovolemia
Consider observing the urine output over a longer period of time
Consider administering furosemide IV, 5–10 mg bolus
If oliguria persists, obtain laboratory data
Send urine sample for measurement of specific gravity (if urine output and specific gravity are both low, this may be due to the kidney's inability to concentrate and excrete electrolytes)
Send samples of urine and plasma for concurrent measurement of osmolality and calculate the urine/plasma osmolality ratio
Less than 1:1 suggests intrinsic renal failure
1:1–2:1 suggests prerenal cause

More than 2:1 suggests physiologic cause
Progressive rises in BUN and creatinine are indicative of acute renal failure

Until acute renal failure has been ruled out
- Restrict K^+ intake unless the patient is symptomatic from hypokalemia
- Use caution in administering drugs that are nephrotoxic or that depend on renal excretion
  - Pancuronium, gallamine
  - Aminoglycoside antibiotics
  - Iodinated radiocontrast agents

Complications

Pulmonary edema from overhydration
Excessive reduction in preload from diuretic therapy
Acute renal failure

Suggested Readings

Conroy PT: Should one treat decreased urine output intraoperatively? Probl Anesth 1:214, 1987
Sweny P: Is postoperative oliguria avoidable? Br J Anaesth 67:137, 1991
Zaloga GP, Hughes SS: Oliguria in patients with normal renal function. Anesthesiology 72:598, 1990

---

41 TRANSFUSION REACTION

Definition

A transfusion reaction is an immunologic reaction directed against red or white blood cells, platelets, or at least one of the immunoglobulins that have been transfused into a patient.

Etiology

Incompatibility between donor and recipient ABO and Rh systems
Incompatibility between donor and recipient minor antibody systems
Allergic reaction to transfused neutrophils, platelets, or other blood component

Typical Situations

When blood products are transfused
- Physician or clerical error in transfusing the correct unit of blood product to the patient
- In emergency situations requiring rapid transfusion of multiple blood products
  - There may be time for a group-specific cross-match only
  - In more urgent situations, un-cross-matched type-specific or O-negative blood may be transfused
  - Human errors are more likely under time pressure

Patients who have previously been exposed to ABO or other antigens

Prevention

Avoid transfusion of blood products when possible by using blood conservation techniques
> Autologous blood donation prior to surgery
>> Use of an intraoperative blood salvage device during surgery where substantial loss of uncontaminated blood is likely
>> Isovolemic withdrawal of blood from the patient at the beginning of surgery for later transfusion back to the patient

Ensure positive identification of the patient and appropriate labeling of the patient's serum sample before sending it to the blood bank for cross-matching

Request blood to be cross-matched in advance of surgery when there is a significant likelihood of a blood transfusion being required
> This allows time for a full cross-match to be performed

Use an appropriate protocol for commencing the transfusion of blood products
> More than one individual should check the patient's name and identification number and the identification number of the blood product against the cross-match report from the blood bank

Monitor the patient for signs of a transfusion reaction when starting a transfusion

Manifestations

The onset of a major ABO transfusion reaction is usually rapid and frequently severe. In patients who have received transfusion products in the past, reactions due to re-exposure to a minor antigen are frequently mild and may be delayed.

In the awake patient, the signs and symptoms may include
> Restlessness or anxiety
> Chest, flank, or lumbar pain
> Tachypnea, tightness of the chest
> Flushing and fever
> Development of a rash or hives

Signs may be concealed during anesthesia but may include
> Hypotension
> Tachycardia
> Bronchospasm
> Hemoglobinuria
> Bleeding from mucous membranes or the operative site secondary to the development of DIC
> Hives or edema of the mucous membranes, which may be apparent after removing the surgical drapes from the patient

Similar Events

Allergic reaction or anaphylaxis (see Event 11, *Anaphylaxis and Anaphylactoid Reactions*)
Bronchospasm from other causes (see Event 24, *Bronchospasm)*
Transfusion of blood or IV fluids contaminated with bacteria
Septic shock secondary to infection with gram-negative organisms
Coagulopathy or other causes of DIC
ARDS
Pulmonary edema secondary to overtransfusion

Management

Stop transfusion of blood products immediately if a transfusion reaction is suspected
>Double check the identity of the recipient and the blood product against the cross-match report from the blood bank
>Save any blood product containers for further compatibility testing

Notify the surgeon that a transfusion reaction may be occurring
>Call for help if symptoms are severe
>>Management of complications may require more than one person
>It may be necessary to abort the surgical procedure

Support the blood pressure with fluids and with vasopressors as needed (see Event 11, *Anaphylaxis and Anaphylactoid Reactions* and Event 7, *Hypotension*)

Treat bronchospasm (see Event 24, *Bronchospasm*)

Administer corticosteroids for severe reactions
>Methylprednisolone IV, 1 mg/kg

If oliguria or frank hemoglobinuria develops (see Event 40, *Oliguria*)
>Insert a urinary catheter if one is not already in place
>Administer 25% mannitol IV, 0.5 g/kg
>Administer low-dose dopamine infusion, 2–3 µg/kg/min, to promote diuresis
>Administer furosemide IV, 5–20 mg

Treat DIC as necessary. Obtain
>Platelet count
>PT/PTT
>Fibrinogen
>Fibrin split products

Avoid further transfusion unless absolutely necessary

Obtain samples of blood and urine and send to the laboratory to establish the diagnosis of a major transfusion reaction
>Demonstration of intravascular hemolysis of RBCs
>>Free hemoglobin in the plasma or urine

Repeat determination of donor and recipient blood types (on pretransfusion specimen if possible)

Coombs' test may assist in diagnosis of delayed antibody-mediated hemolytic reactions but will not help in the acute phase

Complications

The risk of a fatal hemolytic reaction is less than 1:100,000 units of blood product
DIC
Hypotension
Acute renal failure
Cardiac arrest

Suggested Readings

Giblett ER: Blood groups and blood transfusion. p. 1494. In Wilson JD, Braunwald E, Isselbacher KJ et al (eds): Harrison's Principles of Internal Medicine. 12th Ed. McGraw-Hill, New York , 1991
Miller RD: Transfusion therapy. p. 1467. In: Anesthesia. 3rd Ed. Churchill Livingstone, New York, 1990

Chapter Seven
Neurologic Events

42 CENTRAL NERVOUS SYSTEM INJURY

Definition

Any new neurologic deficit presenting after anesthesia that can be localized anatomically to the CNS (brain or spinal cord) is classified here as a CNS injury.

Etiology

Cerebral ischemia
  Global
  Focal
Cerebral hemorrhage
Cerebral embolism
Increased ICP
Direct traumatic or surgical injury to CNS tissue
Injection of neurolytic solutions into the CSF or into CNS tissue
Epidural hematoma

Typical Situations

In patients with pre-existing disease predisposing to cerebral ischemia or embolism
  Atrial fibrillation
  Endocardial mural thrombus following a myocardial infarction
  Known cerebrovascular occlusive disease
    Previous stroke or TIAs
    Hypertension
  Pregnancy-induced hypertension
Following surgery that carries a high risk of CNS injury
  Carotid endarterectomy
  Procedures requiring CPB
  Craniotomy or procedures on or near the spinal cord
Following an intraoperative catastrophe involving profound hypotension or cardiac or respiratory arrest
In patients with raised ICP
When the patient is positioned so that there is traction on the spinal cord or compromise of blood flow to the spinal cord
Procedures in the sitting position
In patients with anatomic abnormalities of the bony covering of the CNS
  Congenital (Down syndrome, Klippel-Feil syndrome)

Acquired (rheumatoid arthritis with cervical instability)

Spinal stenosis

Following epidural anesthesia or continuous spinal anesthesia with a small-bore intrathecal catheter

Prevention

Identify patients with conditions that predispose to CNS injury

Treat patients with correctable disease states

Monitor patients at risk with advanced intraoperative monitoring

EEG

Evoked potentials

TEE

Position the patient carefully

Avoid extreme rotation and flexion of the cervical spine

When the patient is in the sitting position, support the patient's body adequately so that there is no traction on the spinal cord or cervical spine

Maintain an adequate cerebral perfusion pressure

Measure blood pressure at the level of the brain if the patient's head is elevated

Treat patients appropriately who are known to have raised ICP

Avoid obstruction to cerebral venous outflow

Maintain the head in an elevated position

Ventilate the patient so that the arterial pCO_2 is 25–35 mm Hg

Avoid neuraxial regional anesthesia in patients with a coagulopathy

Avoid small-bore catheters for continuous spinal anesthesia (microbore spinal catheters are no longer approved for use by the U.S. Food and Drug Administration)

Manifestations

Cerebral injuries may be manifested by

Delayed recovery from anesthesia (see Event 45, *Postoperative Alteration in Mental Status*)

A new focal motor or sensory deficit

If a subarachnoid hemorrhage has occurred, by a conscious patient complaining of headache, stiff neck, or neurologic deficit

SCI may be manifested by

Motor or sensory deficits in a dermatomal distribution corresponding to the level of injury

Failure of the level of a spinal or epidural block to recede

Cauda equina syndrome

Loss of bowel and/or bladder function

Similar Events

Inadequate reversal of neuromuscular blockade (see Event 46, *Postoperative Failure to Breathe*)

Slow resolution of spinal or epidural blockade

Delayed recovery from general anesthesia (see Event 45, *Postoperative Alteration in Mental Status*)

Psychosomatic neurologic deficit

Transient neurologic deficits secondary to metabolic disorders (see Event 45, *Postoperative Alteration in Mental Status* and Event 44, *Peripheral Nerve Injury*)

Management

Ensure adequate oxygenation and ventilation (see Event 8, *Hypoxemia* and Event 27, *Hypercarbia*)

Mild hypoxemia can cause obtundation but more often causes restlessness, which can be mistakenly treated with further sedation and respiratory depression

Severe hypoxemia can cause coma

Hypercarbia generally causes obtundation

Check that all anesthetics, both volatile and IV, have been turned off

Increase O_2 flow into the anesthesia breathing circuit to enhance the elimination of inhalation anesthetics

Check expired anesthetic gas concentrations (if an agent analyzer is available)

Stimulate the obtunded patient

Use verbal or tactile stimuli and careful suctioning of the upper airway

Avoid excessive physical force

Conduct a neurologic examination

Check pupillary diameter and reaction to light

Anesthetic or ophthalmic drugs may affect pupillary size or response to light

Check for the presence of corneal and gag reflexes

Test the response to physical stimulation or deep pain

Check the limb reflexes and plantar responses (Babinski reflex)

If the neurologic examination is abnormal, obtain a consultation urgently from a neurologist or neurosurgeon

If damage to the CNS or spinal cord is evident

Assume that cerebral ischemia, infarction, embolism, or hemorrhage has occurred

Obtain an immediate consultation from a neurologist or neurosurgeon

Obtain a CT or MRI scan of the head or spinal cord if the patient can be moved safely

Angiography may be needed to determine the nature of cerebrovascular lesions

Further therapy depends on the diagnosis but may include

Anticoagulation for cerebral thromboembolism

Surgical decompression of intracranial hemorrhage

For acute SCI consider administering high-dose corticosteroids

Methylprednisolone IV, 1 g q8h for 3 doses

Rule out a metabolic etiology

Send blood and urine samples to the clinical laboratory

Abnormalities of glucose metabolism

Check Dextrostix and electrolytes in the operating room if test devices are available

Hypoglycemia should be treated with 50% dextrose IV, 25 ml, or rapid infusion of D_5W (see Event 34, *Hypoglycemia*)

Risk of treatment is virtually zero

Hyperglycemia due to DKA or hyperosmolar nonketotic coma will require insulin therapy IV (see Event 32, *Diabetic Ketoacidosis*)

Hyponatremia (see Event 36, *Hyponatremia and Hypo-osmolality*)

Metabolic acidosis (see Event 39, *Metabolic Acidosis*)
Obtain samples of blood and urine for toxicologic analysis
Inform the surgeon of the problem

Complications

Hypoxemia or hypercarbia
Inability to maintain or protect the airway
Aspiration of gastric contents
Permanent CNS injury

Suggested Reading

Mahla M: Nervous system. p. 383. In Gravenstein N (ed): Manual of Complications During Anesthesia. JB
  Lippincott, New York, 1991

---

43 LOCAL ANESTHETIC TOXICITY

Definition

Local anesthetic toxicity consists of the adverse systemic effects of high blood concentrations of local anesthetics.

Etiology

Direct intravascular injection of local anesthetic solution
Excessive amount of local anesthetic absorbed into the circulation over a short period

Typical Situations

During regional anesthesia in which large volumes of local anesthetic are administered or there
    is significant potential for intravascular injection
        Intercostal nerve blocks
        Epidural anesthesia
        Brachial plexus block
        Paracervical block for gynecologic procedures
        IV regional anesthesia (Bier block)
During IV lidocaine infusion
During topicalization of the oropharynx with local anesthetic

Prevention

Pretreat the patient with a benzodiazepine to increase the seizure threshold
Begin monitoring the patient prior to commencing regional block

Administer supplemental O_2 during and after placement of a regional block
Use special techniques during regional blockade to avoid intravascular injection
      Aspirate from the block site immediately prior to injecting local anesthetic
      Assess the patient's response to a test dose of local anesthetic
      Administer local anesthetic in incremental doses
      Do not administer more than the maximum recommended dose of local anesthetic
Monitor the surgeon's use of local anesthetic for infiltration and in surgical packing
Use appropriate bolus doses and infusion rates for IV lidocaine therapy
      Check blood lidocaine levels during prolonged infusions

Manifestations

CNS abnormalities
      Tinnitus
      Circumoral numbness, heavy tongue
      Nystagmus, difficulty in focusing
      Decreased level of consciousness, restlessness
      Preseizure motor irritability, followed by overt seizure
      Coma
Airway and respiratory abnormalities
      Loss of ability to maintain airway patency
      Loss of airway reflexes
      Respiratory depression followed by apnea
Cardiovascular abnormalities
      Increased PR interval
      Bradycardia
      Conduction abnormalities
      Arrhythmias
      Hypotension
      Irreversible cardiovascular collapse
            Bupivacaine is the local anesthetic most likely to produce cardiovascular collapse as the cardiovascular collapse/convulsion dosage ratio is lower for bupivacaine than for lidocaine
            Pregnant patients may be more susceptible to the cardiotoxic effects of bupivacaine
            Acidosis and hypoxia markedly potentiate the cardiotoxicity of bupivacaine

Similar Events

Hyponatremia (see Event 36, *Hyponatremia and Hypo-osmolality*)
Epinephrine reaction
Hypoxemia (see Event 8, *Hypoxemia*)
Inadvertent neuromuscular blockade (see Event 60, *Syringe or Ampule Swap*)
High spinal/epidural block (see Event 74, *Total Spinal Anesthesia*)
Primary seizure disorder (see Event 47, *Seizures*)
Anaphylaxis (see Event 11, *Anaphylaxis and Anaphylactoid Reactions*)
Panic reaction

Management

Intra-arterial injection into the carotid or vertebral arteries will result in CNS signs early, even with small volumes of local anesthetic.

Stop injection of local anesthetic at the first indication of toxicity

If respiratory distress, apnea, or loss of consciousness occurs

    Establish mask airway

    Administer 100% O_2, assist ventilation as necessary

    Do not hyperventilate the patient, as this decreases the seizure threshold

Ensure adequate IV access

If there is preseizure motor irritability or seizure activity

    Administer O_2

        The seizure may terminate but this is unlikely

Administer an anticonvulsant drug

    Thiopental IV, 25–50 mg increments

    Midazolam IV, 0.5–1 mg increments

    Seizures are often exquisitely sensitive to these drugs

If seizures do not resolve rapidly or if there is difficulty ventilating the patient

    Intubate the patient using a short-acting muscle relaxant

    Administer higher doses of thiopental or midazolam

    Administer other anticonvulsant drugs

        Phenytoin IV, loading dose, 10 mg/kg, administered slowly (may cause hypotension)

        Phenobarbital IV, 1–2 mg/kg

        Volatile anesthetic agents, except enflurane

    Initiate neuromuscular blockade to minimize peripheral O_2 consumption during seizures

        Assess ongoing seizure activity using an EEG monitoring device

Treat cardiovascular complications following ACLS protocols

    Lidocaine <u>can</u> be used to treat bupivacaine-induced arrhythmias

Consider CPB for bupivacaine cardiotoxicity

    May take several hours to recover

Obtain a consultation from a neurologist if seizures do not resolve

Complications

Cardiovascular collapse

Hypoxic brain injury

Suggested Reading

Covino BG: Clinical pharmacology of local anesthetic agents. p. 111. In Cousins MJ, Bridenbaugh PO (eds): Neural Blockade. 2nd Ed. JB Lippincott, Philadelphia, 1988

44 PERIPHERAL NERVE INJURY

Definition

A peripheral nerve injury is a new neurologic deficit presenting after anesthesia, which can be localized anatomically to a site distal to the CNS.

Etiology

Peripheral nerve or nerve plexus injury secondary to
      Direct trauma
      Ischemia
      Compression
      Stretch
Idiopathic

Typical Situations

Following surgery in which a support frame, stirrups, airplane, or other mechanical device has maintained the patient's position
Patients with pre-existing dysfunction of peripheral nerves
Following cardiac surgery
Following the use of limb tourniquets
After encountering a sustained paresthesia during regional blockade
Surgical procedures requiring anticoagulation
Administration of excessive amounts of vasoconstrictor
      By local infiltration around a nerve
      By direct application of a vasoconstrictor to a nerve root
Surgical procedures involving prolonged hypotension

Prevention

Ensure proper positioning of the patient
      The anesthetist is responsible for checking the positioning of the patient by other operating room personnel
      Avoid pressure on the ulnar nerve at the elbow or abduction of the arm of more than 90 degrees
      Avoid pressure on the common peroneal and saphenous nerves by leg holders used to maintain the patient in the lithotomy position
      Use axillary rolls for patients in the lateral position
      When the patient is in the steep Trendelenburg position
            Place and protect the arms at the patient's side
            Position shoulder pads over the acromioclavicular joint
      Carefully pad all areas between the patient and support structures
If feasible, relieve pressure on extremities or the head periodically during anesthesia
Use the minimum limb tourniquet pressure required to achieve adequate hemostasis
      Release the tourniquet for at least 15 minutes q2h

Manifestations

The diagnosis of an ongoing intraoperative nerve injury is difficult.

Loss of motor or sensory function in the distribution of a peripheral nerve or nerve plexus
Apparently delayed recovery from regional block or local nerve block
Symptoms are sometimes delayed and may progressively worsen over time

Similar Events

Inadequate reversal of neuromuscular blockade (see Event 46, *Postoperative Failure to Breathe*)
Excessive spread of local anesthetic following regional or local blockade

Management

Evaluate and treat any factors that might cause further nerve injury
    Check the patient's position and padding around affected nerves
Review the patient's history and perform a careful neurologic examination of the patient
    Identify any predisposing factors in the patient's history
        Diabetes
        Pre-existing neurologic disorders
    Assess the anatomic distribution of the injury
        Specific peripheral nerve(s)
        Nerve plexus
    Check for possible intraoperative factors
        Tourniquet time(s) during surgery
        Patient positioning and positioning aids
        Intraoperative hypotension
    Impound and inspect any equipment that might have been involved in the injury
        Tourniquets
        Positioning aids
        Operating table
Inform the surgeon of the problem
Obtain a consultation from a neurologist
Discuss the situation with the patient as soon as possible

Peripheral nerve injuries can be classified into one of three categories
    Neurapraxia is a temporary injury, frequently caused by compression. There is no axonal degeneration and only slight demyelination at the site of trauma. Full and rapid recovery is likely without specific treatment
    Axonotmesis is a destructive injury of the axons but not the supporting matrix. This is a more severe injury than neurapraxia, with degeneration and demyelination of the axon and its myelin sheath distal to the injury. Proximal degeneration of the nerve also occurs, with regeneration beginning in 3 weeks
    Neurotmesis is a severe crushing injury, avulsion, or severing of the nerve. Prognosis is poor without surgical intervention. Consult a neurologist or neurosurgeon about management options

Complications

Permanent loss of function of the distal musculature
Permanent sensory changes
Contractures

Suggested Readings

Britt BA, Joy N, Mackay MB: Positioning trauma. p. 646. In Orkin FK, Cooperman LH (eds): Complications in Anesthesiology. JB Lippincott, Philadelphia, 1983

Kroll DA, Caplan RA, Posner K et al: Nerve injury associated with anesthesia. Anesthesiology 73:202, 1990

Mahla M: Nervous system. p. 383. In Gravenstein N (ed): Manual of Complications During Anesthesia. JB Lippincott, Philadelphia, 1991

Nicholson MJ, McAlpine FS: Neural injuries associated with surgical positions and operations. p. 193. In Martin JT (ed): Positioning in Anesthesia and Surgery. WB Saunders, Philadelphia, 1978

Oliver SB, Cucchiara RF, Warner MA, Muir JJ: Unexpected focal neurologic deficit on emergence from anesthesia: a report of three cases. Anesthesiology 67:823, 1987

Roy RC, Stafford MA, Charlton JE: Nerve injury and musculoskeletal complaints after cardiac surgery: influence of internal mammary artery dissection and left arm position. Anesth Analg 67:277, 1988

45 POSTOPERATIVE ALTERATION IN MENTAL STATUS

Definition

Postoperative changes in mental status include failure to recover consciousness, responsiveness, or baseline mental status within the expected time frame following general anesthesia.

Etiology

Absolute or relative overdose of drugs that impair mental status
    Volatile anesthetics
    Hypnotics, ketamine, scopolamine, benzodiazepines
    Narcotics
    Nonanesthetic CNS-active medications
        Phenothiazines
        Antihypertensive medications (reserpine, methyldopa, clonidine)
        Tricyclic antidepressants
Metabolic abnormalities affecting the level of consciousness
    Hypoxia or hypercarbia
    Endocrinopathies (thyroid, adrenal, glucose/insulin)
    Electrolyte disorders (sodium, potassium, calcium)
    Endogenous toxins (uremia, porphyria, hepatic encephalopathy)

Neurologic abnormalities affecting the level of consciousness
  Cerebral injury due to ischemia, hemorrhage, embolism, or tumor
  Postictal states
  CNS infection, AIDS
Hypothermia
Recent use of or withdrawal from alcohol or street drugs
Overwhelming systemic infection/sepsis
Severe pain

Typical Situations

Following shorter than anticipated surgical procedure
Following cardiac or carotid artery surgery
In patients with compromised renal or hepatic function
Following major trauma, massive fluid resuscitation, or metabolic acidosis
In neonates or the elderly
Following TURP
In patients with pre-existing disorders of the CNS
Organic brain disease
  Alcoholism
  Psychiatric conditions
  Seizure focus

Prevention

Identify and treat patients with metabolic or neurologic abnormalities that might contribute to
  impaired level of consciousness
Avoid excessive preoperative sedation, especially in elderly or compromised patients
Titrate anesthetics, narcotics, hypnotics, and anticholinergics to clinical effect
  Avoid administering narcotics near the end of the anesthetic unless the dose can be titrat-
    ed to the patient's respiratory rate
  Avoid concomitant use of high doses of narcotics and high concentrations of volatile
    anesthetics
Monitor blood sugar carefully during anesthesia when indicated clinically (see Event 34,
  Hypoglycemia)

Manifestations

Failure to recover an appropriate level of consciousness following general anesthesia as evi-
  denced by the lack of one or more of the following
  Protective airway reflexes
  Appropriate response to stimuli
  Alertness
Focal neurologic signs may be associated with impaired consciousness, depending on the etiology
Confusion
  Agitation, restlessness, incoherence
  Hallucinations or lack of orientation to location, identity, or date
  Inability to follow commands or unintentional, uncooperative behavior

Similar Events

Residual neuromuscular blockade (see Event 46, *Postoperative Failure to Breathe*)
Psychiatric disorders
      Post-traumatic stress syndrome
      A psychotic episode
Organic brain syndrome
Anger or resentment against hospital and/or hospital personnel

Management

Ensure adequate oxygenation and ventilation (see Event 8, *Hypoxemia* and Event 27, *Hypercarbia*)
      Mild hypoxemia can cause obtundation but more often causes restlessness, which can be mistakenly treated with further sedation, and respiratory depression
      Severe hypoxemia can cause coma
      Hypercarbia generally causes obtundation
Check that all anesthetics, both volatile and IV, have been turned off
      Increase O_2 flow into the anesthesia breathing circuit to enhance elimination of inhalation anesthetics
      Check expired anesthetic gas concentrations (if an agent analyzer is available)
Stimulate the obtunded patient
      Use verbal or tactile stimuli and careful suctioning of the upper airway
            Avoid excessive physical force
Restrain the combative patient to prevent injury to self and staff
      Mechanical or chemical restraints should only be used to protect the patient or the staff while determining a definitive diagnosis
      Call for help to restrain the patient safely
      Carefully place physical restraints
      Administer a small dose of narcotic if severe pain suspected
      Consider using minor tranquilizers (benzodiazepines) or major tranquilizers (haloperidol) if correctable etiologies have been ruled out
Rule out a metabolic etiology
      Send blood and urine samples to the clinical laboratory
      Abnormalities of glucose metabolism
            Check Dextrostix and electrolytes in the operating room if test devices are available
            Hypoglycemia should be treated with 50% dextrose IV, 1 ml/kg, or rapid infusion of D_5W (see Event 34, *Hypoglycemia*)
                  Risk of treatment is virtually zero
            Hyperglycemia due to DKA or hyperosmolar nonketotic coma will require insulin therapy IV (see Event 32, *Diabetic Ketoacidosis*)
      Hyponatremia (see Event 36, *Hyponatremia / Hypo-osmolality*)
      Metabolic acidosis (see Event 39, *Metabolic Acidosis*)

Review the doses of medications administered and check for syringe or ampule swap
Consider reversing the effects of specific drugs
      Narcotics
            Naloxone IV, 40 µg increments, titrated to effect

Benzodiazepines
> Flumazenil IV, 0.2 mg over 15 seconds, repeat q1min until effective (maximum dose is 1 mg in 5 minutes, 3 mg in 1 hour)

Anticholinergics
> Physostigmine IV, 1 mg q3min to maximum of 4 mg

Conduct a neurologic examination
> Check pupillary diameter and reaction to light
>> Anesthetic or ophthalmic drugs may affect pupillary size or response to light
>
> Check for the presence of corneal and gag reflexes
> Test the response to physical stimulation or deep pain
> Check the limb reflexes and plantar responses (Babinski reflex)
> If the neurologic examination is abnormal, obtain a consultation urgently from a neurologist or neurosurgeon (see Event 42, *Central Nervous System Injury*)

Obtain samples of blood and urine for toxicologic analysis
Inform the surgeon of the problem
If the confused or agitated patient does not recover baseline mental status
> Keep the environment as quiet as possible
> Maintain verbal contact with the patient and provide reassurance
> Repeatedly orient the patient to time, place, and person
> Keep the patient warm and pain free
> Obtain a consultation from a neurologist or psychiatrist

If the patient does not recover consciousness
> Arrange to transfer the patient to an ICU for continuing care
> Obtain a consultation from a neurologist

Complications

Prolonged endotracheal intubation
Self-inflicted injury

Suggested Readings

Denlinger JK: Prolonged emergence and failure to regain consciousness. p. 368. In Orkin FK, Cooperman LH (eds): Complications in Anesthesia. JB Lippincott, Philadelphia, 1983

Feeley TW: The postanesthesia care unit. p. 2113. In Miller RD (ed): Anesthesia. 3rd Ed. Churchill Livingstone, New York, 1990

Kafer ER, Anderson JA, Isley MR: Evaluation of neurologic problems following anesthesia. Probl Anesth 1:245, 1987

46 POSTOPERATIVE FAILURE TO BREATHE

Definition

Postoperative failure to breathe is diminished or inadequate efforts to breathe following anesthesia.

46

E
V
E
N
T

Etiology

Decreased ventilatory response to hypercarbia or hypoxemia
>Narcotics
>Volatile anesthetics
>Hypnotics

Neuromuscular blockade
>Overdosage
>Residual effects of appropriate dose of relaxant
>>Impaired metabolism of drug
>>Co-administration of drugs that potentiate neuromuscular blockade

CNS impairment or injury
>Metabolic abnormality
>Structural abnormality

Neuromuscular disorders

Typical Situations

Shorter than anticipated surgical procedure
Hyperventilated patient
Neonates and elderly patients
Patients with compromised renal or hepatic function
Following major trauma, massive fluid resuscitation, or metabolic acidosis
Parturients receiving $MgSO_4$
Patients receiving aminoglycoside antibiotics
Hypothermic patients

Prevention

Identify patients with metabolic or neurologic abnormalities that might contribute to postoperative failure to breathe
Avoid profound hypocarbia unless clinically necessary
Titrate anesthetics, narcotics, and hypnotics to clinical effect
>Avoid administering narcotics near the end of the anesthesia unless the dose can be titrated to the patient's respiratory rate
>Avoid concomitant use of high doses of narcotics and high concentrations of volatile anesthetics

Use the minimum necessary dose of neuromuscular blocking drugs as determined by peripheral nerve stimulation

Manifestations

Inadequate or absent efforts to breathe
Apparently decreased level of consciousness
>Level of consciousness may be normal if there is residual neuromuscular blockade

If there is residual neuromuscular blockade
>Tetanic fade or fade in the train-of-four (nondepolarizing relaxant)
>Inability to sustain headlift
>Maximum inspiratory force less than 25–30 cm H_2O

Signs of hypercarbia or hypoxemia are late manifestations
  Tachycardia
  Hypertension
  Bradycardia
  Ventricular ectopy

Similar Events

Failure to awaken (see Event 45, *Postoperative Alteration in Mental Status)*
Mechanical obstruction to breathing

Management

Ensure adequate oxygenation and ventilation
  Do not extubate the trachea until adequate ability to breathe is confirmed
  Continue to ventilate the patient
  Maintain normocarbia or moderate hypercarbia
      Ensure that oxygenation is maintained and that significant tachycardia or hypertension does not develop
Check that all anesthetics, both volatile and IV have been turned off
  Increase O_2 flow into the anesthesia breathing circuit to enhance elimination of inhalation anesthetics
  Check expired anesthetic gas concentrations (if an agent analyzer is available)
Stimulate the patient
  Use verbal or tactile stimuli and careful suctioning of the upper airway
      Avoid excessive physical force
Check neuromuscular function
  If residual neuromuscular blockade is present
      Administer additional reversal medications to a maximum neostigmine dose of 70 µg/kg
  If neuromuscular blockade persists after a full dose of reversal agents have been administered
      Reassure the patient that residual drug levels are causing a temporary weakness
      Administer light sedation until there is recovery of neuromuscular function
      Extubate the trachea only when there is full recovery of neuromuscular function
      Consider any synergistic effects of muscle relaxants and aminoglycoside antibiotics or bacitracin (include antibiotics in the irrigation solutions)
          If present, administer calcium chloride IV, 1 g slowly, to promote reversal of neuromuscular blockade
Review the doses of medications administered and check for syringe or ampule swap
  Narcotics
  Hypnotics
  Muscle relaxants
  Anticholinergics
  Local anesthetics and narcotic administered to the epidural space
Consider reversing the effects of specific drugs
  Narcotics
      Naloxone IV, 40 µg increments, titrated to effect
          Monitor for excessive sympathetic response or pulmonary edema

Benzodiazepines
> Flumazenil IV, 0.2 mg over 15 seconds, repeat q1min until effective (maximum dose is 1 mg in 5 minutes, 3 mg in 1 hour)

Anticholinergics
> Physostigmine IV, 1 mg q3min to maximum of 4 mg

Inform the surgeon of the problem
Send blood samples to the laboratory for
> ABG analysis
> Serum electrolyte and Mg^{2+} levels

Conduct a neurologic examination to exclude a focal CNS injury as the cause of failure to breathe (see Event 45, *Postoperative Alteration in Mental Status* and Event 42, *Central Nervous System Injury*)
If failure to breathe persists
> Arrange to transfer the patient to an ICU for mechanical ventilation
> Obtain a consultation from a neurologist
> Follow up the patient postoperatively for underlying abnormalities
>> Pseudocholinesterase deficiency
>> Myasthenia gravis or myasthenic syndrome
>> Abnormalities of metabolism

Complications

Hypercarbia
Hypoxemia
Inability to reintubate the trachea
Postoperative pain on reversal of narcotics

Suggested Readings

Chang J, Fish KJ: Acute respiratory arrest and rigidity after anesthesia with sufentanil: a case report. Anesthesiology 63:710, 1987

Miller RD: How should residual neuromuscular blockade be detected? Anesthesiology 70:379, 1989

Partridge BL, Ward CF: Pulmonary edema following low-dose naloxone administration. Anesthesiology 65:709, 1986

Pavlin EG, Holle RH, Schoene RB: Recovery of airway protection compared with ventilation in humans after paralysis with curare. Anesthesiology 70:381, 1989

---

47 SEIZURES

Definition

Seizures are paroxysmal discharges from abnormally excited neuronal foci, which can be classified as

Tonic-clonic, generalized seizures (grand mal)
Partial focal motor seizures (jacksonian)

Temporal lobe seizures (complex partial)
Absence seizures (petit mal)

Etiology

Intrinsic CNS injury
Hypoxemia
Metabolic abnormality
Drugs
Infection
Pyrexia (especially in children)

Typical Situations

Local anesthetic toxicity
Patients with pre-existing seizure disorders
Parturients with pre-eclampsia (see Event 73, *Pre-Eclampsia and Eclampsia*)
Patients with acute head trauma or raised ICP
Patients who are hypoxemic
Patients who receive insulin
During TURP surgery
Patients who are taking street drugs
Patients who are postdialysis
Febrile children

Prevention

Identify patients with a pre-existing seizure disorders
    Continue preoperative anticonvulsant medications and check that blood levels of anti-convulsants are therapeutic
    Avoid medications that promote abnormal cerebral electrical activity such as enflurane
    Administer benzodiazepines as a preoperative medication to raise the seizure threshold
Avoid local anesthetic toxicity (see Event 43, *Local Anesthetic Toxicity*)
Treat pre-eclamptic patients with magnesium sulfate (see Event 73, *Pre-eclampsia and Eclampsia*)
Monitor for and treat hyponatremia during TURP surgery (see Event 36, *Hyponatremia and Hypo-osmolality*)

Manifestations

Awake patients may report an aura prior to a seizure
Generalized seizures
    Uncontrolled tonic-clonic motor activity involving most or all extremities
    Loss of consciousness
    Loss of bowel or bladder control
    Airway obstruction is common

47 EVENT

Partial focal motor seizures
    Tonic-clonic motor activity restricted to all or part of an isolated limb
Temporal lobe seizures
    Bizarre behavior, motions, or utterances
Absence seizures
    Blank stare
    Unresponsiveness
Following seizures there is often a postictal state of deep "sleep"
    The patient may be slow to awaken from general anesthesia

Similar Events

Nonepileptic myoclonus
Muscle fasciculations secondary to succinylcholine
Partial neuromuscular blockade in the awake patient
Light anesthesia
Loss of consciousness for other reasons
Panic reaction or fictitious seizure disorder (pseudoseizures)

Management

Prevent traumatic injury to the patient
If respiratory distress, apnea, or loss of consciousness occurs
    Establish mask airway
    Administer 100% O_2, assist ventilation as necessary
    Do not hyperventilate the patient as this would decrease the seizure threshold
Ensure adequate IV access
Administer an anticonvulsant drug
    Thiopental IV, 25–50 mg increments
    Midazolam IV, 0.5 mg increments
    Avoid overdoses as they may cause myocardial depression and may prolong the postictal
        state
        Seizures caused by intrinsic disease of the CNS may not respond to small doses of
            these drugs, but seizures due to other etiologies are often exquisitely sensitive
            to them
If seizures do not resolve rapidly or if there is difficulty ventilating the patient
    Administer a short-acting muscle relaxant and intubate the trachea
    Administer higher doses of thiopental or midazolam
    Administer other anticonvulsant drugs
        Phenytoin IV, loading dose 10 mg/kg administered slowly (may cause hypotension)
        Phenobarbital IV, 1–2 mg/kg
        Volatile anesthetic agents, except enflurane
    Initiate neuromuscular blockade if necessary
        To allow adequate ventilation and oxygenation
        To avoid or control complications of excessive muscular activity
            Increased peripheral O_2 consumption
            Risk of injury in the presence of an unstable neck fracture
            Laceration of the tongue
    Assess ongoing seizure activity using an EEG monitoring device

Treat cardiovascular complications following ACLS protocols
Obtain a consultation from a neurologist

Administer $MgSO_4$ to parturients with eclampsia (see Event 73, *Pre-eclampsia and Eclampsia*)
Investigate underlying etiologies if one is not already known
> Check blood glucose to rule out hyper- or hypoglycemia
> Obtain blood samples for serum Na^+ and osmolality (particularly during or after TURP surgery), toxicology screen
> Examine the patient for signs of infection, occult head trauma, drug reaction, or intracranial disaster unrelated to the anesthetic
If seizures are secondary to an acute head injury or increased ICP
> Commence hyperventilation to reduce the arterial pCO_2 to 25–35 mm Hg
> Administer mannitol IV, 1 g/kg rapidly
> Administer dexamethasone IV, 10–20 mg bolus
> Administer furosemide IV, 10–20 mg bolus
> Elevate the patient's head if possible to ensure adequate venous drainage
> If the patient does not regain consciousness and seizures continue despite anticonvulsant treatment, seizures can be controlled by administering volatile anesthetics such as isoflurane 0.5–3.0%

Complications

Aspiration of gastric contents
Hypoxemia
Cerebral injury from
> Prolonged hypoxemia during an uncontrolled seizure
> Too rapid reversal of hyponatremia with hypertonic saline
Hypotension and respiratory depression from anticonvulsant therapy
Side effects of Mg^{2+} therapy, including neuromuscular and CNS depression

Suggested Readings

Kofke WA, Snider MT, Young RSK et al: Prolonged low flow isoflurane anesthesia for status epilepticus. Anesthesiology 62:653, 1985
Modica PA, Tempelhoff R: Seizures during emergence from anesthesia. Anesthesiology 71:296, 1989
Modica PA, Tempelhoff R, White PF: Pro- and anticonvulsant effects of anesthetics (part I). Anesthesiology 70:303, 1990
Modica PA, Tempelhoff R, White PF: Pro- and anticonvulsant effects of anesthetics (part II). Anesthesiology 70:433, 1990

Chapter Eight
Equipment Events

---

48 CIRCLE SYSTEM EXPIRATORY VALVE STUCK CLOSED

Definition

The expiratory valve of a circle system is "stuck closed" when the valve does not open properly during expiration, thus preventing exhalation of gas from the lungs.

Etiology

Valve components are misassembled
Extra parts or foreign bodies are present in the valve assembly
Dirt, blood, moisture, or secretions contaminate the valve assembly

Typical Situations

After cleaning or reassembly of the valve

Prevention

Ensure that only trained individuals assemble the valves
Conduct a thorough pre-use checkout of the circle system and the one-way valves
    Check for normal appearance of the valve assembly
    Check that the valve disc moves appropriately when breathing from the circuit or when
        ventilating a "test lung" (reservoir bag)
    Check that the breathing circuit pressure at end-expiration is zero during mechanical
        ventilation of the test lung

Manifestations

Progressive increase in PIP and PEEP
        The increase in PIP may plateau at a high value owing to the performance envelope of the
            ventilator and to gas escaping through a high-pressure relief valve during inspiration
        The sustained pressure alarm will sound if set appropriately
Hypotension secondary to increased intrathoracic pressure and impaired venous return
        Lack of response to injected vasoactive medications
                They may not reach the arterial circulation because of decreased venous return
Progressive difficulty in ventilating the patient due to apparent low pulmonary compliance (i.e.,
    "stiff lungs")

Decreased or absent end-tidal CO_2
Decreased O_2 saturation
Pulmonary barotrauma
    Pneumothorax
    Pneumomediastinum
    Subcutaneous emphysema

Similar Events

Kinked or obstructed ETT or breathing circuit hose (see Event 5, *High Peak Inspiratory Pressure*)
Obstruction of the scavenging system hose (see Event 59, *Scavenging System Malfunction*)
Bronchospasm (see Event 24, *Bronchospasm*)
Pneumothorax from other causes (see Event 28, *Pneumothorax*)

Management

Disconnect the patient from the anesthesia circuit to release high intrathoracic pressure
Use an alternate ventilation system
    If the apparent pulmonary compliance is still low (stiff lungs), the problem is in the patient, not the breathing circuit (see Event 5, *High Peak Inspiratory Pressure*)
If the circle system must be used
    Reduce the fresh gas flow into the circuit
    Ventilate the patient manually, disconnecting the patient from the breathing circuit as often as necessary to relieve the excess pressure
    Attempt to relieve the obstruction
        Tap the valve dome
        Remove the expiratory valve
        Increase the fresh gas flow to maximum
        Hyperventilate the patient
        Repair or replace the expiratory valve or valve–CO_2 absorber assembly

Complications

Hypotension
Pneumothorax
Following release of the high intrathoracic pressure
    Hypertension and tachycardia due to release of the venous obstruction
    Repeated doses of vasopressors and inotropes that were administered for the treatment of hypotension may finally reach the arterial circulation and cause extreme hypertension

Suggested Readings

March MG, Crowley JJ: An evaluation of anesthesiologists' present checkout method and the validity of the FDA checklist. Anesthesiology 75:724, 1991
Eisenkraft JB, Sommer RN: Hazards of the anesthesia breathing system. p. 321. In Ehrenwerth J, Eisenkraft JB (eds): Anesthesia Equipment: Principles and Applications. Mosby-Year Book, St. Louis, 1993

49 CIRCLE SYSTEM INSPIRATORY VALVE STUCK CLOSED

Definition

The inspiratory valve of a circle system is "stuck closed" when it does not open properly during inspiration, thus preventing ventilation of the lungs.

Etiology

Valve components are misassembled
Extra parts or foreign bodies are present in the valve assembly
Dirt, blood, moisture, or secretions contaminate the valve assembly

Typical Situations

After cleaning or reassembly of the valve

Prevention

Ensure that only trained individuals assemble the valves
Conduct a thorough pre-use checkout of the circle system and the one-way valves
>   Check for normal appearance of the valve assembly
>   Check that the valve disc moves appropriately when breathing from the circuit or when ventilating a "test lung" (reservoir bag)
>   Check that there is a normal PIP during ventilation of the test lung and that there is appropriate flow of gas into the test lung during inspiration

Manifestations

Markedly increased PIP
>   The high pressure alarm may sound
>>   Some high pressure alarms have a pre-set threshold as high as 65 cm H_2O
Apparent low pulmonary compliance
>   The reservoir bag feels "stiff" on manual ventilation
Diminished or absent breath sounds
Decreased expired minute volume
Absent or decreased end-tidal CO_2
>   Elevated arterial pCO_2
Hypoxemia

Similar Events

Kinked or obstructed ETT or breathing circuit hose (see Event 5, *High Peak Inspiratory Pressure*)
Obstruction of the scavenging system hose (see Event 59, *Scavenging System Malfunction*)

Bronchospasm (see Event 24, *Bronchospasm*)
Pneumothorax (see Event 28, *Pneumothorax*)
Endobronchial intubation (see Event 25, *Endobronchial Intubation*)

Management

Use an alternate ventilation system
    Maintain oxygenation and ventilation
    Convert to IV anesthesia if necessary
To diagnose the obstruction in the inspiratory limb of the circle system
    Disconnect the patient from the anesthesia breathing circuit and activate the O_2 flush
        If the breathing circuit pressure rises dramatically but there is no gas flow from the circuit, the inspiratory limb is obstructed
    Inspect the valve assembly
If the circle system must be used
    Remove the disc from the inspiratory valve, effectively making the valve stick open
    Increase the fresh gas flow to maximum
    Hyperventilate the patient

Complications

Hypoventilation
Hypoxemia
Hypercarbia

Suggested Reading

Dorsch JA, Dorsch SE: The breathing system. p. 210. In: Understanding Anesthesia Equipment. 2nd Ed. Williams & Wilkins, Baltimore, 1984

---

50 CIRCLE SYSTEM VALVE STUCK OPEN

Definition

A valve in the circle system is "stuck open" when it does not fully occlude the inspiratory or expiratory limb, thereby causing rebreathing of exhaled gases.

Etiology

The valve disc or valve ring is broken or deformed
Valve components are misassembled
Extra parts or foreign bodies are present in the valve assembly
Components are missing from the valve

Dirt, blood, moisture, or secretions contaminate the valve assembly
Electrostatic force causes the valve disc to stick in the open position

Typical Situations

After cleaning or reassembly of the valve

Prevention

Ensure that only trained individuals assemble the valve systems
Conduct an appropriate pre-use checkout of the circle system and the one-way valves
> Check for normal appearance of the valve assembly
> Check that the valve disc moves appropriately when breathing from circuit or when ventilating a "test lung" (reservoir bag)
> Check for consistent tidal volumes between those set on the ventilator and those delivered and exhaled from the test lung

Manifestations

Increased inspiratory CO_2
> This is pathognomic for rebreathing or for exogenous administration of CO_2
Increased end-tidal CO_2 and arterial pCO_2
> Hypertension, tachycardia, and vasodilation secondary to hypercarbia
Reverse flow may be indicated on a spirometer that can sense the direction of flow
> This will occur only if the spirometer sensor is in the limb of the incompetent valve
A significant disparity may exist between the expired volumes measured by a spirometer in the expiratory limb and the inspiratory movement of the ventilator bellows
> This will occur if the incompetent valve is in the inspiratory limb
Hyperventilation in patients who are breathing spontaneously

Similar Situations

Failure or exhaustion of the CO_2 absorbent
CO_2 absorber bypass valve accidentally left in the bypass position
CO_2 infused into the circuit from a pipeline or tank

Management

Use an alternate ventilation system if the end-tidal CO_2 or arterial pCO_2 is significantly increased or if there are systemic signs of hypercarbia
Repair or replace the valve assembly or anesthesia machine as soon as feasible
> Otherwise continue to use the alternate ventilation system
If the circle system must be used
> Hyperventilate the patient
> Increase the fresh gas flow into the breathing circuit
> > Unlike the situation in which the CO_2 absorber is exhausted, in this case the improvement in arterial CO_2 will be slight unless fresh gas flow is maximized

Complications

Hypercarbia
Tachycardia
Hypertension
Arrhythmias

Suggested Readings

March MG, Crowley JJ: An evaluation of anesthesiologists' present checkout method and the validity of the FDA checklist. Anesthesiology 75:724, 1991

Smith TC: Anesthesia breathing systems. p. 89. In Ehrenwerth J, Eisenkraft JB (eds): Anesthesia Equipment: Principles and Applications. Mosby-Year Book, St Louis, 1993

51 COMMON GAS OUTLET FAILURE

Definition

Common gas outlet failure is the disconnection or obstruction of the fresh gas supply from the common gas outlet of the anesthesia machine to the anesthesia breathing circuit.

Etiology

Disconnection of the connector hose from the common gas outlet
Disconnection of the connector hose from the anesthesia breathing circuit
    Usually at the CO_2 absorber housing
Disconnection of the proximal or distal portion of the connector hose from a coupler in the middle of the hose
Obstruction of the common gas outlet or connector hose

Note: some older anesthesia machines have two common gas outlets, one for spontaneous ventilation and one for controlled ventilation. Although misconnection of the anesthesia breathing circuit to the wrong outlet will not cause a disconnection or obstruction it will result in no anesthetic gas being delivered to the circuit.

Typical Situations

After the connector hose has been disconnected from the common gas outlet to provide a source of O_2 for a face mask or nasal cannulae
After cleaning or service of the anesthesia machine

Prevention

Use locking connectors at each end of the connector hose between the common gas outlet and the anesthesia breathing circuit

Do not connect O_2 nasal cannulae or masks to the common gas outlet or hose
> Connect them to a separate O_2 source or connect them to the Y piece of the breathing circuit

Conduct a thorough pre-use checkout of the anesthesia machine

Discourage nonessential activity in the vicinity of the anesthesia machine and the anesthesia breathing circuit

Manifestations

The reservoir bag or ventilator bellows will progressively empty
> In ventilators in which the bellows falls during expiration ("hanging bellows"), the loss of gas from the circuit may not be apparent

When the O_2 flush is activated, there will be a loud sound of rushing gas but the reservoir bag or ventilator bellows will not fill

The low airway pressure alarm of the ventilator will sound

The low minute ventilation alarm may sound

Increase in the N_2 concentration of the inspired gas

Decrease in the O_2 concentration of the inspired gas

The signs of hypoventilation, hypoxemia, and hypercarbia will appear later

Similar Events

Major leak in the anesthesia circuit from other causes (see Event 57, *Major Leak in the Anesthesia Breathing Circuit*)

Management

See Event 57, Major Leak in the Anesthesia Breathing Circuit.

Increase the fresh gas flow into the anesthesia breathing circuit
> The leak from a disconnection of the common gas outlet or connector hose cannot be fully compensated for in this fashion

Switch to the reservoir bag, close the pop-off valve, and attempt to fill the anesthesia breathing circuit by activating the O_2 flush
> Activating the O_2 flush will not fill the anesthesia circuit
>> If the common gas outlet is not obstructed, there will be a loud sound of rushing gas but the reservoir bag will not fill

Scan for an obvious disconnection or interruption of the hose between the common gas outlet and the anesthesia breathing circuit
> Reconnect the hose in the correct position

Use an alternate ventilation system
> Continue to ventilate the patient using the alternate ventilation system
> Call for help to identify and correct the leak
> If necessary, replace the anesthesia machine if this is feasible

If an alternate ventilation system is used during inhalation anesthesia, maintain anesthesia with IV agents if necessary, or awaken the patient

Inform biomedical engineering of the failure and have the equipment inspected by a biomedical engineer

Complications

Hypoventilation
Awareness

Suggested Readings

Dorsch JA, Dorsch SE: The anesthesia machine. p. 38. In: Understanding Anesthesia Equipment: Construction, Care and Complications. 2nd Ed. Williams & Wilkins, Baltimore, 1984
Raphael DT, Weller RS, Doran DJ: A response algorithm for the low-pressure alarm condition. Anesth Analg 67:876, 1988

---

52 ELECTRICAL POWER FAILURE

Definition

All or part of the electrical power supply, possibly including the emergency power generation system, fails.

Etiology

Power failure external to the hospital
Power failure internal to the hospital
Failure of an electrical circuit within the operating room
Failure of the emergency power generation system or battery backup system

Typical Situations

During severe weather
During or after a fire in the hospital
Following an earthquake
During or after construction work on the electrical power system inside or outside the hospital

Prevention

Ensure that backup batteries in anesthesia equipment are charged and that the batteries continue to hold charge
    Nickel-cadmium batteries may need to be fully discharged occasionally to maintain their ability to hold a full charge
Plug critical electrical equipment into circuits connected to the emergency power generation system
Test the emergency power generation system on a regular basis, and correct any faults that might prevent a rapid switchover to emergency power

Manifestations

Failure of primary <u>and</u> emergency electrical power
> Room lights go off
> All electrical equipment without a battery backup goes off
> Electronically controlled or powered ventilator without battery backup will stop
>> Some anesthesia ventilators are both pneumatically powered and pneumatically controlled and will continue to function
>> Most new anesthesia ventilators are electronically controlled or electrically powered and will stop working
>> Check the operating manual of each anesthesia machine and ventilator
>>> Some newer anesthesia machines have a battery backup, which can power the ventilator for a short time

Failure of primary power only, emergency power on
> When switching to emergency power, microprocessor-based equipment may reset to factory defaults or may even lock up owing to power surge
> Equipment that is not connected to an emergency power <u>outlet</u> will not operate on emergency power

Similar Events

Localized failure of a single outlet or circuit
Failure of an individual monitor, device, or light

Management

Find the emergency flashlight
> Use the laryngoscope light, if necessary, to assist you in finding other lights and in checking out the situation
> Open the operating room door to let in light or daylight from the corridor

Evaluate the patient and the operating room staff to ensure that their electrocution did not trigger the power failure

If emergency power is on, ensure that all critical devices are connected to emergency power outlets

Ensure that the O_2 supply is still intact
> If not, open backup O_2 cylinders on the anesthesia machine, use manual ventilation

If both the primary and emergency power systems have failed
> Check the ventilator to ensure the patient is being mechanically ventilated
>> The backup battery may power the ventilator for a short time
> If the ventilator is not operating, initiate manual ventilation using the anesthesia machine and breathing circuit

Confer with the surgeon
> Consider the status of the surgical procedure and its urgency
> If the surgery is at an irreversible critical point, the highest priority for lighting may go to the surgical field

Establish monitoring of the patient
> Place esophageal or precordial stethoscope and manual blood pressure cuff if not already in use

Palpate peripheral pulses or have the surgeon palpate arterial pulses in the operative field

Check that routine monitors with battery backups are still operating

Pulse oximeter

Circuit O_2 analyzer

Obtain battery-powered ECG and invasive monitor for critically ill patients

An aneroid manometer can be used for monitoring arterial pressure in noncritically ill patients who have arterial lines in place

Ensure that the central desk nurse and engineers are informed and activate the hospital disaster plan if appropriate

Allocate personnel where needed most

Patients undergoing CPB (some CPB pumps have battery backups, all have hand cranks)

Complex or urgent surgical cases

ICU (all ventilators may be inoperative if there has been a large-scale power loss)

Obtain pneumatic ventilators for paralyzed patients during prolonged cases

Assess likely delay until power is restored. If more than a few minutes, terminate all nonemergent cases as soon as possible

Reassess priorities of allocation of personnel as the situation clarifies

Check on status of repairs to determine when the operating room can be reopened

Do not start nonemergent cases until a reliable electrical power supply is ensured

Complications

Hypoxemia

Surgical mishap

Hemodynamic instability

Suggested Reading

Welch RH, Feldman JM: Anesthesia during total electrical failure, or what would you do if the lights went out? J Clin Anesth 1:358, 1989

53 FAULTY OXYGEN SUPPLY

Definition

The O_2 supply to the anesthesia machine does not contain 100% O_2.

Etiology

Crossing of pipelines during construction or repair of the central O_2 delivery system

Incorrect connector on the O_2 hose to the central O_2 outlet

Connection of the O_2 hose and connector to the wrong gas outlet

Another gas source connected to the O_2 supply with a Y connector
Substitution of a non-O_2 cylinder at the O_2 yoke
   Failure of or misuse of the Pin Index Safety System
O_2 cylinders contain another gas

Typical Situations

Following construction or repair of the piped gas delivery system
Following initial installation or maintenance of the anesthesia machine
Following disconnection of the O_2 supply hose from the O_2 outlet in the operating room
Following delivery of bulk O_2 to the central O_2 supply system

Prevention

Analyze medical gases at all outlets following any construction or repair of the piped gas supply
Use an O_2 analyzer with a low O_2 alarm in the anesthesia breathing circuit
   Calibrate the O_2 analyzer before each case
Conduct a thorough preanesthesia checkout of the anesthesia machine
Use DISS connectors on high-pressure medical gas supply hoses
Utilize the Pin Index Safety System on all gas cylinders and cylinder yokes
   Do not force a cylinder onto the yoke
   Do not attempt to bypass the Pin Index Safety System
Use appropriately color-coded gas cylinders
   Color codes differ in different countries

Manifestations

The anesthesia breathing circuit O_2 analyzer indicates an abnormally low O_2 concentration for
   the setting of the flowmeters
   The low O_2 concentration alarm should sound
Hypoxemia that
   Occurs in the absence of another cause
   Occurs rapidly and quickly becomes severe
   Is worsened by increasing the flow of O_2
The O_2 concentration in the anesthesia breathing circuit cannot be increased by increasing the
   O_2 flow
Late manifestations of hypoxemia
   Arrhythmias
   Bradycardia
   Cardiac arrest

Similar Events

Hypoxemia secondary to other causes (see Event 8, *Hypoxemia*)
Artifact or malfunction of O_2 analyzer or pulse oximeter
Anaphylaxis (see Event 11, *Anaphylaxis and Anaphylactoid Reactions*)
Pulmonary embolism (see Event 18, *Pulmonary Embolism*)

Management

Ventilation with a non-O$_2$-containing gas causes hypoxemia more rapidly than does apnea or airway obstruction.

Verify that the O$_2$ concentration is abnormally low
  Check the O$_2$ analyzer and respiratory gas analyzer
  Check the settings of flowmeters on the anesthesia machine
Open an O$_2$ cylinder on the anesthesia machine AND disconnect the O$_2$ pipeline hose
  With the O$_2$ cylinder open, most anesthesia machines will preferentially draw O$_2$ from the pipeline if there is sufficient pressure in the pipeline
  Activate the O$_2$ flush valve and fill the anesthesia breathing circuit with O$_2$ from the cylinder
Verify that the circuit O$_2$ concentration rises appropriately
  Check the O$_2$ analyzer and the respiratory gas analyzer
  Maintain ventilation with 100% O$_2$ until the patient's oxygenation is normal
If the O$_2$ concentration in the anesthesia breathing circuit does not rise appropriately
  Ventilate the patient with an alternate ventilation system, using a new O$_2$ cylinder as the O$_2$ source
  If no other O$_2$ cylinder is available, ventilate with a self-inflating bag using room air, or perform mouth-to-ETT ventilation
Immediately alert personnel in other parts of the hospital to the problem
  Instruct the circulating nurse to use the telephone or intercom to contact the operating room main desk or hospital operator
  The desk personnel or operator should contact other operating rooms, ICUs, PACUs, emergency room, and hospital engineering

If significant hypoxemia has occurred, terminate the case as soon as possible
Consider observation of the patient in an ICU following recovery from anesthesia

Complications

Hypoxemia
Hypoxic injury to the heart or brain
Cardiac arrest

Suggested Readings

Eichhorn JH, Ehrenwerth J: Medical gases: storage and supply. p. 1. In Ehrenwerth J, Eisenkraft JB (eds): Anesthesia Equipment: Principles and Applications. Mosby-Year Book, St Louis, 1993
Krenis LJ, Berkowitz DA: Errors in installation of a new gas delivery system found after certification. Anesthesiology 62:677, 1985

54 FLOWMETER MALFUNCTION

Definition

Failure of a flowmeter in the anesthesia machine to function properly.

Etiology

Leak
  Broken or cracked flowmeter
  Leaking seal between the flowmeter and the anesthesia machine
  Leaking flowmeter valve
Obstruction
  Foreign body or dirt in the flowmeter tube
  Bobbin stuck at the top of the flowmeter tube
Misleading reading
  Bobbin stuck at the bottom, top, or inside of the flowmeter without obstructing flow
  Worn, distorted, or damaged bobbins
  Wrong gas for the flowmeter in use
  Interchange of parts during repair
  Improper alignment of the flowmeter
  Artifact induced by high pressure in the breathing circuit

Typical Situations

After installation or repair of the anesthesia machine
Mechanical damage to the anesthesia machine
When initially turning on the gas supply to the anesthesia machine or flowmeter

Prevention

Provide appropriate routine maintenance of anesthesia machine
  Some flowmeters are sealed units and require no preventive maintenance
Turn flowmeters off before turning off the gas supply to the anesthesia machine
Check that flowmeters are turned off before connecting pipeline hoses to the machine or before
  opening cylinders on the anesthesia machine
Conduct appropriate pre-use checkout of the anesthesia machine
Monitor FIO_2 throughout each case

Manifestations

Hypoxemia (if O_2 flowmeter leaks)
Abnormal readings on respiratory gas analyzer
  Different concentrations than those set on flowmeters
  Presence of an unexpected gas in the inspired gases
    CO_2, N_2, helium
Light anesthesia (if N_2O flowmeter is obstructed or leaks)

Similar Events

Incorrect calibration of the respiratory gas analyzer
Operator error in adjusting the flowmeter control valve
O_2/N_2O pipeline crossover (see Event 53, *Faulty Oxygen Supply*)

Management

Check FiO_2 and O_2 saturation

If FiO_2 is abnormally low, check for O_2 flowmeter leak or inappropriate flow through another flowmeter

Check that the appropriate O_2 concentration can be maintained with mechanical ventilation

If unable to ventilate manually or if O_2 saturation is low, switch to backup ventilation system with a separate source of O_2

Call for help to assist in identifying and correcting the problem

If the FiO_2 is appropriate and the patient can be mechanically ventilated, consider continuing with the surgical procedure

Arrange to replace the anesthesia machine

Have an alternate ventilation system ready

Monitor the FiO_2, O_2 saturation, anesthetic gas concentrations, and airway pressures carefully

Check for a leak in the low-pressure circuit

Visually check each flowmeter bobbin for free rotation and for appropriate rise and fall with changes in gas flow

If there is any question about the anesthesia machine and its operating condition, remove it from service immediately and have it tested and repaired by a qualified technician

Complications

Anesthetic overdose
Hypoxemia

Suggested Readings

Dorsch JA, Dorsch SE: The anesthesia machine. p. 38. In: Understanding Anesthesia Equipment. 2nd Ed. Williams & Wilkins, Baltimore, 1984

Eisenkraft JB: The anesthesia machine. p. 27. In Ehrenwerth J, Eisenkraft JB (eds): Anesthesia Equipment: Principles and Applications. Mosby-Year Book, St Louis, 1993

55 INTRAVENOUS LINE FAILURE

Definition

An intravenous line failure is a previously functioning IV line that fails for any reason.

Etiology

Obstruction of the IV catheter or tubing
      Stopcock turned in the wrong direction
      Roller clamp on the IV tubing closed
      Precipitation of incompatible drugs in the IV tubing
      Tip of the IV catheter up against a valve in the vein
      Thrombus in IV catheter or IV tubing and filters
Disconnection of, or leak from, the IV catheter or tubing
Migration of the IV catheter outside the vein
External compression of the vein at a site between the IV insertion and the heart
      Due to limb position
      Due to surgical compression on the arm
      Due to compression by surgical retractor (e.g., Favallaro retractor)

Typical Situations

IV catheter was inserted by ward staff prior to surgery
After repositioning the patient
      From one bed or table to another
      On the operating table
      Rotating the operating table relative to the anesthesia machine
During induction of anesthesia
      Failure to turn stopcocks after administering drugs
When large amounts of fluid are infused through a small vein
When the tip of a CVP catheter is in the right atrium
After a difficult IV placement
When using an unfamiliar IV administration set

Prevention

Carefully assess IV catheters placed by other personnel
      Determine how well the IV runs
      Look for signs of erythema or infiltration
      Observe for pain if IV is forcibly flushed or on injection of a test dose of thiopental
Check all IV lines after placement and after repositioning the patient
Use Luer-Lok IV connectors
Ensure that all IV connections are tight
Secure the IV catheter to the patient

Manifestations

Obstruction to flow or external compression of the vein
    IV infusion stops running
    High resistance to injection or forcible flush
    No blood return when the tubing is open to the atmosphere below the level of the heart
Disconnection
    IV infusion runs excessively fast
    Unusually low resistance to injection
    A pool of fluid or blood accumulates on the drapes or on the floor
Subcutaneous migration of the IV catheter
    Hematoma, swelling, or pain at the IV site or on injection through the IV
Lack of patient response to drug or fluid administration

Similar Events

Irrigation fluid or blood from the wound on the surgical drapes or pooling on the floor
Excessively small-gauge IV catheter

Management

If the IV infusion stops
    Check for a high resistance to the injection of IV fluid
    Trace the IV from the solution bag to the catheter hub
        Check that all stopcocks and roller clamps are open
        Check for kinks in the IV tubing
        Look for surgical clamps or surgical retractors that may be obstructing the IV tubing
    Inspect the IV catheter insertion site for signs of extravasation
    Check for external compression of extremity
        Check for a blood pressure cuff that may not have fully deflated
        Check for compression of the arm by a surgical retractor attached to the side of
            the operating room table
    If the cause cannot be found or cannot be alleviated, insert a new IV line
        If access is limited and the need is urgent, ask the surgeons whether they have
            direct access to a vein in the surgical field
If there is suspicion of a disconnection of the IV line
    Trace the IV tubing to exclude disconnection
        Check that stopcocks are in the correct position
        Check that all connections are tight
        Check that the IV catheter is still in the patient
If a disconnection has occurred, reconnect or replace the appropriate components
    Decontaminate connectors as thoroughly as possible with alcohol or iodine
**If no disconnection is found and there is pooling of blood on the drapes or floor, rule out
    the surgical site as the source**

Complications

Hypovolemia
Local tissue necrosis, ulceration, or compartment syndrome due to extravasation of vasoactive
    medications or large volumes of fluid

Light anesthesia
Patient paralyzed but awake

56 LOSS OF PIPELINE OXYGEN

Definition

Pipeline O_2 has been lost when pipeline O_2 pressure drops to zero or below the operating threshold of the anesthesia machine.

Etiology

Exhaustion of the hospital's central O_2 storage supply
Rupture or obstruction of O_2 piping connecting the central O_2 storage to the operating room
O_2 shutoff valve in operating room or zone turned off
Obstruction or disconnection of O_2 hose coupler within the operating room
Failure of O_2 regulator in anesthesia machine

Typical Situations

When pipeline system or central O_2 storage is under repair
During disasters that damage the central O_2 storage or delivery system
     Electrical power, water, and vacuum may fail simultaneously
     The building may suffer structural damage
After disconnecting the pipeline hose to the machine to check "fail-safe" system
When quick-connect hose couplers are used
During delivery of O_2 to the central storage supply tank

Prevention

Before beginning each case conduct a thorough pre-use check of the anesthesia machine and O_2 supply system
     Verify a normal pipeline pressure
     Check that O_2 couplers and hoses are tightly connected
     Check that backup O_2 tanks are full
Arrange for hospital engineering department to notify the anesthesia department and the operating room when the O_2 delivery system requires service

Manifestations

Manifestations will vary depending on how quickly pressure is lost and the type of anesthesia machine in use.

Pipeline O_2 pressure gauge indicates a fall in line pressure

Audible low O_2 supply pressure alarm (if present) will sound when the threshold is reached

O_2 flow falls to zero (bobbin drops)

Flows of all other gases (N_2O and air) fall to zero if the anesthesia machine contains an operational fail-safe system

O_2 flush becomes inoperative

Bag or ventilator fails to fill completely

Loss of ventilator pneumatic drive

Hiss from leak or partial disconnection in O_2 couplers or hoses

Late signs

    Apnea alarms on spirometer, capnograph

    Decrease in FiO_2 as remaining O_2 in circuit is metabolized

    Signs of hypoxemia and hypercarbia

Similar Events

Major leak from the anesthesia breathing circuit (see Event 57, *Major Leak in the Anesthesia Breathing Circuit*)

Isolated N_2O failure

Failure of the O_2 flush valve

Failure of the O_2 flowmeter or gauge (see Event 54, *Flowmeter Malfunction*)

Management

Verify loss of O_2 supply

    Check function of O_2 flush

    Check pipeline pressure gauge

    Check O_2 flowmeter

    Check O_2 analyzer for hypoxic gas mixture

Open O_2 tank on the anesthesia machine

If O_2 tank is empty

    Close the breathing circuit pop-off valve (converts to closed circuit)

    Ventilate manually using reservoir bag with gas contained in circle system

        Refill the volume of reservoir bag as necessary with your own breath

    Switch to self-inflating bag or Jackson-Rees circuit if a separate O_2 tank is available

    Use self-inflating bag with room air or mouth-to-ETT ventilation only if absolutely necessary

    Call for new O_2 tanks; use on anesthesia machine or with self-inflating bag

    Switch to IV agents to maintain anesthesia if anesthesia machine cannot be used

    Notify surgeon of problem

    Notify operating room desk personnel and have them check other operating rooms for O_2 failure

If O_2 tank is full

    Use manual ventilation to conserve O_2

    Call for additional O_2 tanks as backups

Check hoses, couplers, anesthesia machine, and in-room shutoff valve

    Hoses may be kinked by the wheels of the anesthesia machine or other equipment

57 E
V
E
N
T

Couplers may be partially disconnected
Notify biomedical engineering or machine service technician if there is a failure in an anesthesia machine, hose, coupler, or in-room shutoff valve
If the failure is not isolated to a single anesthesia machine, hose, or coupler
Notify hospital engineering
Do not start elective cases until the problem is resolved

Complications

Hypoxemia
Hypercarbia
Light anesthesia, patient recall of intraoperative events

Suggested Readings

Eichhorn JH, Ehrenwerth J: Medical gases: storage and supply. p. 3. In Ehrenwerth J, Eisenkraft JB (eds): Anesthesia Equipment: Principles and Applications. Mosby-Year Book, St Louis, 1993
Eisenkraft JB: The anesthesia machine. p. 27. In Ehrenwerth J, Eisenkraft JB (eds): Anesthesia Equipment: Principles and Applications. Mosby-Year Book St Louis, 1993

57 MAJOR LEAK IN THE ANESTHESIA BREATHING CIRCUIT

Definition

A major leak has occurred when the loss of gas from the anesthesia machine or breathing circuit is significant.

Etiology

Leak in the low-pressure side of the anesthesia machine
Component failure
Disconnection
Leak in the anesthesia breathing circuit
Ventilator/bag selector switch or pop-off valve in the wrong position for positive pressure ventilation
Disconnection
Structural failure of or defect in an anesthesia breathing circuit component
Leak in or around the ETT
ETT not in the trachea (see Event 4, *Esophageal Intubation*)
ETT cuff does not seal the trachea
Hole or laceration in the ETT itself
Placement of a nasogastric tube in the trachea
Leak from the lungs
Pneumothorax (see Event 28, *Pneumothorax*)
Bronchopleural-cutaneous fistula

Typical Situations

When the patient's position is changed by
> Moving the operating table relative to the anesthesia machine
> Moving the patient from one bed or table to another

During manipulation of the head and neck
When the airway is shared with the surgeon
When manipulating the anesthesia breathing circuit hoses or surgical drapes
After changing components of the anesthesia breathing circuit
When first initiating positive pressure ventilation
After a difficult endotracheal intubation or the use of Magill forceps to guide the endotracheal
> intubation

After the common gas outlet has been disconnected to provide a source of O_2 for a face mask or
> nasal cannula

After service of the anesthesia machine

Prevention

Perform a thorough pre-use checkout of the anesthesia machine and breathing circuit
> Conduct a <u>high-pressure leak test</u> on the anesthesia breathing circuit
>> Repeat the test after any component of the breathing circuit has been changed
> Conduct a <u>low-pressure</u> leak test on the anesthesia machine and ventilator
>> Turn on any vaporizer and flowmeter that may be used during anesthesia
> Test the ETT cuff for leaks and examine the integrity of the ETT

Following endotracheal intubation, inflate the ETT cuff to minimal occlusion volume and
check carefully for leaks around the cuff
> Check again for leaks around the cuff and for changes in the position of the ETT after
> any movement of the patient or the ETT

Check the position of the ventilator/bag selector switch and pop-off valve before initiating
mechanical ventilation
Have an appropriate range of ETT sizes available for pediatric patients

Manifestations

During spontaneous ventilation
> An abnormally high fresh gas flow is required to fill the reservoir bag between each
> breath
> Signs of light anesthesia
>> Tachycardia
>> Hypertension
>> Movement
> Strong odor of volatile anesthetic agent
> Increase in inspired and end-tidal N_2 (if measured)
> The capnograph waveform may appear normal

During positive pressure ventilation
> Leaking gas may be heard
> No breath sounds or abnormal breath sounds heard through the esophageal or precordial
> stethoscope

Decreased or zero PIP

Decreased or zero expiratory gas flow measured by a spirometer in the anesthesia breathing circuit

Expired volume will be significantly less than inspired volume

Little or no expired CO_2

Patient's chest does not rise with inspiration

Ventilator bellows either does not refill at an appropriate rate during expiration or collapses (only for a bellows that normally ascends during expiration)

Abnormally high fresh gas flow required to prevent bellows collapse

Alteration of tone of the ventilator if the bellows empties completely and is compressed against the bottom of the housing

Strong odor of volatile anesthetic agent

ETT may be visualized outside the trachea

Similar Events

Low fresh gas flow in the presence of a small leak from the anesthesia circuit

Failure of the ventilator or bellows to operate correctly (see Event 61, *Ventilator Failure*)

Tracheobronchial gas leak during thoracic surgery (see Event 28, *Pneumothorax*)

Management

Maintain adequate ventilation and oxygenation of the patient at all times. Switch to an alternate system for ventilation and call for help early if the leak cannot be resolved quickly.

During Spontaneous Ventilation

Close the pop-off valve

Increase the fresh gas flow into the circuit

The reservoir bag should fill

If the reservoir bag does not fill

Activate the O_2 flush

A major leak should become apparent

Check for and tighten loose connections

Switch to an alternate system for ventilation if the leak cannot be identified or corrected quickly

During Positive Pressure Ventilation

Increase the fresh gas flow into the anesthesia breathing circuit

If the leak can be compensated for, continue positive pressure ventilation while determining the cause of the leak

Switch to the reservoir bag, close the pop-off valve, and attempt to fill the anesthesia circuit by activating the O_2 flush

If the reservoir bag fills, squeeze it to give a breath

Check the compliance of the reservoir bag and look for the rise of the chest on inspiration

Listen for breath sounds and look for a CO_2 waveform on the capnograph

If manual ventilation is possible

Continue manual ventilation

Call for help to identify the leak, which is probably in the ventilator

If the reservoir bag fills but positive pressure ventilation cannot be maintained due to loss of gas from the circuit

Use an alternate ventilation system

Call for help

Listen for a leak around the ETT during inspiration

If there is a leak, add air to the ETT cuff to determine whether the leak can be stopped

If there is still a leak

Assess the position of the ETT and the integrity of the ETT (see Event 30, *Unplanned Extubation*)

Consider removing the ETT, ventilating the patient by mask with the alternate ventilation system, and replacing the ETT

Test the mechanical components of the anesthesia breathing circuit by occluding the Y piece of the breathing circuit and activating the O_2 flush

If the breathing circuit pressurizes and holds a sustained pressure, the problem is either in the ETT, in the ETT cuff, or in the patient

If the leak persists after all mechanical components have been checked, evaluate the patient for a possible pneumothorax or bronchopleural-cutaneous fistula

A bronchopleural fistula may only be apparent after chest tubes are connected to suction

If the reservoir bag does not fill when the O_2 flush is activated

Scan for an obvious disconnection

The connection of the anesthesia breathing circuit to the ETT

The connection of the anesthesia breathing circuit to the common gas outlet

Sites at which external devices such as humidifiers, spirometers, respiratory gas analyzers, and temperature probes are connected to the anesthesia breathing circuit

Use an alternate ventilation system

Call for help to identify the leak

Check the O_2 pipeline pressure and the function of the O_2 flowmeter

If the pipeline pressure is low, open the O_2 cylinder on the anesthesia machine

Check for a vaporizer leak

Feel for a gas leak around the vaporizer mountings

Turn off the vaporizer and check for a persistent leak

If all the above is normal, consider an internal malfunction in the anesthesia machine

Continue to ventilate the patient using the alternate ventilation system

Replace the anesthesia machine if this is feasible

If an alternate ventilation system is used during inhalation anesthesia, maintain anesthesia with IV agents if necessary, or awaken the patient

Inform biomedical engineering of the failure and have the equipment inspected by a biomedical engineer

Complications

Hypoventilation

Hypoxemia

Hypercarbia

Selector switch of breathing circuit bag or ventilator selector valve set incorrectly for the desired mode of ventilation
Inadvertent extubation

Suggested Reading

Raphael DT, Weller RS, Doran DJ: A response algorithm for the low-pressure alarm condition. Anesth Analg 67:876, 1988

58 POP-OFF VALVE FAILURE

Definition

A pop-off valve (adjustable pressure limitation valve) in the anesthesia breathing circuit or in the ventilator fails.

Etiology

Pop-off valve inappropriately left open or closed by the user
Failure of the pop-off valve control knob
Internal failure in the pop-off valve mechanism
Failure of the internal pop-off valve of the ventilator

Typical Situations

After switching from manual ventilation to the mechanical ventilator or vice versa (user error)
After service of breathing circuit components or the ventilator

Prevention

Conduct a thorough pre-use checkout of the anesthesia breathing circuit
  Set the ventilator/bag selector switch to BAG and occlude the breathing circuit
  Close the circuit pop-off valve, and pressurize the anesthesia circuit. Ensure that pressure builds up in the circuit (this discloses a stuck <u>open</u> pop-off valve)
  Open the circuit pop-off valve fully and ensure that there is a decrease in circuit pressure to 1–2 cm H_2O (this checks for a circuit pop-off valve that is stuck closed or a failure of the control knob)
  Increase the fresh gas flow rate to 10 L/min and check for any increase in circuit pressure (an increase in pressure would indicate either a faulty pressure gauge or a partially closed circuit pop-off valve)
  Set the ventilator/bag selector switch to VENTILATOR, maintain the fresh gas flow at 10 L/min, and ventilate a test lung (reservoir bag). Check for any increase in circuit pressure during the expiratory phase (an increase in pressure indicates either a faulty pressure gauge or a closed <u>ventilator</u> pop-off valve)

Observe the anesthesia circuit while preoxygenating the patient and maintaining a tight seal between the mask and the patient's face

Ensure that inspiratory and expiratory valves move appropriately and that circuit pressure does not rise to more than 1–2 cm H_2O

Manifestations

Circuit Pop-Off Valve Stuck Closed or Inappropriately Set to CLOSED

If the ventilator/bag selector switch is on BAG (the relevant pop-off valve is in the breathing circuit)

Progressive increase in PIP and PEEP

The increase in PIP may plateau at a high value owing to gas escaping through a high-pressure relief valve

The sustained pressure alarm will sound if set appropriately

Increasing distention of the reservoir bag

Hypotension secondary to increased intrathoracic pressure and impaired venous return

Lack of response to injected vasoactive medications

Drugs may not reach the arterial circulation because of decreased venous return

Progressive difficulty in ventilating the patient due to apparent low pulmonary compliance (i.e., stiff lungs)

Decreased or absent end-tidal CO_2

Decreased O_2 saturation

Pulmonary barotrauma

Pneumothorax

Pneumomediastinum

Subcutaneous emphysema

If the ventilator/bag selector switch is on VENTILATOR (the relevant pop-off valve is internal to the ventilator)

The same manifestations listed above, PLUS

Unusual sound of the ventilator as it works against the increased circuit pressure

Decreased tidal volume (the performance of most ventilators degrades as the circuit pressure increases)

Circuit or Ventilator Pop-Off Valve Stuck Open or Inappropriately Set to OPEN

IF the patient is breathing spontaneously

The reservoir bag may fail to fill adequately

IF the patient is being mechanically ventilated

There will be a major leak during inspiration (see Event 57, *Major Leak in the Anesthesia Breathing Circuit*)

The ventilator bellows will fall or the reservoir bag will collapse, making ventilation impossible

Tidal volume and minute ventilation will decrease

Similar Events

Closed Pop-Off Valve

Expiratory valve stuck in the closed position (see Event 48, *Circle System Expiratory Valve Stuck Closed*)

Scavenger system malfunction (see Event 59, *Scavenging System Malfunction*)
Obstruction of the expiratory limb of the anesthesia circuit
Pneumothorax (see Event 28, *Pneumothorax*)
Bronchospasm (see Event 24, *Bronchospasm*)

Open Pop-Off Valve
Major leak from other circuit component (see Event 48, *Major Leak in the Anesthesia Breathing Circuit*)

Management

If Pop-Off Valve Stuck Closed or Inappropriately Set to CLOSED
Check that the pop-off and selector valves are set appropriately for the desired mode of ventilation
If the circuit pressure is high, switch the selector valve to its alternative setting (from bag to ventilator or vice versa)
>   This will change the relevant pop-off valve
>   If the high airway pressure does <u>not</u> resolve
>>   Interrupt (disconnect) the circuit to relieve the high airway pressure
>>   Use an alternate ventilation system
>>   Call for help to repair or replace defective components in circuit or ventilator
>   If the high airway pressure resolves, but the original pop-off valve is stuck closed
>>   Maintain ventilation using the ventilator or bag as appropriate
>>   Get help to correct the pop-off valve problem
>>   If the <u>ventilator</u> pop-off valve is stuck closed but mechanical ventilation is necessary
>>>   Call for help to manage the patient's ventilation
>>>   Lower the fresh gas flow
>>>   Intermittently relieve circuit pressure by "breaking" the circuit
>>   If there is sufficient help, replace or repair the defective pop-off valve or replace the CO_2 absorber, ventilator, or anesthesia machine

If Pop-Off Valve Stuck Open or Inappropriately Set to OPEN
Check that the pop-off and selector valves are set appropriately for the desired mode of ventilation
Ensure adequate oxygenation and ventilation
>   Use an alternate ventilation system if controlled ventilation is in use and there is a large, uncorrectable leak through the circuit pop-off valve
>   Consider converting to spontaneous ventilation
>   Increase the fresh gas flow to keep the reservoir bag adequately filled during spontaneous ventilation
>   If there is sufficient help, replace or repair the defective pop-off valve or replace the CO_2 absorber, ventilator, or anesthesia machine

Complications

Hypotension
Hypoxemia
Hypercarbia
Pulmonary barotrauma
Gas embolism

Pneumothorax
Cardiac arrest
Following release of high intrathoracic pressure
  Hypertension and tachycardia due to release of the venous obstruction
  Repeated doses of vasopressors and inotropes, administered for the treatment of hypotension, may finally reach the arterial circulation and cause extreme hypertension

Suggested Reading

Dorsch JA, Dorsch SE: The breathing system. I. General considerations. p. 136. In: Understanding Anesthesia Equipment. 2nd Ed. Williams & Wilkins, Baltimore, 1984

59 SCAVENGING SYSTEM MALFUNCTION

Definition

The anesthetic gas scavenging system does not function properly.

Etiology

Internal obstruction or external compression of the scavenging system hose
Mechanical failure of components of the scavenging system
Incorrect assembly of the scavenging system

Typical Situations

When the anesthesia machine or other heavy equipment is rolled over scavenging system hoses lying on the operating room floor
Following service of the scavenging system or the anesthesia machine

Prevention

Use of a scavenging system that incorporates safety devices
  Positive- and negative-pressure relief mechanisms
  In-line breathing circuit pressure gauges and alarms to indicate and warn of excessive positive or negative pressure
Avoid external compression of scavenging system hoses
  Use scavenging system hoses that are constructed to be resistant to kinking or twisting
  Keep scavenging system hoses off the floor
  Move anesthesia machines and carts carefully to avoid obstructing scavenging system hoses
  Visually inspect the scavenging system hoses during the routine pre-use machine check and after the anesthesia machine has been moved

Confirm that scavenging system hoses are connected to the correct ports on the scavenging
   system
During the pre-use machine check, occlude the anesthesia breathing circuit
      Activate the O_2 flush and ensure that the gas pressure can be relieved through the pop-off
         valve (tests both the valve and the scavenging system)
      With zero fresh gas flow, occlude the anesthesia breathing circuit and ensure that nega-
         tive pressure does not develop in the circuit (active scavenging)

Manifestations

Excessive end-expiratory pressure (either positive or negative) is observed in the anesthesia
   circuit
      When passive scavenging is used, only positive pressure should develop
      When active scavenging (vacuum) is in use, a failure of the scavenging interface can
         cause either positive or negative pressure to develop
Inability to ventilate the patient
Possible difficulty in keeping the circuit filled
Hypotension due to increased intrathoracic pressure
Hypoxemia
Odor of volatile anesthetic gas may be detected by operating room personnel

Similar Events

Closed or obstructed pop-off valve (see Event 58, *Pop-Off Valve Failure*)
Expiratory valve of a circle system stuck in the closed position (see Event 48, *Circle System
   Expiratory Valve Stuck Closed*)
Stuck closed pop-off valve inside the ventilator bellows (see Event 61, *Ventilator Failure*)
Faulty pressure gauge
Pneumothorax (see Event 28, *Pneumothorax*)
Loss of anesthetic gas from the anesthesia breathing circuit (see Event 57, *Major Leak in the
   Anesthesia Breathing Circuit*)

Management

Confirm a fault in the scavenging system
      Observe the pressure in the anesthesia breathing circuit
      If excessive pressure (either positive or negative) is observed, disconnect the patient
         from the anesthesia breathing circuit
            Use an alternate ventilation system
Check for an obstruction of the scavenger hoses
      Between the CO_2 absorber and the scavenging interface
      Between the ventilator and the scavenging interface
      Between the scavenging interface and the operating room scavenging exhaust
**If there is an obstruction of the scavenging system hose between the scavenging interface
and either the CO_2 absorber or the ventilator**
            Relieve any obvious obstruction
            Consider switching from the ventilator to the reservoir bag or vice versa for posi-
               tive pressure ventilation

Use the alternate ventilation system if there is any doubt

If the patient is breathing spontaneously, either the reservoir bag or the ventilator bellows can be used as a gas reservoir

If the obstruction of the scavenging system hose is between the scavenging interface and the operating room exhaust point

Relieve any obvious obstruction

Continue to use the alternate ventilation system if the obstruction cannot be relieved

If there is no immediate resolution

Continue to use the alternate ventilation system

Alternatively, disconnect the scavenging interface from the anesthesia breathing system, venting the waste gases into the operating room

Check for other causes of high airway pressure

Get help to repair and replace the faulty scavenging system components

Complications

Pneumothorax

Subcutaneous emphysema

Hypotension due to increased intrathoracic pressure

Hypoventilation due to loss of anesthetic gases from the circuit

Exposure of operating room personnel to waste anesthetic gases

Suggested Readings

Andrews JJ: Inhaled anesthetic delivery systems. p. 171. In Miller RD (ed): Anesthesia. 3rd Ed. Churchill Livingstone, New York, 1990

Dorsch JA, Dorsch SE: Controlling trace gas levels. p. 247. In: Understanding Anesthesia Equipment. 2nd Ed. Williams & Wilkins, Baltimore, 1984

60 SYRINGE OR AMPULE SWAP

Definition

Administration of the wrong drug may occur in the following ways:

Ampule swap: The incorrect drug is drawn up into a labeled syringe or infusion pump
Syringe swap: Medication from the wrong syringe is administered to the patient
Infusion pump swap: The wrong infusion pump is adjusted by the clinician

Etiology

Failure to label syringes or infusion pump

Incorrect matching of labels on syringes and drug ampules

Failure to read the label on the syringe

Failure to read the label on the infusion pump

Typical Situations

When the anesthetist is working in unfamiliar settings
When drug packaging or ampules are changed
When there is time pressure
When ampules have a similar appearance, especially if they are located close to each other in a
    drug cart
When syringe and infusion pump labels are written by hand
When syringes are prepared by other personnel
When there is minimal illumination in the operating room

Prevention

Check the drug name and concentration on each drug ampule carefully
Use drug ampules whose labels conform to ASTM standard D 6267-88
Label syringes carefully
        Use preprinted, color-coded adhesive syringe labels
                There is an ASTM standard on adhesive syringe labels (ASTM D 4774-88)
        For emergency drugs use "ready to use" syringes that conform to the syringe labeling
            standard ASTM D 4775-88
        Discard unlabeled syringes
        Discard syringes if there is any doubt about their actual contents

Manifestations

Unusual response or lack of response to drug administration
        The awake patient may complain of an unusual sensation
                Pounding heart or palpitations
                Change in mental status
                Muscle weakness
                Visual disturbance
        Unusual increase or decrease in blood pressure or heart rate
        Unexpected occurrence or persistence of muscle relaxation
        Unexpected change, or lack of change, in level of consciousness
Incorrect ampule found to be open in the anesthetist's work area

Similar Events

Seizures (see Event 47, *Seizures*)
Airway obstruction
Hypotension from other causes (see Event 7, *Hypotension*)
Failure to awaken or breathe from other causes (see Event 46, *Postoperative Failure to Breathe*
    and Event 45, *Postoperative Alteration in Mental Status)*
Anaphylaxis (see Event 11, *Anaphylaxis and Anaphylactoid Reactions*)
Failure of the IV infusion (see Event *55, Intravenous Line Failure)*

Management

If the error in drug administration is recognized immediately after injection
        Stop the IV line carrying the drug

Attempt to aspirate or drain the IV tubing from the patient back to the point of injection

If there is a blood pressure cuff on the same arm as the IV catheter, inflate it to slow down the entry of the drug into the central circulation

Maintain the patient's airway and ensure adequate oxygenation and ventilation

If the medication error involved administration of a muscle relaxant

If appropriate, reassure the patient and provide sedation with a short-acting IV agent

Assess neuromuscular function with a nerve stimulator and reverse neuromuscular blockade when sufficient recovery has occurred

If the patient is hypotensive (see Event 7, *Hypotension*)

Expand the circulating fluid volume rapidly

Administer a vasopressor (e.g., phenylephrine IV, 50–100 μg bolus)

Treat any associated bradycardia with atropine IV, 0.6 mg bolus; or glycopyrrolate IV, 0.2–0.4 mg bolus, repeated as necessary

If the patient is hypertensive (see Event 6, *Hypertension*)

Administer a short-acting vasodilator (sodium nitroprusside by IV infusion, 0.25–2 μg/kg/min)

Treat any associated tachycardia with esmolol IV, 0.5 mg/kg loading dose, followed by an infusion as necessary to control the heart rate

Attempt to determine what drug was actually administered

Check the syringes and ampules used during the case

Check the label on the syringe just used to determine whether it was the desired one

Check to see whether one syringe has an unexpectedly low volume of drug remaining

Inspect opened ampules to determine whether an incorrect ampule was opened

Have the trash and "sharps" containers impounded to allow inspection of ampules and syringes at a later time

Treat any additional side effects of the medications that were administered

Complications

Awareness, with or without concomitant muscle paralysis

Hypoventilation, hypoxemia, or hypercarbia

Myocardial ischemia or infarction secondary to hypotension, hypertension, or tachycardia

Cerebral hypoperfusion or hemorrhage

Suggested Reading

Cooper JB, Newbower RS, Kitz RJ: An analysis of major errors and equipment failures in anesthesia management: considerations for prevention and detection. Anesthesiology 60:34, 1984

61 VENTILATOR FAILURE

Definition

A ventilator failure is defined as an inability of the ventilator to deliver the required inspired gas volume to the patient.

Etiology

Stuck bellows or other ventilator malfunction
Improper assembly of ventilator or connecting hoses
Lung compliance outside the performance envelope of the ventilator
Failure of fresh gas flow to the anesthesia circuit and ventilator
Electrical power failure of an electrically controlled ventilator (see Event 52, *Electrical Power Failure*)

Typical Situations

When the user is unfamiliar with the anesthesia machine or ventilator controls
Following anesthesia machine service or disconnection
In patient with severe lung disease and low lung compliance
During interruptions of electrical power or O_2 supply
> Severe weather
> Earthquake

Prevention

Provide appropriate routine maintenance for the anesthesia machine and ventilator
Conduct a thorough preoperative check of the anesthesia machine and ventilator
> Place a breathing bag on the end of the Y piece and use it as a test lung for the ventilator
Ensure that the ventilator power is turned <u>on</u> and that the bag/ventilator selector valve is set properly

Manifestations

Ventilator bellows moves inadequately or sticks in a tilted position
Ventilator fails to cycle, bellows does not move at all
Abnormal sound of the ventilator during inspiration
Ventilator malfunction alarm sounds
Signs of hypoventilation of the patient
> Decreased or absent chest movement on inspiration
> Reduced or absent breath sounds heard via a precordial or esophageal stethoscope
> Little or no end-tidal CO_2 present on capnograph waveform
> As arterial pCO_2 rises, the patient may make respiratory efforts if not fully paralyzed
> Low or zero tidal volume measured by spirometry
> Apnea alarm may sound
> Low pressure alarm may sound
> Hypoxemia (see Event 8, *Hypoxemia*)
If there has been a loss of electrical power, other devices may lose power or operating room lights may go out
If the main O_2 supply to the operating room fails, the bobbins will fall to the bottom of the flowmeters and an alarm should sound

Similar Events

Ventilator never turned on

Pop-off valve failure (see Event 58, *Pop-Off Valve Failure*)

Inspiratory valve stuck closed (see Event 49, *Circle System Inspiratory Valve Stuck Closed*)

Obstruction of the inspiratory tubing of the anesthesia circuit or the ETT

Major leak from the anesthesia circuit (see Event 57, *Major Leak in the Anesthesia Breathing Circuit*)

Breathing circuit bag/ventilator selector switch set incorrectly

Management

Attempt to manually ventilate the patient using the breathing circuit

Switch to manual ventilation using the reservoir bag on the anesthesia machine

Activate the O_2 flush device to fill the reservoir bag

If ventilation is restored, continue manual ventilation

Call for help to identify the problem in the ventilator and to assist you in caring for the patient

If unable to fill the anesthesia breathing circuit using the O_2 flush

Ventilate the patient using a backup ventilation system (Jackson-Rees circuit, self-inflating bag, or mouth-to-ETT)

Visually check for a major circuit disconnection, checking the ETT, Y piece, hoses, and reservoir bag

Ensure that the bag/ventilator selector switch is set to <u>BAG</u> for manual ventilation

Check the flowmeters and pipeline O_2 pressure gauge

Switch to O_2 cylinders if the external O_2 supply has failed

If the anesthesia breathing circuit fills but the patient cannot be ventilated manually

Ventilate the patient using a backup ventilation system (Jackson-Rees circuit, self-inflating bag, or mouth-to-ETT)

Check the inspiratory limb of the anesthesia breathing circuit for obstruction

If unable to ventilate with backup ventilation system

Check for kinked ETT, bronchospasm, endobronchial intubation, pneumothorax

Once you have established adequate ventilation, call for help

Check the circuit hoses, bag/ventilator selector switch and the ventilator ON switch again

Find and correct the fault in the ventilator

Maintain anesthesia with IV agents, if necessary

In the event of an electrical power failure, the emergency power system should automatically activate

The emergency power generator may fail or may itself be damaged by an event that cuts the main power supply (see Event 52, *Electrical Power Failure*)

Make sure that the ventilator is plugged into an emergency power outlet

If electrical power cannot be restored quickly, obtain a pneumatically controlled ventilator

Suggested Readings

Marks JD, Schapera A, Kraemer RW et al: Pressure and flow limitations of anesthesia ventilators. Anesthesiology 71:403, 1989

Raphael DT, Weller RS, Doran DJ: A response algorithm for the low-pressure alarm condition. Anesth Analg 67:876, 1988

Sommer RM, Bhalla GS, Jackson JM et al: Hypoventilation caused by ventilator valve rupture. Anesth Analg 67:999, 1988

62 E V E N T

62 VOLATILE ANESTHETIC OVERDOSE

Definition

An excessively high inspired concentration of a volatile anesthetic constitutes either an absolute or a relative overdose:

Absolute overdose: concentration of anesthetic substantially greater than that desired
Relative overdose: desired concentration of anesthetic causes cardiopulmonary compromise

Etiology

Error in setting the anesthetic vaporizer to deliver the desired concentration of volatile anesthetic
Vaporizer accidentally left on after a previous case
Failure to decrease a high concentration of volatile anesthetic used for induction of anesthesia
Malfunction of the anesthetic vaporizer
Vaporizer filled with the wrong agent
Vaporizer has been tilted, causing liquid anesthetic to enter the bypass portion of the vaporizer
    or the anesthesia machine piping

Typical Situations

After conducting an inhalation induction with a volatile anesthetic
In patients who have pre-existing cardiovascular or pulmonary compromise
When using a measured flow vaporizer (Copper Kettle or Verni-Trol)
        If the practitioner is not appropriately trained in the use of a measured flow vaporizer
        If an error is made in calculating the correct setting of the vaporizer flowmeter
        If the vaporizer flowmeter is not set at the intended setting
        When there are two vaporizer flowmeters (low range and high range) operating in parallel
                If the vaporizer high-range flowmeter is inadvertently set instead of the low-range
                    flowmeter
                If there is flow through a flowmeter that was intended to be off
When a vaporizer has just been installed on the anesthesia machine

Prevention

Use an anesthesia agent analyzer
        Set appropriate alarm limits for excessive concentration of volatile anesthetic
Use care when administering high concentrations of volatile anesthetic
        Ensure that the concentration is lowered as necessary
Use care when using a Copper Kettle or Verni-Trol vaporizer
        Double check calculations and vaporizer flowmeter settings
        If in doubt as to the proper setting, do not use the vaporizer
Maintain vaporizers in the upright position at all times

Manifestations

Both a high fresh gas flow and mechanical ventilation will result in more rapid equilibration of the anesthesia breathing circuit and the patient to the administered concentration of volatile anesthetic.

Volatile anesthetic overdose should be included in the differential diagnosis of any unexpected hypotension or bradycardia during anesthesia.

If the vaporizer is accidentally left on from a previous case

    The patient may complain of the smell during preoxygenation

    The patient may become unresponsive during preoxygenation

A high concentration of volatile anesthetic measured by an anesthetic agent analyzer

Respiratory depression or apnea in the spontaneously ventilating patient

Hypotension

Bradycardia

Electromechanical dissociation or cardiac arrest

Failure to breathe or to awaken at the end of the anesthesia

Similar Events

Hypotension and cardiovascular collapse from other causes (see Event 7, *Hypotension*)

Respiratory depression or apnea from other causes (see Event 46, *Postoperative Failure to Breathe*)

Overdose of intravenous medication(s)

Management

Confirm a volatile anesthetic overdose

    Check the vaporizer and flowmeter settings

    Check the anesthetic agent analyzer to determine whether volatile anesthetic concentrations measured in the anesthesia breathing circuit are appropriate

        If there is no anesthetic agent analyzer, smell the gas in the anesthesia breathing circuit

Turn off all volatile anesthetic vaporizers

Ensure adequate oxygenation and ventilation

Check vital signs frequently

Increase the FIO$_2$ to 100% with a high flow rate of O$_2$ into the anesthesia breathing circuit

Purge volatile anesthetic from the breathing circuit by activating the O$_2$ flush between breaths

    Confirm that the concentration of volatile anesthetic in the anesthesia breathing circuit has decreased

    If the anesthetic concentration does not decrease, ventilate the patient with an alternate ventilation system

        There may be an internal fault in the anesthesia machine or vaporizer

Support the circulation

    Check for cardiac ejection since EMD can occur

        Palpate the peripheral pulses

        Pulse oximetry

        Auscultate the heart sounds

    Call for help if there is severe hemodynamic compromise

    Administer vasopressors or inotropes as necessary to maintain the blood pressure (see Event 7, *Hypotension* and Event 13, *Sinus Bradycardia*)

    If cardiac arrest occurs, follow ACLS guidelines (see Event 2, *Cardiac Arrest*)

Arrhythmias may occur when using catecholamines in the setting of a volatile anesthetic overdose

Terminate the surgery as soon as possible if there has been profound hypotension or cardiac arrest

Impound the anesthesia machine if there is any possibility of misfilling or malfunction of the vaporizer or of a fault in the anesthesia machine (see Appendix of Ch. 2)

Complications

Respiratory arrest
Cardiac arrest

Suggested Readings

Chilcoat RT: Hazard of mis-filled vaporizers: summary tables. Anesthesiology 63:726, 1985

Eisenkraft JB, Sommer RM: Hazards of the anesthesia delivery system. p. 321. In Ehrenwerth J, Eisenkraft JB (eds): Anesthesia Equipment: Principles and Applications. Mosby-Year Book, St. Louis, 1993

Sinclair A: Vaporizer overfilling. Can J Anaesth 40:77, 1993

Chapter Nine

Cardiac Anesthesia Events

63 CARDIAC LACERATION

Definition

A cardiac laceration is an inadvertent incision into the right atrium, right ventricle, great vessels, or vein graft(s) during sternotomy.

Etiology

Adhesion of scar tissue and/or myocardial tissue to the sternum

Typical Situations

Patients who have had a previous sternotomy ("redo" sternotomy)
Inexperienced surgeon
When the lungs are ventilated during sternotomy
Emergency sternotomy
Patients with ascending aortic aneurysms or multivessel aortic arch disease
Patients with an anatomic abnormality of the chest wall (kyphoscoliosis, pectus excavatum)
Patients who have received mediastinal radiation

Prevention

Do not ventilate the lungs during sternotomy
Reduce myocardial chamber size during sternotomy
      Place the patient in reverse Trendelenburg position
      Vasodilate the patient with an IV infusion of sodium nitroprusside
      Consider instituting femoral artery-to-femoral vein CPB
Suggest that sternotomy be performed following deep hypothermia and complete circulatory arrest if an aortic aneurysm is adherent to the underside of the sternum

Manifestations

Large volumes of blood welling out of the surgical field
Hypotension
      May be due to blood loss
      Acute cardiac failure may occur if a critical vein or internal mammary artery graft to a coronary artery is lacerated

Similar Events

Bleeding from other intrathoracic structures (see Event 1, *Acute Hemorrhage*)
Hypotension from other causes (see Event 7, *Hypotension*)

Management

Cardiac laceration may occur during any sternotomy.

Be prepared for major hemorrhage during sternotomy
Ensure adequate IV access in place for reoperations
A minimum of two 14-gauge IV catheters
If a blood salvage device is to be used during surgery, have it set up prior to sternotomy
Stop ventilating the lungs prior to sternotomy
Ensure that cross-matched blood is available in the operating room prior to sternotomy
Especially important for a redo sternotomy
Observe the operative field carefully during sternotomy

If major hemorrhage is apparent during sternotomy
Stop administering volatile anesthetics and flush the anesthesia breathing circuit with 100% O_2
Stop administering vasodilators
Increase the FiO_2 to 100% and resume ventilation

Maintain the circulating fluid volume
Administer IV fluid (crystalloid, colloid, blood)
Get help to administer volume rapidly

Maintain perfusion pressure
Administer vasopressors as required (see Event 7, *Hypotension*)
Phenylephrine IV, 50–100 µg
Epinephrine IV, 10–50 µg
Get help to set up a rapid infusion device

Conserve the patient's blood
Ensure that the blood salvage device is used by the surgeons

If surgical repair without CPB is impossible
Heparin should be administered by the anesthesiologist through the distal lumen of the PA catheter (if in place) or the CVP catheter
Check ACT as soon as feasible
Administer more heparin if ACT is less than 400 seconds
After heparinization, blood can be salvaged by the cardiotomy suction line of the CPB pump
The femoral artery may have to be cannulated for the arterial perfusion line
A right ventriculotomy and the cardiotomy suction can be used as venous return for bypass

Complications

Myocardial ischemia
Arrhythmias
Cardiac arrest

ARDS
Hypothermia
Systemic air embolism

Suggested Readings

Croughwell N: Reoperation for coronary artery bypass. p. 337. In Reves JG, Hall KD (eds): Common Problems in Cardiac Anesthesia. Year Book Medical Publishers, Chicago, 1987

Estafanous FG: Management of emergency revascularization or cardiac reoperations. p. 833. In Kaplan JA (ed): Cardiac Anesthesia. 2nd Ed. WB Saunders, Philadelphia, 1987

Romanoff ME, Rung GW: Anesthetic management in the precardiopulmonary bypass period. p. 202. In Hensley FA, Martin DE (eds): The Practice of Cardiac Anesthesia. Little, Brown, Boston, 1990

Tinker JH: Cardiopulmonary bypass: technical aspects. p. 378. In Thomas SJ (ed): Manual of Cardiac Anesthesia. Churchill Livingstone, New York, 1984

64 HYPOTENSION DURING CARDIOPULMONARY BYPASS

Definition

A mean arterial pressure of less than 50 mm Hg during CPB is considered hypotension.

Etiology

Low blood viscosity secondary to hemodilution
Decreased flow from the pump
      Roller pump malocclusion
      Error in calculating the required flow rate for a patient
      Reduced venous return to the oxygenator reservoir
      Hypovolemia
Difficulty with aortic cannulation
      Aortic dissection by the aortic cannula
      Aortic cannula advanced too far into the aorta
            Carotid artery or innominate artery cannulation
Clamping of the aortic cannula by the aortic cross-clamp
Decreased SVR
      Vasodilator overdose
      Hyperthermia

Typical Situations

Acute reduction of viscosity when instituting CPB
Aortic cannula advanced too far into the aorta
      More likely to be occluded by the aortic cross-clamp
      Cannula may kink

Roller pump malocclusion
Reversal of tubing in the roller pump
Administration of vasodilator
 Infusion pump or IV administration device
  Accidentally turned on
  Not set correctly
  Malfunctioning
During the rewarming phase following hypothermia
Anticoagulation in the presence of
 A gastric or duodenal ulcer or other potential site for major hemorrhage
 Recent cannulation of a major blood vessel

Prevention

Control the blood pressure (MAP of 60–80 mm Hg) at the time of aortic cannulation and when
 the aortic cross-clamp is applied or removed
Observe the cannulation, initiation of CBP, and cross-clamp processes and inform the surgeon
 if abnormalities are seen
 Aortic dissection
 Aortic cannula advanced too far
 Occlusion of the aortic cannula with the aortic cross-clamp
When using vasodilators, use care in setting infusion pumps and IV administration devices
Maintain a minimum hematocrit of 20% during routine CPB
Monitor temperature from at least two sites during CPB

Manifestations

Decreased MAP while on CPB
Signs of organ hypoperfusion
 Oliguria
 Slowing or "flat line" EEG
  May be seen normally during CPB secondary to hypothermia or barbiturate
  administration
If aortic dissection occurs, there may be
 Acute dilation and bluish discoloration of the aorta
 Low MAP
 Increase in the aortic line perfusion pressure
 Decrease in venous return
Insertion of the tip of the aortic cannula into one of the arch vessels will be manifested by
 Increase in the pressure of the arterial side of the CPB pump circuit
 Low MAP
 Otorrhea, rhinorrhea, conjunctival edema, and facial edema from cerebral hyperperfusion
Unexpectedly rapid administration of vasodilator
 Manifested by
  Rapid flow in the drip chamber
  Excessive movement of the moving parts of the infusion pump mechanism
 May be temporally related to connection of a new vasodilator drug infusion to the
  administration port of the CVP catheter or to a recent change in administration rate of
  a vasodilator

Similar Events

Artifacts of invasive blood pressure measurement (see Event 7, *Hypotension*)
Anaphylaxis (see Event 11, *Anaphylaxis and Anaphylactoid Reactions*)

Management

Confirm the low blood pressure
> Flush the arterial line
> Check the transducer, tubing, and arterial line for obstruction, kinking, loose connections, or air bubbles
> Check the calibration and zero of the transducer
> Check the pressure of the arterial side of the CPB pump circuit
> If there is pulsatile flow, measure blood pressure using an NIBP device

Inform the surgeon of the hypotension
> Have the surgeon palpate the aorta to assess the intra-aortic pressure
> Inspect the aorta to exclude dissection
> Check the position of the tip of the aortic cannula to confirm that it is in the aorta

Have the perfusionist check for and correct CPB circuit problems
> Inspect the CPB tubing for kinks, obstruction, or venous airlock
> Check the flow setting on the CPB pump
> Inspect the occlusion settings on the CPB roller pump

Inspect all vasodilator infusions
> If a vasodilator is being infused
>> Check the rate setting on the infusion pump or IV control device
>> Check the concentration of vasodilator
> If a vasodilator is not being infused
>> Turn stopcocks to the OFF position to exclude accidental administration of vasodilator

Stop administration of all vasodilators
> Effects of IV infusion of nitroprusside or NTG are short acting
>> Turning them off may be all that is necessary to correct hypotension
> Ensure that vaporizers are off or turned down

Restore the blood pressure
> Have the perfusionist transiently increase the CPB pump flow rate
> Administer phenylephrine IV (or directly into the oxygenator reservoir), 50–200 µg bolus
> If hypotension is persistent, consider instituting a phenylephrine or norepinephrine infusion

Check the hematocrit
> If the hematocrit is below 20%, add PRBCs to raise hematocrit and blood viscosity

Check ABGs and mixed venous blood gases
> If mixed venous O_2 tension is low or marked metabolic acidosis is present, tissue hypoperfusion is present
>> Increase the FIO_2 to 100%
>> Increase the pump flow rate
>> Administer $NaHCO_3$ to reverse severe metabolic acidosis

If aortic dissection has occurred
> Immediately terminate CPB

Recannulate the true aortic lumen distal to the dissection or cannulate the femoral artery
Surgical repair of the aortic dissection may be required

Complications

Aortic or great vessel dissection
Neurologic injury
Acute renal failure
Myocardial ischemia or infarction

Suggested Readings

DiNardo JA: Management of cardiopulmonary bypass. p. 217. In DiNardo JA, Schwartz MJ (eds):
Anesthesia for Cardiac Surgery. Appleton & Lange, East Norwalk, CT, 1990

Johnston WE: Aortic dissection with cardiopulmonary bypass arterial cannula. p. 21. In Reves JG, Hall
JD (eds): Common Problems in Cardiac Anesthesia. Year Book Medical Publishers, Chicago, 1987

Larach DR: Anesthetic management during cardiopulmonary bypass. p. 223. In Hensley FA, Martin DE
(eds): The Practice of Cardiac Anesthesia. Little, Brown, Boston, 1990

65 COAGULOPATHY FOLLOWING CARDIOPULMONARY BYPASS

Definition

Bleeding diathesis following CPB may be due to deficiency or dysfunction of platelets or of the coagulation cascade.

Etiology

Circulating anticoagulant
     Inadequate heparin neutralization
     Heparin rebound
     Protamine overdose
Thrombocytopenia
Impaired platelet function
Low plasma concentrations of coagulation factors
DIC
Primary fibrinolysis
Pre-existing congenital or acquired coagulopathy

Typical Situations

Patients who have had cardiac surgery previously

Prolonged time on CPB
> Increased platelet activation
> Consumption of coagulation factors

Surgery associated with major blood loss
Vigorous cardiotomy suction
Patients requiring a circulatory assist device
Patients undergoing deep hypothermia (core temperature below 20°C)
Pre-existing coagulopathy
> Drug therapy inhibiting platelet function (aspirin, dipyridamole)
> Hepatic dysfunction
> Anticoagulant therapy
> Thrombolytic therapy
> Chronic renal failure
> Myeloproliferative disorders
> Thrombocytopenia

Prevention

Identify patients with pre-existing clinical or subclinical coagulation disorders
> Obtain preoperative laboratory studies of coagulation function
>> PT, PTT
>> Platelet count, bleeding time

Keep CPB time as short as possible
Use a membrane oxygenator to minimize blood trauma and platelet activation
Minimize the negative pressure applied to the cardiotomy suction
Administer heparin and protamine in appropriate doses
> Monitor coagulation during CPB
> Maintain adequate anticoagulation (ACT above 400 seconds)

Use acute normovolemic hemodilution (remove whole blood pre-CPB for retransfusion post-CPB)
Discontinue medications preoperatively that are known to cause platelet dysfunction
Consider administering experimental pharmacologic therapy in high-risk cases
> Aprotinin
> ε-Aminocaproic acid
> Tranexamic acid

Have blood products available at the end of CPB for patients at high risk of a coagulopathy
> Patients who have had previous cardiac surgery
> Duration of CPB longer than 3 hours

Manifestations

Bleeding into the surgical field from multiple sites and from wound edges after administration of an adequate dose of protamine
Increased mediastinal chest tube output after the chest has been closed
Bleeding from IV insertion sites, wounds, or mucous membranes
Abnormalities in laboratory tests of coagulation function
> Prolonged ACT that does not correct with additional protamine
> Thrombocytopenia
> Prolonged PT and PTT

Increased thrombin time, reptilase time
Decreased fibrinogen level
Increased levels of fibrin split products
Hypotension, tachycardia
Pericardial tamponade

Similar Events

Surgical bleeding from an identifiable site
Acute hemorrhage (see Event 1, *Acute Hemorrhage*)
Transfusion reaction (see Event 41, *Transfusion Reaction*)
Erroneous laboratory results
Pericardial tamponade from other causes (see Event 16, *Pericardial Tamponade*)

Management

Surgical exploration is indicated if
The mediastinal chest tube drainage exceeds 300–400 ml in 1 hour, drainage is continuing, and laboratory tests of coagulation are normal
Signs of pericardial tamponade are occurring (see Event 16, *Pericardial Tamponade*)
Provide supportive therapy until bleeding is controlled
Maintain the circulating fluid volume
Infuse crystalloid, colloid, and blood as necessary
Use vasopressors as necessary to maintain the blood pressure (see Event 7, *Hypotension*)
Maintain normothermia (see Event 37, *Hypothermia*)
Use heating blankets and/or a forced-air warming device
Warm all IV fluids
Prevent hypertension
Maintain adequate sedation
Administer vasodilator agents
Consider judicious use of PEEP to decrease the amount of venous mediastinal bleeding following chest closure
Assess laboratory tests of coagulation function
Check the ACT
Administer additional protamine until the ACT returns to control or until there is no further reduction in the ACT
Check a bleeding time
Send samples to the clinical laboratory for
Platelet count
PT
PTT
Fibrinogen
Fibrin split products
Begin empirical therapy while waiting for laboratory results if bleeding is severe
Restore platelet numbers and function
Reinfuse any fresh whole blood removed from the patient prior to CPB after administration of protamine

Administer platelets (1–1.5 units/10 kg) should be administered and will increase platelet count by 50,000–80,000/mm^3

Infuse 4 units of fresh frozen plasma (adults)

Further use of blood products should be guided by laboratory results if practical

Consult a hematologist for further management of a coagulopathy that does not resolve

If primary fibrinolysis is thought to be the cause of bleeding

Administer ε-aminocaproic acid (5 g bolus infusion followed by 1 g/hr for 6 hours)

Complications

Transfusion reaction
Bloodborne virus infection
Hypervolemia
Mediastinitis following re-exploration

Suggested Readings

Campbell FW, Jobes DR, Ellison N: Coagulation management during and after cardiopulmonary bypass. p. 546. In Hensley FA, Martin DE (eds): The Practice of Cardiac Anesthesia. Little, Brown, Boston, 1990

Comunale ME, Lisbon A: Postoperative care of the cardiac surgical patient. p. 313. In DiNardo JA, Schwartz MJ (eds): Anesthesia for Cardiac Surgery. Appleton & Lange, East Norwalk, CT, 1990

Mammen EF, Koets EF, Washington BC et al: Hemostasis changes during cardiopulmonary bypass surgery. Semin Thromb Hemost 11:281, 1985

66 LOW CARDIAC OUTPUT STATE POST-CARDIOPULMONARY BYPASS

Definition

Inadequate cardiac output that occurs after separation from CPB.

Etiology

Poor ventricular function prior to surgery (ejection fraction less than 0.40)
Inadequate surgical repair or revascularization
Long aortic cross-clamp time
Inadequate myocardial protection while on CPB, especially when there has been
    Prolonged ventricular fibrillation before or after application of the aortic cross-clamp
    Inadequate myocardial cooling
    Ventricular distention
Myocardial ischemia or infarction in the preoperative or pre-CPB period
Arrhythmias

Typical Situations

Severe CAD
Severe valvular disease of the heart
Coronary embolism (particulate matter or air)
Acute pericardial tamponade
Acidosis
Hypoxemia
Hypovolemia
Increased SVR (from hypothermia or injudicious use of vasopressor agents)
Inadequate inotropic support
Surgically induced structural changes
      Residual intracardiac shunting
      Residual valvular obstruction or insufficiency (in prosthetic or native valve)
      Coronary artery dissection
Following administration of protamine

Prevention

Observe the techniques used for myocardial preservation and inform the surgeon of any compromise in their implementation
Control the patient's hemodynamic status carefully
Optimize the patient's condition prior to terminating CPB
      Commence IV infusions of inotropes and/or vasopressors or vasodilators as indicated clinically
      Correct metabolic acidosis, if present
      Ensure that there is sufficient blood volume in the oxygenator reservoir to restore the patient's circulating blood volume as CPB is terminated

Manifestations

Decreased cardiac output
Hypotension
Small increases in fluid volume cause disproportionate elevations of CVP and PCWP
Increased SVR
Reduced tissue perfusion
      Decreased peripheral perfusion
      Decreased mixed venous O_2 saturation
      Oliguria
      Acidosis

Similar Events

Artifact of blood pressure measurement system
      Faulty blood pressure transducer
      Transducer at inappropriate height
Spasm of radial artery or other lack of correlation between radial and central arterial pressure

Management

Optimize the cardiac rate and rhythm

    Maintain the heart rate at 70–100 bpm

        Epicardial pacemaker

            Sequential AV pacing will improve ventricular filling and increase stroke volume, especially if atrial contraction is required for maintenance of adequate cardiac output (e.g., aortic stenosis, low compliance of left ventricle)

        Pharmacologic assistance (e.g., dopamine, dobutamine, epinephrine, amrinone)

    Optimize heart rhythm

        Convert or control atrial fibrillation or junctional rhythms (see Event 19, *Supraventricular Arrhythmias*)

        Suppress arrhythmias (see Event 15, *Nonlethal Ventricular Arrhythmias*)

            Lidocaine IV, 1 mg/kg bolus, followed by an infusion of 1–4 mg/min

            Bretylium IV, 5 mg/kg, followed by an infusion of 1–2 mg/min

            Mg^{2+} IV, 1–2 g, by slow infusion

Optimize the cardiac filling pressures

    Administer fluid boluses to raise the PCWP by 10–20 mm Hg

    An even higher PCWP may be required in patients with a very low-compliance left ventricle preoperatively

Ensure adequate oxygenation and ventilation

    Ventilate the patient with an FIO_2 of 100%

    Check ABG measurement to ensure that the arterial pCO_2 is not increased

        Respiratory acidosis will compromise right ventricular function

Ensure that vasoactive drugs are reaching the circulation

    Check that infusion pumps are in fact administering vasoactive agents

    Check calculations to ensure that the appropriate dose is set on each infusion pump

Do not allow the heart to become overdistended

    Administer small boluses of epinephrine IV, 5–20 μg

    Be prepared to go back on CPB emergently

If low cardiac output state persists, consider placement of a mechanical device to augment cardiac output

    IABP

    Left ventricular assist device

Complications

Myocardial ischemia or infarction

Cerebral ischemia

Renal failure

Pulmonary edema

Complications of IABP or left ventricular assist device

    Impaired perfusion of lower extremity

    Thrombocytopenia

    Gas embolization

    Renal failure

    Causalgia

Suggested Reading

Comunale ME, Lisbon A: Postoperative care of the cardiac surgical patient. p. 318. In DiNardo JA, Schwartz MJ (eds): Anesthesia for Cardiac Surgery. Appleton & Lange, East Norwalk, CT, 1990

67 MASSIVE SYSTEMIC AIR EMBOLISM

Definition

Large volumes of air in the patient's arterial circulation during or after CPB is a massive systemic air embolism.

Etiology

Air pumped into the aorta through the aortic cannula from the CPB pump
Air sucked into the heart through the aorta cannulation site or from other sites when active suction has been applied to the left ventricle or PA for venting of the heart

Typical Situations

Air pumped into the aorta from the CPB pump
      Vortexing in an oxygenator with a low blood level
      Failure to set the oxygenator low-volume alarm during CPB
      When blood is being returned to the patient from the oxygenator following CPB
      When the perfusionist is distracted by the operation of other devices
            Intraoperative RBC salvage equipment
            IABP
            Blood gas analyzer
      Use of "hard shell" oxygenator or cardiotomy suction reservoirs
Urgent/emergent CPB requiring rapid setup of the oxygenator and CPB pump circuit
Reversal of vent or perfusion lines in pump head
      Flow would occur in the opposite direction to that intended
      The cardiotomy suction reservoir might become pressurized with air

Prevention

Ensure that the perfusionist takes appropriate care in the setup and pre-bypass check of the oxygenator and circuit
      Prime and remove all air from the oxygenator and lines prior to CPB
      Set the oxygenator low-volume alarm
      Incorporate an arterial line filter with a continuous vent to the oxygenator
Check that there is an adequate blood volume in the oxygenator reservoir during CPB
      Add volume to the circuit as necessary

An air lock in the atrial lines will cause venous return to the oxygenator to stop acutely
    The blood volume in the oxygenator will fall dramatically in seconds
Use extreme care when returning blood back to the patient following CPB
    The perfusionist typically disables the oxygenator low-volume alarm at this time
    If possible, return the blood through the venous line
    During reinfusion of blood through an aortic line, the surgeon should visually monitor the line for bubbles of air
        The surgeon should have a clamp available immediately to occlude the aortic line should air become visible in the tubing
    The perfusionist should clamp the blood return line when not in use in case the CPB pump head becomes activated inadvertently
Avoid the use of N_2O during and after CPB

Manifestations

Air may be visible
    In the aortic cannula from the oxygenator to the patient
    In the vein grafts
    In the chambers of the heart when TEE is used
    If the tubing in the roller pumps is reversed, air may be visible in other portions of the CPB pump circuit tubing
The oxygenator reservoir may be empty or may have an abnormally low air/blood level
Signs of myocardial ischemia or infarction may occur
    Air emboli are more likely to enter the vein grafts if the site of the proximal anastomosis is the anterior portion of the aorta
    Abnormalities of ECG morphology or rhythm
        ST elevation, often on the inferior leads II, III, AVF
        Heart block
        Ventricular arrhythmias
        Asystole
    Regional wall motion abnormalities
    Low cardiac output state after CPB
EEG activity may slow or become quiescent
The patient may be slow to awaken (see Event 45, *Postoperative Alteration in Mental Status*)
There may be major focal or diffuse cerebral dysfunction

Similar Events

Hypotension due to other causes (see Event 7, *Hypotension*)
Systemic embolization of particulate matter from the operative field

Management

Have the perfusionist stop the CPB pump
Place the patient in the steep Trendelenburg position

E
V
E
N
T

67

This will reduce embolization to the cerebral circulation

Remove as much air as possible from the circulation

The surgeon should immediately make a stab incision into the ascending aorta to allow air to escape

The surgeon should remove the aortic cannula

This allows more air to escape

This makes it easier to reprime the CPB pump

If CPB is to be continued, the surgeon must replace the aortic cannula

The surgeon should massage the heart and great vessels to dislodge trapped air

The surgeon can vent air from vein grafts using a small (25-gauge) needle and syringe, massaging the vein grafts

Have the perfusionist reprime the oxygenator and CPB pump circuit immediately

The surgeon may elect to attempt retrograde perfusion of the cerebral circulation through a superior vena cava cannula to backwash air out of the cerebral arteries

If retrograde cerebral perfusion is to be attempted, it must be instituted quickly, especially if the patient is normothermic

The heart can be perfused in a retrograde manner via a coronary sinus catheter

CPB must be reinstituted emergently if there has been significant coronary air embolization and the patient is unable to maintain an adequate cardiac output

Begin CPB gradually, increasing the flow rate up to twice normal

Partial aortic clamping distal to the aortic perfusion cannula may help force remaining air through the coronary arteries

Provide 100% O_2 to the patient

The goal is to denitrogenate the patient

If CPB is terminated, ventilate the lungs with 100% FIO_2

When CPB is reinstituted, use only O_2 and CO_2 in the gases supplied to the oxygenator

Increase the arterial pressure and support the heart

Use vasopressors as necessary (see Event 7, *Hypotension*)

Consider the use of mechanical assist device (IABP or left ventricular assist device) to aid separation from CPB

For treatment of cerebral air embolism, consider administering medications to attempt to reduce cerebral injury

The likelihood of cerebral injury is high, and these medications theoretically may be protective, but there is no definitive evidence that they can reduce the extent of cerebral injury when given <u>after</u> the event

Thiopental IV, 10–20 mg/kg

May have significant negative inotropic effects on the heart

Dexamethasone IV, 10–20 mg

Institute hypothermia to increase the solubility of air in the tissues

Compression in a hyperbaric chamber has been reported to reverse the adverse cerebral effects of a major systemic air embolus

This therapy is only available in a few medical centers

Most patients are too sick to be transported to a hyperbaric chamber

Complications

Stroke

Myocardial ischemia or infarction

Difficulty in separation from CPB
Arrhythmias
Renal failure
Cardiac arrest

Suggested Readings

Cooper JR: Air in the aortic perfusion cannula at conclusion of cardiopulmonary bypass. p. 75. In Reves JG, Hall KD (eds): Common Problems in Cardiac Anesthesia. Year Book Medical Publishers, Chicago, 1987

Lell WA, Huber S, Buttner EE: Myocardial protection during cardiopulmonary bypass. p. 932. In Kaplan JA (ed): Cardiac Anesthesia. 2nd Ed. WB Saunders, Philadelphia, 1987

Mills NL, Ochsner JL: Massive air embolism during cardiopulmonary bypass. J Thorac Cardiovasc Surg 80:708, 1980

Nussmeier NA, McDermott JP: Air embolism and subsequent central nervous system dysfunction. p. 187. In Reves JG, Hall KD (eds): Common Problems in Cardiac Anesthesia. Year Book Medical Publishers, Chicago, 1987

Profeta J, Silvay G: Postoperative right ventricular failure due to air in a coronary vein graft. p. 304. In Reves JG, Hall KD (eds): Common Problems in Cardiac Anesthesia. Year Book Medical Publishers, Chicago, 1987

Stoney WS, Alford WC, Burrus GR et al: Air embolism and other accidents using pump oxygenators. Ann Thorac Surg 80:708, 1980

Chapter Ten
Obstetric Events

68 AMNIOTIC FLUID EMBOLISM

Definition

An amniotic fluid embolism results from entry of amniotic fluid through the uteroplacental or endocervical veins into the maternal circulation, causing profound cardiopulmonary compromise.

Etiology

Direct communication of open uteroplacental and endocervical veins with amniotic fluid, allowing the fluid to enter the maternal venous and pulmonary circulation

Typical Situations

During labor and delivery
    Short or tumultuous labor or delivery
    Large fetus
    Cephalopelvic disproportion
In older parturients
When uterine stimulants are used during labor
In multiparous parturients
When placenta previa is present

Prevention

Avoid inappropriate use of uterine stimulants during labor

Manifestations

Respiratory distress
    Decreased O_2 saturation and cyanosis
    Dyspnea, pleuritic chest pain, coughing, or hemoptysis
Cardiovascular collapse
    Hypotension
    Pulmonary hypertension with right ventricular failure
        ECG signs of right heart strain
    Cardiac arrest
        EMD
        Asystole

Hyperreflexia, convulsions, coma

Chest x-ray may show diffuse pulmonary edema

If the patient survives the initial event, further complications may develop

       Uterine atony

       Left ventricular failure

       DIC

Similar Events

Thrombotic or venous air pulmonary embolism (see Event 18, *Pulmonary Embolism* and Event 20, *Venous Air or Gas Embolism*)

Aspiration of gastric contents (see Event 23, *Aspiration of Gastric Contents*)

Eclampsia (see Event 73, *Pre-eclampsia and Eclampsia*)

Toxic reaction to local anesthetic (see Event 43, *Local Anesthetic Toxicity*)

Hemorrhagic, septic, or anaphylactic shock (see Event 1, *Acute Hemorrhage* and Event 11, *Anaphylaxis and Anaphylactoid Reactions*)

Acute heart failure secondary to previous cardiac disease or tocolytic therapy

Intracranial hemorrhage

Management

Inform the obstetrician and call for help

       The obstetric team should apply fetal monitors

       Prompt delivery of the fetus and placenta is indicated

Ensure adequate oxygenation and ventilation

       Administer 100% O_2 by non-rebreathing face mask to the awake patient

       Intubate the trachea if there is loss of consciousness, respiratory failure, or cardiovascular collapse

              Initiate mechanical ventilation using 100% FIO_2

       Monitor oxygenation by pulse oximetry

       Consider other more common causes of hypoxemia (see Event 8, *Hypoxemia*)

Support the circulation

       Expand the circulating fluid volume

              Secure adequate IV access, preferably with two large-bore IV catheters

              Infuse boluses of 0.9% NS, 250–500 ml; or 5% albumin, 100–250 ml

       Administer vasopressors IV as indicated to maintain blood pressure

              Ephedrine, 5–20 mg bolus

              Phenylephrine, 50–200 µg bolus

              Epinephrine, 10–100 µg bolus

       Consider using IV infusions of inotropic agents for blood pressure support (see Event 7, *Hypotension*)

       Place an arterial line and a PA catheter for monitoring, blood sampling, and infusion of vasoactive medications

If the patient has no pulse, begin CPR

       Follow ACLS guidelines and see Event 2, *Cardiac Arrest* and Event 69, *Cardiac Arrest in the Parturient*

       Maintain left uterine displacement during CPR and until after delivery of the fetus

       If the patient is not already intubated

Ventilate the patient using 100% FiO_2, with cricoid pressure

Intubate the trachea as soon as possible

If CPR is unsuccessful within 5 minutes, consider immediate cesarean section

Send blood samples to the clinical laboratory for

ABG analysis

Treat acidosis as necessary (see Event 39, *Metabolic Acidosis*)

PT, PTT, fibrinogen, and fibrin split products

Type and cross-match for at least 4 units of blood if DIC develops or if cesarean section is likely

Prepare to administer blood, FFP, and/or platelets as necessary

Place a urinary catheter to monitor urine output

Perform a bleeding time if appropriate help is available

Consider administering corticosteroids

Hydrocortisone IV, 1–2 g

The diagnosis of amniotic fluid embolism is very difficult to make

The definitive diagnosis is frequently one of exclusion

Send samples of blood drawn from a CVP or PA line to pathology to check for fetal debris in blood samples

Complications

Fetal distress or death

Cardiac arrest

Cerebral hemorrhage

Cerebral anoxia

Aspiration pneumonitis

Suggested Readings

Kotelko DM: Amniotic fluid embolism. p. 377. In Shnider SM, Levinson G (eds): Anesthesia for Obstetrics. 3rd Ed. Williams & Wilkins, Baltimore, 1993

Sprung J, Cheng EY, Patel S, Kampine J: Understanding and management of amniotic fluid embolism. J Clin Anesth 4:235, 1992

69 CARDIAC ARREST IN THE PARTURIENT

Definition

The absence of effective mechanical activity of the heart and, in the spontaneously ventilating patient, cessation of effective ventilation in a parturient indicate cardiac arrest.

Etiology

Hypovolemia

Hypoxemia
Drug overdose or toxicity
Pre-existing cardiac disease
Trauma
Anaphylaxis
Pulmonary embolism

Typical Situations

Difficult tracheal intubation
Overdose of medication
      Total spinal
      Local anesthetic toxicity
      Tocolytic agent toxicity
Parturients with a high risk of major hemorrhage
      Placenta previa, accreta, increta, or percreta
      Abruptio placentae
      Uterine atony
Parturients with acquired or congenital heart disease
Parturients with a history of a previous thromboembolic event

Prevention

Evaluate the parturient's airway carefully
Place epidural catheters carefully and use appropriate tests and doses of local anesthetic during
    regional anesthesia
Anticoagulate patients with previous thromboembolic events
Manage parturients with cardiac disease carefully
      Obtain a consultation by a cardiologist
      Treat chronic arrhythmias
      Consider placing invasive monitors during labor
Careful administration of all medications to parturients with a history of drug allergies (see
    Event 11, *Anaphylaxis and Anaphylactoid Reactions*)
Use β-mimetic tocolytic agents with caution

Manifestations

No palpable peripheral pulses
Loss of consciousness or seizure in the awake parturient
Absence of heart tones on auscultation
Cessation of respiration in the spontaneously ventilating parturient
Cyanosis
Arrhythmias
      Ventricular fibrillation
      Complete AV block without escape rhythm
      Sinus arrest
      EMD
      Asystole
Bradycardia followed by asystole on the fetal heart rate monitor

Similar Events

Hypotension (see Event 7, *Hypotension*)
    May be caused or exacerbated by lack of left uterine displacement
Hypoxemia or cyanosis (see Event 8, *Hypoxemia*)
ECG artifact
Seizures (see Event 47, *Seizures* and Event 73, *Pre-eclampsia and Eclampsia*)

Management

Verify that there is a cardiac arrest
    Check peripheral pulses
    Check for respiration
    Check ECG if available
If cardiac arrest is present
    Inform the obstetrician and call for help
    Start CPR
    Follow management according to ACLS protocol (see Event 2, *Cardiac Arrest*) with the
        following caveats
Pregnant patients are always considered to have full stomachs
    Bag-and-mask ventilation should be performed with cricoid pressure
    The trachea should be intubated as quickly as possible
Maintain left uterine displacement during resuscitation
    Parturients are very difficult to resuscitate because aortocaval compression causes
        decreased venous return
If the fetus is viable and immediate resuscitative efforts are not successful, cesarean section should be performed quickly
    To maximize the chances for maternal and fetal survival, this decision should be made
        within 5 minutes of the arrest
    The mother is easier to resuscitate after delivery of the infant because aortocaval compression is relieved

Complications

CNS injury of mother or fetus
Death of mother or fetus

Suggested Readings

Emergency Cardiac Care Committee and Subcommittees, American Heart Association: Special resuscitation situations. JAMA 268:2242, 1992
Shnider SM, Levinson G, Ralston D: Regional anesthesia for labor. p. 135. In Shnider SM, Levinson G (eds): Anesthesia for Obstetrics. 3rd Ed. Williams & Wilkins, Baltimore, 1993

70 EMERGENCY CESAREAN SECTION

Definition

Emergency cesarean section is the immediate or urgent operative delivery of the fetus through an abdominal incision.

Etiology

Fetal or maternal emergency that in the opinion of the obstetrician requires an immediate or urgent cesarean

Typical Situations

Immediate cesarean section
      Severe fetal distress
      Prolapsed umbilical cord
      Massive hemorrhage
      Uterine rupture
Urgent, but not immediate, surgery
      Pre-eclampsia or eclampsia
      Malpresentation in labor
      Failure to progress in labor
      Mild fetal distress
      Chorioamnionitis
      Failed induction or trial of labor
      Repeat cesarean section, with unfavorable scar
      Failed forceps delivery

Prevention

Identify high-risk parturients
Optimize the volume status of the parturient
Maintain left uterine displacement to prevent aortocaval compression
Correct coagulopathy if present

Manifestations

The obstetrician declares an emergency requiring an immediate or urgent cesarean section

Similar Events

None

Management

In most patients presenting for <u>immediate</u> cesarean section, <u>general anesthesia</u> is the most suitable anesthetic technique.

Before induction of anesthesia

Call for help

Administer sodium citrate PO, 30 ml

Maintain left uterine displacement

Preoxygenate with 100% FiO_2

Check the fetal heart tones

If the fetal heart rate is normal, immediate surgery may <u>not</u> be necessary or there may be time to institute regional anesthesia

At induction of anesthesia

Apply cricoid pressure until the ETT is <u>confirmed</u> to be in the trachea

Perform a rapid-sequence induction

Sodium thiopental IV, 3–5 mg/kg (reduce the dose in patients who are hypotensive or have had an antepartum hemorrhage)

An alternative induction agent (especially for the hypotensive patient) is ketamine IV, 0.5–1.5 mg/kg

To produce complete muscle relaxation rapidly, administer succinylcholine IV, 1–2 mg/kg

Intubate the trachea and inflate the ETT cuff as quickly as possible

Confirm the position of the ETT

Check the capnograph waveform

Auscultate the breath sounds bilaterally

Observe chest movement

Allow the obstetrician to begin

Maintain general anesthesia

Ventilate the patient with 50% O_2/50% N_2O and a low dose of volatile anesthetic

Administer a short- or medium-duration nondepolarizing muscle relaxant after recovery from neuromuscular blockade with succinylcholine

After delivery of the neonate

Commence pitocin IV infusion, 20–30 units/L

Infuse IV fluid rapidly to maintain circulating fluid volume

Confirm adequate uterine contraction

Maintain general anesthesia with 30% O_2/70% N_2O

Discontinue the volatile anesthetic and administer IV narcotics for analgesia

After completion of the surgical procedure

Reverse neuromuscular blockade

Suction the oropharynx

Extubate the patient after the return of laryngeal reflexes, muscle strength, and consciousness

In patients who have a working epidural in place and in whom <u>immediate</u> cesarean section is indicated, it may be possible to avoid general anesthesia by following the directions for <u>urgent</u> cesarean section below, with the following modifications.

Increase the IV infusion rate immediately

Infuse 1500–2000 ml of non-glucose-containing crystalloid

Administer local anesthetic via the epidural catheter

Use 3% chloroprocaine or 2% lidocaine with epinephrine (1:200,000) and $NaHCO_3$ (1 ml of 8.4% $NaHCO_3$ per 10 ml of lidocaine)

Administer 10 ml of local anesthetic, then check fetal heart tones

If fetal heart tones are normal, the cesarean section may be canceled or postponed
If the cesarean section will proceed, administer an additional 5–10 ml of local anesthetic
Check the level of sensory block prior to incision
Be prepared to induce general anesthesia immediately if epidural anesthesia is inadequate at the time of surgical incision
Treat hypotension from epidural blockade by
Rapid infusion of non-glucose-containing IV fluid
Ephedrine IV, 5–25 mg

For cesarean section that is urgent but not emergent, it is not necessary to induce anesthesia in the most rapid fashion. Regional anesthesia is chosen most commonly in this situation.

Prior to establishing a major regional block
Infuse a 1500–2000 ml IV bolus of non-glucose-containing crystalloid
Administer sodium citrate PO, 30 ml
Administer metoclopramide IV, 10 mg bolus
Administer O_2 via nasal cannula
Maintain left uterine displacement
Place routine monitors on the patient
For spinal anesthesia
Perform a lumbar puncture using a small-gauge spinal needle
Administer 12 mg of hyperbaric 0.75% bupivacaine
This dose is appropriate except for patients at the extremes of height
Administer ephedrine IV, 5–10 mg, prophylactically when the spinal anesthetic is injected
Check the level of sensory block immediately after the patient has been positioned in the supine position with left uterine displacement
Trendelenburg position may be necessary to achieve adequate spread of local anesthetic to a T4 level
For epidural anesthesia
Insert an epidural catheter if not already in place
Administer a test dose of lidocaine 1.5%, 3 ml, with epinephrine 1:200,000
Check the level of sensory block before administering the full dose of local anesthetic
Administer 2% lidocaine with 1:200,000 epinephrine and $NaHCO_3$ (1 ml 8.4% $NaHCO_3$ per 10 ml of lidocaine)
15–25 ml administered in divided doses is adequate to achieve a T4 level of surgical anesthesia in most parturients
Convert to a general anesthetic if
The parturient does not have adequate surgical anesthesia with incision
Fetal distress is present
For general anesthesia
See the section above on general anesthesia for immediate cesarean section

Complications

Difficult endotracheal intubation
Local anesthetic toxicity
Failed epidural or subarachnoid block
Total spinal anesthesia

Suggested Readings

Hartwell BL: General anesthesia. p. 154. In Ostheimer GW (ed): Manual of Obstetric Anesthesia. Churchill Livingstone, New York, 1992

Shnider SM, Levinson G: Anesthesia for cesarean section. p. 211. In: Anesthesia for Obstetrics. 3rd Ed. Williams & Wilkins, Baltimore, 1993

71 HYPOTENSION FOLLOWING CONDUCTION BLOCKADE

Definition

Hypotension following conduction blockade is a decrease in arterial blood pressure of more than 25% below baseline, an absolute value of systolic pressure below 90 mm Hg, or MAP below 60 mm Hg.

Etiology

Sympathetic blockade from regional anesthesia
Aortocaval compression

Typical Situations

High level of conduction blockade
Inadequate hydration prior to instituting conduction blockade
Failure to treat with a vasopressor prior to induction of spinal anesthesia
Parturients in the supine position without left uterine displacement

Prevention

Maintain left uterine displacement at all times
Administer a fluid bolus of non-glucose-containing crystalloid prior to instituting conduction blockade
Administer vasopressor prophylactically in patients undergoing spinal anesthesia for cesarean section

Manifestations

Fall in or low arterial pressure (systolic, diastolic, or mean)
Nausea and vomiting in the conscious patient
Mental status changes
Arrhythmias
Weak or absent peripheral pulses
Inability of pulse oximeter or NIBP device to give a satisfactory reading

Decreased end-tidal CO_2 or decreased O_2 saturation
Decreased urine output
Diminished heart sounds

Similar Events

Artifact of blood pressure measurement system (see Event 7, *Hypotension*)
> Motion artifact with NIBP measurement
> Incorrect NIBP cuff size
> Transducer height artifact
> Faulty blood pressure transducer

Aortocaval compression
Hemorrhage (see Event 1, *Acute Hemorrhage* and Event 72, *Obstetric Hemorrhage*)
Amniotic fluid embolism (see Event 68, *Amniotic Fluid Embolism*)
Pulmonary or venous air embolism (see Event 18, *Pulmonary Embolism* and Event 20, *Venous Air or Gas Embolism*)
Total spinal anesthesia

Management

Expand the circulating fluid volume prior to initiating conduction blockade
> One large-bore IV line is usually adequate
> For a labor epidural or saddle block (spinal block to T10 level), infuse a bolus of at least 500 ml NS or LR
> For a high epidural or spinal anesthetic (T4 level) for cesarean section, infuse 1500–2000 ml NS or LR
> Alternatively, infuse 500 ml of colloid (e.g., Hetastarch 6%) with 1000 ml of crystalloid

Monitor the parturient frequently after initiating conduction blockade
> Blood pressure
> Level of sensory block

Administer prophylactic vasopressor if the parturient has a spinal anesthetic placed
> Administer ephedrine IV, 5–10 mg, at the time of administration of local anesthetic

Immediately check the blood pressure to rule out hypotension if
> The parturient complains of nausea or feeling faint
> The parturient is unresponsive to verbal stimuli
> The parturient complains of nasal congestion
> Fetal bradycardia or decelerations are observed
>> Persistent fetal distress will require immediate cesarean section (see Event 70, *Emergency Cesarean Section*)

If hypotension is diagnosed
> Place the parturient in the Trendelenburg position (10–20 degrees head down)
> Ensure adequate IV access
> Rapidly administer non-glucose-containing crystalloid IV fluid
> Administer a vasopressor
>> Ephedrine IV, 5–25 mg bolus
>> Phenylephrine IV, 25–100 µg bolus
>> Epinephrine IV, 5–100 µg bolus

Ensure adequate oxygenation and ventilation
>Administer 100% O$_2$ by non-rebreathing face mask to the awake patient
>Intubate the trachea if there is loss of consciousness, respiratory failure, or cardiovascular collapse
>>Initiate mechanical ventilation using 100% FiO$_2$
>Monitor oxygenation by pulse oximetry

If the blood pressure cannot be obtained
>Check for peripheral pulses
>If peripheral pulses are absent, commence CPR (see Event 69, *Cardiac Arrest in the Parturient*)

Complications

Cerebral or myocardial ischemia
Cardiac arrest
Aspiration of gastric contents
Pulmonary edema
Acute renal failure
Hypertension from treatment of artifact

Suggested Reading

Wright S, Shnider SM: Regional anesthesia in obstetrics. p. 397. In Shnider SM, Levinson G (eds): Anesthesia for Obstetrics. 3rd Ed. Williams & Wilkins, Baltimore, 1993

72 OBSTETRIC HEMORRHAGE

Definition

An obstetric hemorrhage is an episode of acute blood loss related to pregnancy.

Etiology

Placental pathology
Uterine pathology
Obstetric trauma
Coagulopathy

Typical Situations

Placenta previa: placenta located in the lower uterine segment over the cervix
>Parturients who have had a previous cesarean section or uterine surgery
>Multiparous or older parturients

Abruptio placentae: premature separation of the placenta after the 20th week of gestation
> Pre-eclampsia
> Trauma

Placenta accreta, increta, and *percreta:* abnormal placentation in which the placenta attaches *to, into,* or *through* the myometrium
> Parturients with placenta previa, especially with a history of previous cesarean section

Uterine rupture
> In patients who have had a previous cesarean section or uterine surgery
> Following prolonged labor
> Secondary to instrumentation during delivery

Uterine inversion
> May be caused by traction on the umbilical cord after delivery without careful abdominal pressure on the uterus

Uterine atony
> Multiparous patients
> Multiple gestation
> Polyhydramnios
> Macrosomia

Retained placenta

Lacerations of the cervix or vagina during delivery
> In forceps deliveries
> Large fetal weight

Coagulopathy
> Pre-existing bleeding diathesis
> Anticoagulant therapy
> Pre-eclampsia

Structural anomalies in the cervix or uterus

Prevention

Identify parturients at high risk of obstetric hemorrhage
> Ensure adequate IV access and the availability of blood for transfusion
> Prepare for pharmacologic treatment of uterine atony if necessary

Monitor parturients carefully when oxytocin is administered

Observe parturients carefully during forceps delivery

Monitor for and treat coagulopathies during labor and delivery

Manifestations

Abnormal bleeding (see Event 1, *Acute Hemorrhage*)
> From the vagina
> From the surgical site during a cesarean section

Decrease in blood pressure (See Event 7, *Hypotension*)

Increase in heart rate

Fetal bradycardia or decelerations

Decreased hemoglobin and hematocrit

Evidence of coagulopathy or DIC
> Oozing from puncture sites
> Abnormal coagulation studies

Similar Events

Anaphylactic or septic shock (see Event 11, *Anaphylaxis and Anaphylactoid Reactions*)
Hypotension from other causes (see Event 7, *Hypotension*)
Maternal dehydration
Fetal bleeding

Management

Check and verify blood pressure
Inform the obstetrician and call for help (see Event 1, *Acute Hemorrhage*)
>The obstetric team should consider monitoring the fetal heart rate

Maintain left uterine displacement
Ensure adequate oxygenation and ventilation
>Administer 100% O_2 by non-rebreathing face mask to the awake patient
>Intubate the trachea if there is loss of consciousness, respiratory failure, or cardiovascular collapse
>>Apply cricoid pressure until the position of the ETT is confirmed
>>Initiate mechanical ventilation using 100% FiO_2
>Monitor oxygenation by pulse oximetry
>Monitor ETT position and adequacy of ventilation by capnography
>Consider other more common causes of hypoxemia (see Event 8, *Hypoxemia*)

Support the circulation
>Treat severe hypotension with IV bolus of ephedrine, 5–50 mg; repeat as necessary to maintain an acceptable blood pressure
>>Phenylephrine IV, 50–200 µg; or epinephrine, 10–100 µg, <u>can</u> be administered if hypotension is severe and does not respond to other measures
>Expand the circulating fluid volume
>>Ensure adequate IV access, at least two large-bore IV cannulae
>>Infuse blood, colloid, or crystalloid rapidly
>>>Use a warmer for all IV fluids
>>Prepare for massive transfusion
>>>Send for blood products if they are not already in the room
>>>Inform the blood bank that more blood and blood products may be needed emergently
>>>Have an assistant set up a cell saver or rapid transfusion device, if available. This will occupy one person full-time

If the patient is under general anesthesia
>Decrease or discontinue volatile anesthetics until hypotension has responded to therapy
>Administer scopolamine IV, 0.2–0.4 mg, for amnesia
>Opiates and benzodiazepines may be given if hypotension has resolved

Treat uterine atony
>Oxytocin IV
>>Administer a 2–3 unit bolus
>>Add oxytocin 20–30 units/L of crystalloid for rapid infusion
>Methylergonovine
>>Administer 0.2 mg IM if uterine atony continues
>>Administer 0.2 mg IV, only in life-threatening situations
>>>Administer <u>slowly</u> in divided doses
>>>May cause severe hypertension and intracranial hemorrhage

The obstetrician may administer prostaglandin $F_2\alpha$ via intrauterine injection or IM, 250 μg
    May cause bronchospasm, nausea, vomiting, hypotension, and hypertension
Keep the obstetrician informed of the parturient's hemodynamic status
    If possible, the obstetrician should hold pressure on the bleeding site
    If there is profound shock, the obstetrician may need to clamp the uterine or iliac
        vessels, or perform a hysterectomy

If hemorrhage continues or is severe problem, send samples to the clinical laboratory for
    ABG
    Hematocrit
    PT, PTT, platelet count, fibrinogen, and fibrin split products
    Ionized Ca^{2+}, serum K^+

Complications

Cerebral or myocardial ischemia or injury
Aspiration pneumonitis
Transfusion reaction
Acute renal failure
Hypocalcemia
Hyperkalemia
Hypothermia
Coagulopathy
Volume overload
ARDS
Bloodborne infection

Suggested Readings

Bannon L: Obstetric hemorrhage. p. 228. In Ostheimer GW (ed): Manual of Obstetric Anesthesia.
    Churchill Livingstone, New York, 1992
Biehl DR: Antepartum and postpartum hemorrhage. p. 385. In Shnider SM, Levinson G (eds): Anesthesia
    for Obstetrics. 3rd Ed. Williams & Wilkins, Baltimore, 1993

---

73 PRE-ECLAMPSIA AND ECLAMPSIA

Definition

Pre-eclampsia is a multisystem syndrome of parturients, involving hypertension, peripheral
edema, and proteinuria:

The diagnosis requires at least two of these three signs in a parturient whose pregnancy is
    beyond 20 weeks' gestation or who has a molar pregnancy
If seizures have occurred, the syndrome is termed eclampsia

Etiology

Uncertain

Typical Situations

Parturients with pre-existing medical conditions
    Hypertension
    Renal disease
    Sickle cell anemia or other hemoglobinopathies
    Systemic lupus erythematosus or other collagen vascular diseases
Parturients who have received no prenatal care
Parturients with a history of pre-eclampsia
Molar pregnancy
Extremes of maternal age
Nulliparous parturient

Prevention

Identify patients at risk of pre-eclampsia
    The obstetrician may elect to treat the patient with aspirin to prevent pre-eclampsia

Manifestations

Hypertension, defined as
    Systolic blood pressure higher than 140 mm Hg or more than 30 mm Hg above baseline
    Diastolic blood pressure above 90 mm Hg or more than 15 mm Hg above baseline
Proteinuria, defined as
    More than 0.3 g of protein/L of urine in a 24-hour period (1–2+ on a "dipstick")
Edema
    Must be generalized (facial and upper extremity) as opposed to the dependent edema
        seen frequently in the lower extremities of normal pregnant women
As pre-eclampsia becomes more severe, systemic manifestations become more pronounced
    Cardiopulmonary
        Severe hypertension, pulmonary hypertension, decreased cardiac output, and CHF
        Pulmonary edema
            Secondary to CHF
            Secondary to pulmonary capillary leak, which can be exacerbated by a
                decrease in colloid oncotic pressure
    Renal
        Increased proteinuria
        Decreased renal blood flow, decreased glomerular filtration rate, elevated serum
            creatinine, elevated uric acid, proteinuria, oliguria, and acute renal failure
    CNS
        Hyperreflexia, clonus, headache, visual changes, somnolence, CNS irritability,
            cerebral edema, and ultimately seizures (eclampsia), intracranial hemorrhage
    Hematologic
        Platelet dysfunction with or without thrombocytopenia
        Elevated PT, PTT, and fibrin split products
        An elevated hematocrit reflects a decreased intravascular volume
    HELLP syndrome
    Obstetric complications
        Increased uterine irritability, decreased uterine blood flow, preterm labor, placen-
            tal abruption, intrauterine growth retardation, and fetal distress
    Epigastric pain

Similar Events

Hypertension
    Essential hypertension
    Pregnancy-induced hypertension without pre-eclampsia
Pre-existing congenital or acquired cardiac disease
Pre-existing renal disease (see Event 40, *Oliguria*)
Seizures from other causes (see Event 47, *Seizures*)
Coagulopathy or DIC from other causes
Pre-existing pulmonary disease

Management

These patients are at higher risk of fetal distress and may require urgent or emergent cesarean section. Early evaluation of the patient's airway, cardiac, pulmonary, and coagulation status will allow preparation for possible anesthetic intervention.

For labor, consider epidural analgesia
    Epidural analgesia will decrease catecholamine release and may improve uterine blood flow
    Use epidural analgesia cautiously in parturients who may not tolerate fluid loading
        If cerebral edema is present
        If cardiac, pulmonary, or renal function is compromised
            A PA catheter may assist in fluid management
    Check the platelet count and bleeding time prior to placing a lumbar epidural catheter
        The interpretation of bleeding time results is controversial
    Slow initiation of epidural blockade will minimize the hypotensive effects of sympathectomy
    The test dose of local anesthetic should <u>not</u> contain epinephrine
    If cesarean section becomes necessary, surgical anesthesia can be provided via the existing epidural catheter
Control the progression of pre-eclampsia, control the blood pressure, and protect the fetus
    Expand the circulating fluid volume
    Administer $MgSO_4$ IV, 4–6 g bolus, over 15 minutes followed by an infusion of 1–3 g/hr
        Mg^{2+} has anticonvulsant and tocolytic actions and is also a mild vasodilator
        Mg^{2+} enhances neuromuscular blockade of both nondepolarizing and depolarizing muscle relaxants
    Administer antihypertensive medications as necessary to maintain diastolic blood pressure at approximately 100 mm Hg
        Nifedipine SL, 10 mg
        Labetolol IV, 5–10 mg bolus
        Hydralazine IV, 5–10 mg bolus
        Sodium nitroprusside IV infusion, 0.25–2 µg/kg/min
        NTG IV infusion, 0.5–3 µg/kg/min
        Intra-arterial pressure monitoring is indicated if infusions of NTG or sodium nitroprusside are administered
If the patient is oliguric
    If O_2 saturation is low or the patient has signs of CHF, place a PA catheter prior to fluid administration

Optimize myocardial filling pressure
If O$_2$ saturation is normal and there are no symptoms or signs of CHF
Administer crystalloid or colloid in 250 ml boluses
If urine output does not increase after 1000–2500 ml, place a CVP or PA catheter to aid fluid management

If seizures occur (see Event 47, *Seizures*)
Administer 100% O$_2$ by face mask
If mask ventilation is necessary, apply cricoid pressure
Mask ventilation may be difficult if facial or upper airway edema is present
Intubate the trachea
A small ETT may be required
Administer an anticonvulsant
Thiopental IV, 50–100 mg
Diazepam IV, 2.5–5 mg
Midazolam IV, 1–2 mg
MgSO$_4$ IV, 2–4 g
Continue MgSO$_4$ by infusion
Maintain left uterine displacement

If general anesthesia is required for cesarean section
Consider placing an arterial line if not already present
Consider aggressive control of hypertension prior to induction and emergence
Sodium nitroprusside by infusion
Labetolol IV, 5–10 mg bolus
Esmolol IV, by bolus (10–50 mg) or infusion
Fentanyl IV, 50–150 µg
Small ETTs and equipment for difficult intubation should be in the operating room, ready for use (see Event 3, *Difficult Tracheal Intubation*)

Complications

Fetal distress
Coagulopathy
Severe hemorrhage
Difficult endotracheal intubation
Intracranial hemorrhage
Cerebral edema
Myocardial, respiratory, renal, or hepatic failure
Subcapsular hematoma of the liver

Suggested Readings

Gutsche BB, Cheek TG: Anesthetic considerations in preeclampsia. p. 305. In Shnider SM, Levinson G (eds): Anesthesia for Obstetrics. 3rd Ed. Williams & Wilkins, Baltimore, 1993
Moran DH: Pregnancy-induced hypertension. p. 25. In Ostheimer GW (ed): Manual of Obstetric Anesthesia. Churchill Livingstone, New York, 1992
Ramanathan J: Anesthetic considerations in preeclampsia. Clin Perinatol 18:875, 1991
Ramos-Santos E, Devoe L, Wakefield M et al: The effects of epidural anesthesia on the Doppler velocimetry of umbilical and uterine arteries in normal and hypertensive patients during active term labor. Obstet Gynecol 77:20, 1991

74 TOTAL SPINAL ANESTHESIA

Definition

Total spinal anesthesia is the production of excessive cephalad spread of local anesthetics in the CSF.

Etiology

Excessive dose of local anesthetic injected into the subarachnoid space during spinal or epidural anesthesia
Unrecognized dural puncture during placement of an epidural anesthetic
Migration of an epidural catheter into the subarachnoid space, with subsequent subarachnoid injection of local anesthetic

Typical Situations

Parturients who have a lower requirement for local anesthetic for conduction blockade
Difficult epidural needle or catheter placement

Prevention

Use the appropriate dose of local anesthetic
Administer a test dose of local anesthetic prior to administration of additional local anesthetic via an epidural catheter
    The test dose should be 3 ml lidocaine 1.5% with epinephrine 1:200,000
Use dilute solutions of local anesthetic solutions
Monitor parturients carefully during conduction blockade

Manifestations

Symptoms may develop very rapidly after inadvertent subarachnoid injection of a large volume of local anesthetic.

Hypotension
Nausea and vomiting
Nasal congestion
Bradycardia
Unresponsiveness
Respiratory arrest
Cardiac arrest

Similar Events

Hypotension from other causes (see Event 7, *Hypotension*)
Seizures (see Event 47, *Seizures* and Event 73, *Pre-eclampsia and Eclampsia*)
Local anesthetic overdose (see Event 43, *Local Anesthetic Toxicity* and Event 71, *Hypotension Following Conduction Blockade*)

Vasovagal episode
Medication error (see Event 60, *Syringe or Ampule Swap*)

Management

Resuscitation equipment and medications should be immediately at hand at all sites where conduction blockade is performed.

Call for help
Ventilate the parturient with 100% FIO$_2$ via bag and mask
  Apply cricoid pressure immediately
Check the blood pressure
Perform endotracheal intubation
  If the parturient has not lost consciousness and is not hypotensive, administer thiopental IV, 50–200 mg, for amnesia
  Succinylcholine IV, 1–1.5 mg/kg, may be necessary prior to intubation for adequate muscle relaxation
  Maintain left uterine displacement
Treat hypotension aggressively
  Administer a bolus of IV fluids, 250–500 ml rapidly
  Administer ephedrine IV, 5–25 mg boluses
  Treat bradycardia with atropine IV, 0.5–2 mg and/or ephedrine
  If hypotension does not respond rapidly to these measures, administer epinephrine IV, 10–100 µg
If cardiac arrest occurs
  Commence CPR immediately (see Event 69, *Cardiac Arrest in the Parturient*)
  If the fetus is viable and immediate resuscitative efforts are not successful, cesarean section should be performed quickly
    To maximize the chances for maternal and fetal survival, this decision should be made within 5 minutes of the arrest
    The mother is easier to resuscitate after delivery of the infant because aortocaval compression is relieved

Complications

Aspiration of gastric contents
Cerebral or myocardial ischemia or injury

Suggested Readings

Bussell GM, Levinson G: Anesthesia related mortality. p. 455. In Shnider SM, Levinson G (eds): Anesthesia for Obstetrics. 3rd Ed. Williams & Wilkins, Baltimore, 1993
Shnider SM, Levinson G, Ralston D: Regional anesthesia for labor. p. 135. In Shnider SM, Levinson G (eds): Anesthesia for Obstetrics. 3rd Ed. Williams & Wilkins, Baltimore, 1993

Chapter Eleven
Pediatric Events

75 ASPIRATION OF A FOREIGN BODY

Definition

A foreign body that is aspirated into the respiratory tract.

Etiology

Foreign body aspirated by the child
Tooth dislodged during airway manipulation enters the trachea
Surgical material left in the airway after a surgical procedure

Typical Situations

In children between 7 months and 4 years of age
   Foreign body aspiration is a leading cause of death in children younger than 1 year of age
   Food is the most common foreign body; however, beads, pins, tacks, coins, and parts of
      toys are also common
After a surgical procedure

Prevention

Encourage home-safety programs to keep small objects out of the reach of toddlers
Perform laryngoscopy carefully
Consider extracting loose teeth prior to laryngoscopy
Double check that all surgical materials placed in the airway are removed before extubation

Manifestations

Cough
Dyspnea
Cyanosis
Decreased breath sounds
Tachypnea
Stridor
Wheezing
Hemoptysis
Hoarseness
Fever
Aphonia

Radiographic visualization of the foreign body or of air trapping, infiltrates, or atelectasis

The most frequent site for a foreign body to lodge is a mainstem bronchus, the right mainstem being slightly more common than the left

Similar Events

Recurrent pneumonia not related to aspiration of a foreign body

Foreign body in the esophagus

Croup

Management

Confirm the diagnosis of foreign body aspiration

Check the O_2 saturation

Ensure adequate oxygenation and ventilation before proceeding further

Perform a physical examination of the airway and chest

Check for uniformity and symmetry of breath sounds, bronchospasm

Obtain a chest x-ray, looking for

The presence and location of a foreign body

Air trapping

Atelectasis

Pneumonia

Anesthetic Induction Protocol for the Patient with a Foreign Body Aspiration

Preoxygenate the lungs thoroughly before beginning induction of anesthesia

Complete airway obstruction may occur at any time; if so, rigid bronchoscopy must be performed <u>immediately</u> to remove the obstructing body or dislodge it to another site that permits ventilation of all or part of the lungs

Perform an inhalation induction with a volatile anesthetic and 100% O_2

Maintain spontaneous ventilation

Maintain the FIO_2 at 100%

Following induction of anesthesia the bronchoscopist typically intubates the trachea with a ventilating bronchoscope in order to remove the foreign body

There may be increased ventilatory resistance when a telescopic lens is inserted through the bronchoscope and controlled ventilation is attempted

Ventilation may need to be alternated with attempts to locate and remove the foreign body

Facilitate passage of the foreign body through the laryngeal inlet

Maintain an adequate depth of anesthesia to prevent patient movement or coughing

Consider administering a small dose of a short-acting muscle relaxant just prior to removing the foreign body

If the foreign body cannot be removed through the bronchoscope and ventilation is inadequate, an emergency thoracotomy and bronchotomy may be necessary

Following removal of the foreign body, the tracheobronchial tree should be examined for evidence of trauma or mucosal damage

Following endoscopic examination, intubate the trachea with an ETT and awaken the patient

The usual criteria for extubation should be applied

Complications

Pneumonia
        Chemical pneumonitis
        Bacterial infection
Airway rupture
Hypoxemia
Hypercarbia
Massive hemoptysis
Severe bronchospasm
Pneumothorax

Suggested Readings

Holzman RS: Advances in pediatric anesthesia: implications for otolaryngology. Ear Nose Throat J 71:99, 1992
Keon TP: Bronchoscopy for a foreign body. p. 203. In Stehling L (ed): Common Problems in Pediatric Anesthesia. 2nd Ed. Mosby-Year Book, St. Louis, 1992
Maze A, Bloch E: Stridor in pediatric patients. Anesthesiology 50:132, 1979
McGuirt WF, Holmes KD, Feehs R, Browne JD: Tracheobronchial foreign bodies. Laryngoscope 98:615, 1988
Pasaoglu I, Dogan R, Demircin M, et al: Bronchoscopic removal of foreign bodies in children: retrospective analysis of 822 cases. Thorac Cardiovasc Surg 39:95, 1991

76 EPIGLOTTITIS (SUPRAGLOTTITIS)

Definition

Epiglottitis (supraglottitis) is an infection of the epiglottis and supraglottic structures (arytenoid cartilage mucosa and aryepiglottic folds).

Etiology

Bacterial infection
        Haemophilus influenzae type B was the most common infecting organism prior to the use of the *Haemophilus influenzae* vaccine
        Group A streptococci
Viral infection
        Parainfluenza virus

Typical Situations

In children 3–5 years of age
        Epiglottitis can occur at any age, including infants, adolescents, or adults
        The frequency of occurrence of epiglottitis peaks in the spring and fall seasons

Prevention

Ensure that infants receive prophylactic vaccination against *Haemophilus influenzae*
Recognize and treat the infection early before significant airway compromise occurs

Manifestations

A convenient mnemonic consists of the "four d's": dysphagia, dysphonia, dyspnea, and drooling.

Abrupt presentation of symptoms of severe infection
>   The patient appears quite ill or toxic
>>   Tachycardia, flushing, and prostration may be observed
>   High fever
>   Severe sore throat and dysphagia

Stridor
>   If present, it is usually during inspiration only

No hoarseness is present
>   It is primarily the lingual surface of the epiglottis that is inflamed; the laryngeal surface of the epiglottis and the subglottic space are typically not involved

The patient often is sitting bolt upright, leaning forward in a sniffing position
>   This improves airflow past the swollen epiglottis
>   The mouth may be open with the tongue protruding
>   Drooling may be prominent because of dysphagia

Laryngeal tenderness to external palpation
Laboratory findings consistent with bacterial infection
>   Leukocytosis with an exaggerated number of immature leukocytes

Lateral radiograph of the neck shows a swollen "thumb sign" at the level of the epiglottis

Similar Events

Croup
>   Subglottic location
>   Younger age group
>   Gradual onset (days instead of hours)
>   Less acute and abrupt symptoms
>   "Steeple" sign on radiograph of anterior neck

Bacterial tracheitis
>   Barking cough atypical for supraglottitis (epiglottitis)
>   Gradual onset
>   No dysphagia, dyspnea, sore throat

Retropharyngeal abscess
>   Airway obstruction or stridor is common

Management

Early recognition of patients who may have epiglottitis is crucial so that the patient may be attended by personnel with appropriate airway management skills until definitive airway management or diagnosis is made.

Administer supplemental O₂ as early as possible

Establish IV access prior to induction of anesthesia ONLY if this can be done without exacerbating the airway compromise

If the patient is not in extremis, obtain a lateral and an anteroposterior radiograph of the neck

The patient should be attended by personnel with appropriate airway management skills

Secure the airway in the operating room if the patient requires immediate airway management or following a radiologic diagnosis of epiglottitis

Protocol for Securing the Airway in the Patient with Epiglottitis

Check that all anesthetic and surgical equipment is in place and is functioning correctly

Laryngoscopes

ETTs

Monitoring equipment

Rigid bronchoscope

Tracheostomy set

Induce general anesthesia by inhalation of halothane and 100% O₂ with the patient in the sitting position

When the patient loses consciousness

Maintain spontaneous ventilation

Begin CPAP (5–10 cm H₂O)

Change the patient's position from sitting to supine

Establish IV access if not already present

Establish an adequate depth of anesthesia for laryngoscopy, as judged by

Eye signs

Blood pressure and heart rate

Loss of prominence of intercostal muscle respiratory efforts and conversion to quiet diaphragmatic breathing

Perform direct laryngoscopy to assess the ease of intubation

Some clinicians prefer to topically anesthetize the airway at this point with lidocaine, 2–4%

Re-establish an appropriate depth of anesthesia for intubation

Intubate the trachea by direct laryngoscopy using either an oral or nasal ETT one-half to one size (0.5–1 mm internal diameter) smaller than normal

Once the airway is secure, blood cultures should be drawn and antibiotic therapy administered immediately

The patient may need to remain intubated for the next 24–48 hours in the ICU, although there is some evidence that two doses of antibiotics with a short (e.g., 6-hour) course of invasive airway support may be efficacious in many cases.

Complications

Systemic infection with the organism causing the epiglottitis

Hypoxemia

Hypercarbia

Pulmonary edema due to negative pressure inspiration with an obstructed airway

Suggested Readings

Adair JC, Ring WH: Management of epiglottitis in children. Anesth Analg 54:622, 1975

Crockett DM, Healy GB, McGill TJ, Friedman EM: Airway management of acute supraglottitis at the Children's Hospital, Boston: 1980–1985. Ann Otol Rhinol Laryngol 97:114, 1988

Davis HW, Gartner JC, Galvis AG et al: Acute upper airway obstruction: croup and epiglottitis. Pediatr Clin North Am 28:859, 1981

Gerber AC, Pfenninger J: Acute epiglottitis: management by short duration of intubation and hospitalization. Intensive Care Med 12:407, 1986

Goldhagen JL: Supraglottitis in three young infants. Pediatr Emerg Care 5:175, 1989

Hannallah RS: Epiglottitis. p. 277. In Stehling L (ed): Common Problems in Pediatric Anesthesia. 2nd Ed. Mosby-Year Book, St. Louis, 1992

Holbrook PR, Zaritsky AL: Pediatric intensive care. p. 661. In Motoyama EK, Davis PJ (eds): Smith's Anesthesia for Infants and Children. 5th Ed. CV Mosby, St. Louis, 1990

Morrison JE Jr, Pashley NR: Retropharyngeal abscesses in children: a 10-year review. Pediatr Emerg Care 4:9, 1988

Novotny W, Faden H, Mosovich L: Emergence of invasive group A streptococcal disease among young children. Clin Pediatr 31:596, 1992

Travis KW, Todres ID, Shannon DC: Pulmonary edema associated with croup and epiglottitis. Pediatrics 59:695, 1977

---

77 INABILITY TO VENTILATE A PATIENT WITH A MEDIASTINAL MASS

Definition

Tracheal or bronchial obstruction during or after anesthesia in a patient with an anterior mediastinal mass that results in an inability to ventilate the lungs.

Etiology

Extrinsic compression of the trachea
Erosion of tracheal cartilage (tracheomalacia)

Note: During normal spontaneous ventilation, a patient with an anterior mediastinal mass compensates for tumor encroachment on the trachea. The effects of volatile anesthetics and muscle relaxants decrease the muscular tone supporting the trachea. The supine position may cause a further increase in tumor blood volume and size. Even in the absence of extrinsic compression of the trachea, the cartilage's support of the trachea may be so weakened that the trachea will collapse.

Typical Situations

In patients with Hodgkin's lymphoma or (less commonly) non-Hodgkin's lymphoma
> The mediastinum is the primary site of involvement in 16–36% of non-Hodgkin's lymphoma and 54–81% of Hodgkin's lymphoma cases

In patients with known mediastinal masses due to teratomas, cystic hygromas, thymomas, hemangiomas, sarcomas, desmoid tumors, pericardial cysts, and Morgagni diaphragmatic hernias

Prevention

Carefully evaluate the patient for signs and symptoms of symptomatic tracheal compromise
> Intolerance of the supine position

Obtain flow-volume loops in the upright and supine position to evaluate for dynamic compression of the trachea

Obtain anteroposterior and lateral chest x-rays and a CT scan of the thorax in patients who are believed to have a mediastinal mass
> The size of a mediastinal mass and the degree of tracheal compression should be compared with age- and sex-adjusted normal subjects. In patients with tracheal cross-sectional areas less than 50% of predicted, consideration should be given to use of local anesthesia ONLY for performing biopsy
> Preoperative radiation treatment (with shielding of a biopsy site) may have to be considered, even prior to tissue diagnosis, if the airway risk outweighs the immediate need for tissue diagnosis

Have a rigid bronchoscope available during induction of anesthesia

Consider lifesaving maneuvers such as changes in position or CPB for those at highest risk

Manifestations

Preoperative symptoms of patients with a mediastinal mass
> Cough
> Dyspnea or orthopnea
> Cyanosis
> Stridor or wheezing
> Fatigue
> Syncope
> Headache

Superior vena cava syndrome also suggests a mediastinal mass
> Facial edema
> Jugular distention
> Papilledema
> Pulsus paradoxus

Intraoperative manifestations
> Inability to maintain a patent airway
> Difficulty in advancing an ETT
> Inability to ventilate through an ETT
> Hypoxemia
> Hypercarbia

Patients with masses compressing the PA may be relatively asymptomatic while awake and yet may develop severe, life-threatening hypoxemia during anesthetic induction or even with sedation, requiring emergency extracorporeal bypass.

Similar Events

Upper airway obstruction at the level of the laryngeal inlet producing stridor

Anatomic pathology in the neck producing extrinsic <u>extrathoracic</u> tracheal compression, tracheomalacia, or laryngomalacia

Stridor due to tracheobronchitis or bacterial tracheitis
Pneumonia
CHF
Bronchospasm (see Event 24, *Bronchospasm*)

Management

In Patients At Risk of Tracheal Collapse Who Must Undergo General Anesthesia
Preoxygenate the lungs
Use an anesthetic technique that preserves spontaneous ventilation
>   Awake intubation followed by gradual induction with a volatile anesthetic or an IV anesthetic
>   Inhalation induction by mask with a volatile anesthetic and 100% O_2

If Tracheal Obstruction Occurs
Maintain oxygenation at all costs
Intubate the trachea with a rigid bronchoscope and advance it beyond the level of the obstruction
Change the patient's position
>   Left or right decubitus position
>   Sitting upright position
>   Semi-Fowler's position

Extubation of Patients at Risk of Tracheal Collapse
Proceed with caution
>   Tachypnea on emergence may worsen airflow and aggravate pre-existing airway obstruction
>   Tracheomalacia may first reveal itself postoperatively, and it may persist for some time after tumor resection
>   The trachea may have to be reintubated postoperatively
>   Airway support and mechanical ventilation may have to continue in the ICU during the postoperative period

Complications

Complete airway obstruction with inability to ventilate
Hypoxemia
Lack of pulmonary blood flow with encroachment of tumor on the pulmonary circulation and right heart, resulting in sudden hypoxemia, hypotension, and cardiac arrest

Suggested Readings

Bray RJ, Fernandes FJ: Mediastinal tumour causing airway obstruction in anaesthetized children. Anaesthesia 37:571, 1982
Ferrari LR: Supraclavicular node biopsy and mediastinal mass. p. 457. In Stehling L (ed): Common Problems in Pediatric Anesthesia. 2nd Ed. Mosby-Year Book, St. Louis, 1992
Froese AB, Bryan AC: Effects of anesthesia and paralysis on diaphragmatic mechanics in man. Anesthesiology 41:242, 1974
Griscom NT: Computed tomographic determination of tracheal dimensions in children and adolescents. Radiology 145:361, 1982

78 E
V
E
N
T

Griscom NT, Wohl MEB: Dimensions of the growing trachea related to age and gender. AJR 146:233, 1986

Hanagiri T, Shirakusa T, Okabayashi K et al: Resection of tracheal carcinoma using partial cardiopul-monary bypass—report of a case. Nippon Kyobu Geka Gakkai Zasshi 40:1285, 1992

Keon TP: Death on induction of anesthesia for cervical node biopsy. Anesthesiology 55:471, 1981

Levin H, Bursztein S, Heifetz M: Cardiac arrest in a child with a mediastinal mass. Anesth Analg 64:1129, 1985

Loeffler JS, Leopold KA, Recht A et al: Emergency prebiopsy radiation for mediastinal masses: impact on subsequent pathologic diagnosis and outcome. J Clin Oncol 4:716, 1986

Piro AJ, Weiss DR, Hellman S: Mediastinal Hodgkin's disease: a possible danger for intubation anaesthe-sia. Int J Radiat Oncol Biol Phys 1:415, 1976

Price SL, Hecker BR: Pulmonary oedema following obstruction in a patient with Hodgkin's disease. Br J Anaesth 59:518, 1987

Pullerits J, Holzman R: Anaesthesia for patients with mediastinal masses. Can J Anaesth 36:681, 1989

Shamberger RC, Holzman RS, Griscom NT et al: CT quantitation of tracheal cross-sectional area as a guide to the surgical and anesthetic management of children with anterior mediastinal masses. J Pediatr Surg 26:138, 1991

Sibert KS, Biondi JW, Hirsch NP: Spontaneous respiration during thoracotomy in a patient with a mediasti-nal mass. Anesth Analg 66:904, 1987

78 INFANTILE STRIDOR

Definition

Stridor in an infant younger than 6 months of age that results from partial obstruction or nar-rowing of the upper airway, producing airflow turbulence.

Etiology

Narrowing of the subglottic region due to
    Congenital narrowing
    Acquired disease
    Inflammation and edema from mechanical irritation by an ETT

Typical Situations

Congenital or acquired laryngeal, subglottic, or tracheal stenosis
    Laryngeal webs
    External compression by cysts, tumors, or vascular rings
    Laryngocele, laryngeal cyst
    Laryngotracheoesophageal cleft
Laryngeal edema
Laryngomalacia or tracheomalacia
Vocal cord paralysis
Hereditary angioneurotic edema

Prevention

Use the correct size ETT in infants
> Use an uncuffed ETT
> A small air leak at 20–25 cm H_2O PIP should be present around the ETT

Conduct an extensive evaluation of the entire airway when the patient has congenital malformations, cysts, or tumors

Manifestations

Noisy respirations, particularly during inspiration
Paradoxical inward chest wall movement during inspiration
Decreased or low O_2 saturation measured by pulse oximetry
> Pulse oximetry may not function properly in the presence of hypothermia or poor peripheral circulation

Cyanosis
Hypercarbia

Similar Events

Reflex laryngospasm (see Event 79, *Laryngospasm*)
Bronchiolitis
Acute respiratory distress syndrome
Asthma (see Event 24, *Bronchospasm*)
Cystic fibrosis
Bronchopulmonary dysplasia
Vocal cord dysfunction secondary to Arnold-Chiari type II malformation (myelomeningocele)

Management

Increase FiO$_2$ to 100%
> Administer 100% O_2 by mask
> Verify that FiO$_2$ approaches 100%

Attempt to open the airway
> Use standard airway maneuvers (jaw thrust, oral or nasal airway insertion)
> Apply positive airway pressure with a tight seal between the face and mask
> Preserve spontaneous breathing if at all possible, since this maintains laminar flow in the distal airways better than controlled ventilation
> Clear the airway of secretions

Assume that low O_2 saturation indicates actual hypoxemia until proven otherwise. If the patient's clinical condition is stable, verify that the pulse oximeter is functioning correctly
> Assess the adequacy of the pulse amplitude
> Check the probe position
> Change the site of the probe (from finger to ear)
> Correlate oximeter readings with activation of electrocautery
> Shield the probe from ambient light
> Test the oximeter probe on yourself

Prepare to establish an airway by invasive means; move aggressively to invasive procedures if oxygenation cannot be maintained

Endotracheal intubation

Consider the use of a rigid bronchoscope if tracheomalacia or external airway compression is the etiology

Cricothyrotomy with transtracheal jet ventilation

Tracheostomy

Complications

Hypoxemia

Hypercarbia

Myocardial arrhythmias

Aspiration of gastric contents

Cardiac arrest

Suggested Readings

Holinger LD: Etiology of stridor in the neonate, infant and child. Ann Otol Rhinol Laryngol 89:397, 1980

Holzman RS: Advances in pediatric anesthesia: implications for otolaryngology. Ear Nose Throat J 71:99, 1992

Kanter RK, Pollack MM, Wright WW, Grundfast KM: Treatment of severe tracheobronchomalacia with continuous positive airway pressure (CPAP). Anesthesiology 57:54, 1982

Maze A, Bloch E: Stridor in pediatric patients. Anesthesiology 50:132, 1979

79 LARYNGOSPASM

Definition

Laryngospasm is occlusion of the glottis and laryngeal inlet by action of the laryngeal muscles.

Etiology

The mechanism of glottic spasm is uncertain

Glottic closure reflex by intrinsic adductor muscles

This reflex does not usually persist beyond the initiating stimulus, whereas laryngospasm does

Glottic closure by extrinsic muscles of the larynx, primarily the thyrohyoid muscles

This may shorten the larynx and create a "ball valve" mechanism

Typical Situations

During the excitement phases of anesthetic induction or emergence

During light anesthesia relative to the surgical stimulus

When there are mechanical irritants in the airway
    Blood or secretions
    Airway instrumentation
In patients with gastroesophageal reflux
In patients with active upper respiratory tract infection
    This is controversial; one study showed an incidence of 0.85%, another an incidence of 5%

Prevention

Ensure an adequate depth of anesthesia prior to laryngeal manipulation
Extubate the trachea when the patient is either deeply anesthetized or is fully awake
Clear all secretions from the airway prior to and after extubation
Use muscle relaxants to facilitate tracheal intubation
Consider the use of topical local anesthetics to "de-afferent" the larynx

Manifestations

Stridor
Hypoxemia
Tachypnea
Tachycardia
Increase in pharyngeal secretions
Retractions (sternal, intercostal)
No airflow despite ventilatory efforts
Inability to phonate

Similar Events

Extrathoracic respiratory tract obstruction from other causes
Postextubation croup (see Event 83, *Postextubation Croup*)
Intratracheal foreign bodies (see Event 75, *Aspiration of a Foreign Body*)
Infectious croup
Subglottic hemangioma
Webs
Vocal cord dysfunction or tumor
Arytenoid dislocation from traumatic instrumentation of the larynx
Pharyngeal edema or abcess
Angioneurotic edema
Pneumothorax or pneumomediastinum (see Event 28, *Pneumothorax*)

Management

Institute CPAP with an FIO_2 of 100% using a bag and mask
    CPAP may break laryngospasm by lowering the pressure gradient across the obstructed
        segment and possibly by pneumatically stenting the pharyngeal and laryngeal muscles
Use maximum efforts to open the airway
    Jaw thrust, head tilt, oral or nasal airway

Monitor oxygenation carefully

Suction the oropharynx

If helium or heliox is available, consider ventilating the patient with a helium and O_2 mixture

> Helium/O_2 mixtures have a lower density than O_2 alone
>
> During turbulent flow, gas density determines flow characteristics

If laryngospasm does not break, administer succinylcholine IV, 0.1–0.3 mg/kg; or IM, 0.2–0.6 mg/kg

> Establish positive pressure ventilation with PEEP by bag and mask
>
> Maintain a patent airway
>
> Allow spontaneous ventilation to return after muscle relaxation resolves

Prepare for more invasive maneuvers to establish an airway; move to the next invasive maneuver if oxygenation cannot be maintained

> Reintubation
>
> > Have a wide selection of ETT sizes available
>
> Cricothyrotomy with transtracheal jet ventilation
>
> Tracheostomy

Complications

Hypoxemia

Hypercarbia

Bradycardia

Arrhythmias

Cardiac arrest

Pulmonary edema

Suggested Readings

Burton DM, Pransky SM, Katz RM et al: Pediatric airway manifestations of gastroesophageal reflux. Ann Otol Rhino Laryngol 101:742, 1992

Lee KW, Downes JJ: Pulmonary edema secondary to laryngospasm in children. Anesthesiology 59:347, 1983

Lorch DG, Sahn SA: Post-extubation pulmonary edema following anesthesia induced by upper airway obstruction. Are certain patients at increased risk? Chest 90:802, 1986

McConachie IW, Day A, Morris P: Recovery from anaesthesia in children. Anaesthesia 44:986, 1989

Olsson GL, Hallen B: Laryngospasm during anaesthesia: a computer-aided incidence study in 136,929 patients. Acta Anaesthesiol Scand 28:567, 1984

Patel RI, Hannallah RS, Norden J et al: Emergence airway complications in children a comparison of tracheal extubation in awake and deeply anesthetized patients. Anesth Analg 73:266, 1991

Rex M: A review of the structural and functional basis of laryngospasm: nerve pathways and clinical significance. Br J Anaesth 42:891, 1970

Rolf N, Cote CJ: Frequency and severity of desaturation events during general anesthesia in children with and without upper respiratory infections. J Clin Anesth 4:200, 1992

Sasaki CT, Suzuki M: Laryngeal spasm: a neurophysiologic redefinition. Ann Otol Rhino Laryngol 86:150, 1977

80 LATEX ANAPHYLAXIS

Definition

Anaphylaxis that is caused by exposure to latex-containing products in a sensitized patient.

Etiology

Low molecular weight polypeptides from natural latex have the ability to bind to specific human IgE and cause an anaphylactic (type I hypersensitivity) response (see Event 11, *Anaphylaxis and Anaphylactoid Reactions*)

Typical Situations

Children with myelomeningocele (spina bifida) who return to the operating room for multiple surgical procedures

Patients with congenital genitourinary abnormalities or multiple reconstructive surgical procedures

Health care or other personnel, especially those with a history of atopy, who work with or around latex

Prevention

Obtain a careful history of previous allergic reactions, atopy, or asthma
    Specifically inquire of any history of allergy to balloons, household gloves, rubber dental dams, or condoms
If there is a history of latex allergy, establish a latex-free environment
    Avoid contact with or manipulation of latex devices
    Use nonlatex surgical gloves
    Use syringe/stopcock methods or unidirectional valves for injecting medications
    Do not use natural rubber stoppers with multiple-dose vials
        Take the top of the vial completely off
        Use the same medication from a glass ampule
        Use glass syringes as an alternative to rubber-plunger plastic syringes

Manifestations

All manifestations may not be present simultaneously.

Hypotension
Tachycardia
Bronchospasm
Flushing
Urticaria

Similar Events

Transfusion reaction (see Event 41, *Transfusion Reaction*)
Cutaneous allergy (rapid urticarial reactions)
Bronchospasm (see Event 24, *Bronchospasm*)

Hypotension from other causes (see Event 7, *Hypotension*)

Pulmonary edema from other causes (see Event 17, *Pulmonary Edema*)

Cutaneous manifestations of mastocytosis, carcinoid syndrome, hereditary angioedema

Anesthetic overdose (see Event 62, *Volatile Anesthetic Overdose*)

Pericardial tamponade (see Event 16, *Pericardial Tamponade*)

Stridor (see Event 78, *Infantile Stridor*)

Pulmonary embolism (see Event 18, *Pulmonary Embolism*)

Aspiration of gastric contents (see Event 23, *Aspiration of Gastric Contents*)

Pneumothorax (see Event 28, *Pneumothorax*)

Management

Remove the antigenic stimulus
> Identify all latex products and remove from contact with the patient

Administer epinephrine IV, 0.1 µg/kg (1 µg to a 10-kg child)
> Repeat as necessary

Inform the surgeons
> Check to see whether they have injected or instilled other potential antigens into a body cavity
> Prepare to terminate the surgical procedure if there is no response to treatment

Maintain the patient's airway and support oxygenation and ventilation
> Increase the FiO_2 to 100%
> Intubate if necessary
> The airway and larynx can become very edematous

Decrease or stop the administration of anesthetic agents if hypotension is present
> If bronchospasm is present and the patient is normotensive, volatile anesthetic agents may be administered to counteract bronchospasm

Expand the circulating fluid volume rapidly
> Immediate fluid needs may be <u>massive</u>
> Insert a large-bore IV catheter

Administer corticosteroids
> Dexamethasone IV, 0.2 mg/kg bolus
> Methylprednisolone IV, 1 mg/kg bolus

Doses of epinephrine recommended for resuscitation during cardiac arrest are higher than those required for the treatment of anaphylaxis and, if administered to patients with anaphylaxis, may lead to severe hypertension, supraventricular tachycardia, or ventricular arrhythmias.

Complications

Inability to intubate, ventilate, or oxygenate

Cardiac arrest

Hypertension, tachycardia from vasopressors

Suggested Readings

Gerber AC, Jorg W, Zbinden S et al: Severe intra-operative anaphylaxis to surgical gloves: latex allergy, an unfamiliar condition. Anesthesiology 71:800, 1989

Gold M, Swartz JS, Braude BM et al: Intraoperative anaphylaxis an association with latex sensitivity. J Allergy Clin Immunol 87:662, 1991

Holzman RS: Latex allergy: an emerging operating room problem. Anesth Analg 76:635, 1993

Holzman RS, Sethna NF: A "latex-safe" environment prevents allergic reactions in latex-allergic patients. Anesth Analg 76:S148, 1993

Holzman RS, Sethna NF: Preoperative profile of latex-allergic patients. Anesth Analg 76:S149, 1993

Kwittken PL, Becker J, Oyefara B et al: Latex hypersensitivity reactions despite prophylaxis. Allergy Proc 13:123, 1992

Meeropol E, Frost J, Pugh L et al: Latex allergy in children with myelodysplasia: a survey of Shriners hospitals. J Pediatr Orthop 13:1, 1993

Mostello LA: Myelomeningocele and orthopedic surgery. p. 450. In Stehling L (ed): Common Problems in Pediatric Anesthesia. 2nd Ed. Mosby-Year Book, St. Louis, 1992

Slater JE: Allergic reactions to natural rubber. Ann Allergy 68:203, 1992

Slater JE: Rubber anaphylaxis. N Engl J Med 320:1126, 1989

Slater JE, Chabra SK: Latex antigens. J Allergy Clin Immunol 89:673,1992

Slater JE, Mostello LA, Shaer C: Rubber-specific IgE in children with spina bifida. J Urol 146:578, 1991

Yassin MS, Sanyurah S, Lierl MB et al: Evaluation of latex allergy in patients with meningomyelocele. Ann Allergy 69:207, 1992

81 MASSETER MUSCLE SPASM

Definition

Masseter muscle spasm is a tightening of the masseter muscle during induction of anesthesia.

Etiology

The etiology is uncertain
> It is unclear why a depolarizing relaxant can produce a persistent increase in muscle tension in the muscles of mastication while producing relaxation in other skeletal muscles

Typical Situations

Following administration of succinylcholine during induction of anesthesia in children using a volatile anesthetic

Prevention

Avoid using succinylcholine during anesthesia with a volatile anesthetic

Administer the correct dose of succinylcholine and wait a sufficient time for it to produce muscle relaxation prior to attempting laryngoscopy

Manifestations

Subjective difficulty in opening the mouth
> This can range from a slight increase in masseter muscle resistance to apparent active tetany

Administration of additional succinylcholine does not result in relaxation of the masseter muscles

Other skeletal muscles are typically relaxed

In some cases other muscles may be in spasm as well

The masseter spasm persists until neuromuscular function begins to return in the peripheral musculature

Increased tension of the masseter muscle may last as long as 30 minutes

Myalgia and weakness may be present for as long as 36 hours following the acute episode

Elevation of CK and myoglobinuria can follow masseter muscle spasm within 24 hours

Some patients will go on to develop MH (see Event 38, *Malignant Hyperthermia*)

Halothane–caffeine contracture testing for MH susceptibility is positive in more than 50% of patients with a history of succinylcholine-induced masseter muscle spasm

Similar Events

Congenital or acquired anatomic abnormalities that restrict mouth opening

Hemifacial microsomia, diseases of the temporomandibular joint, prior surgical procedures producing contractures

Light anesthesia

Normal increase in masseter muscle tension during induction of anesthesia and administration of succinylcholine

Malignant hyperthermia (see Event 38, *Malignant Hyperthermia*)

Inadequate level of neuromuscular blockade

Management

Maintain positive pressure ventilation with bag and mask until the masseter muscles relax

Even though it is difficult to open the mouth, positive pressure ventilation is typically not a problem

Intubate the trachea whenever it becomes feasible to do so

Observe the patient carefully for the signs of MH

Skeletal muscle rigidity

Increased CO_2 production and O_2 consumption

Metabolic acidosis

Tachycardia or arrhythmias

Increase in body temperature

Myoglobinuria

If MH is developing or is strongly suspected

Declare an MH emergency (see Event 38, *Malignant Hyperthermia*)

If there is no evidence of MH, recent studies suggest that continuing the anesthetic does not result in the later evolution of a MH crisis. However, this approach is controversial. Triggering agents can be replaced by other anesthetics and muscle relaxants, although there is no evidence that this will prevent the development of MH. If the surgery is elective and there is any doubt, it may be appropriate to abort the surgery.

Complications

Inability to intubate the trachea

Difficulty maintaining ventilation by mask

Hypoxemia

Suggested Readings

Brandom BW: Masseter spasm. p. 337. In Stehling L (ed): Common Problems in Pediatric Anesthesia. 2nd Ed. Mosby-Year Book, St. Louis, 1992

Brandom BW, Carroll JB, Rosenberg H: Malignant hyperthermia. p. 763. In Motoyama EK, Davis PJ (eds): Smith's Anesthesia for Infants and Children. 5th Ed. CV Mosby, St. Louis, 1990

Holzman RS: Mass spectrometry for early diagnosis and monitoring of malignant hyperthermia crisis. Anesth Rev 15:31, 1988

Kosko JR, Brandom BW, Chan KH: Masseter spasm and malignant hyperthermia: a retrospective review of a hospital-based pediatric otolaryngology practice. Int J Pediatr Otorhinolaryngol 23:45, 1992

Ryan JF: Malignant hyperthermia. p. 421. In Cote CJ, Ryan JF, Todres ID, Goudsouzian NG (eds): A Practice of Anesthesia for Infants and Children. 2nd Ed. WB Saunders, Philadelphia, 1993

Van der Spek AF: Triggering agents continued after masseter spasm: there is proof in this pudding! Anesth Analg 73:364, 1991

Van der Spek AF, Fang WB, Ashton-Miller JA et al: Increased masticatory muscle stiffness during limb muscle flaccidity associated with succinylcholine administration. Anesthesiology 69:11, 1988

Van der Spek AF, Fang WB, Ashton-Miller JA et al: The effects of succinylcholine on mouth opening. Anesthesiology 67:459, 1987

Van der Spek AF, Reynolds PI, Fang WB et al: Changes in resistance to mouth opening induced by depolarizing and nondepolarizing neuromuscular relaxants. Br J Anaesth 64:21, 1990

82 NEONATAL ASPHYXIA

Definition

Asphyxia in a neonate is a reduction in arterial pO_2 and increase in arterial pCO_2 as a result of inadequacy of the placenta or lung for gas exchange.

Etiology

Failure of neonatal ventilation
Neonatal heart failure

Typical Situations

Neonatal asphyxia frequently accompanies fetal distress or asphyxia in utero, which can be caused by maternal hypoxia, decreased placental-umbilical blood flow, or fetal heart failure due to

  Obstetric emergencies (abruptio placentae, placenta previa, antepartum hemorrhage)
  Maternal hypotension
  Adverse conditions of labor and delivery (forceps delivery, breech presentation and delivery, prolonged labor, prolapsed cord)
  Chronic maternal systemic illness (diabetes, hypertension, pre-eclampsia, and eclampsia)
  Respiratory or myocardial depressant medications administered to the mother
    Narcotics
    Barbiturates

Fetal conditions, such as multiple births, small-for-gestational-age, meconium staining, acidosis, or prematurity

The presence of meconium in amniotic fluid is a general, rather than a specific, indicator of fetal distress. It is of greatest risk to the fetus during the fetus' transition to neonatal life if it is aspirated into the tracheobronchial tree

Prevention

Treat underlying causes of maternal, fetal, and/or neonatal distress

Assist in the prompt delivery and resuscitation of the fetus when fetal or maternal conditions warrant urgent or emergent delivery

If the parturient is under anesthesia, her condition is the primary concern of the anesthetist

Avoid administering respiratory or myocardial depressant drugs to the parturient unless absolutely necessary

Use the minimum dose possible

Use drugs that do not cross the placenta

Maintain adequate maternal blood pressure

Apply left uterine displacement to allow adequate venous return

Fluid load prior to instituting a regional anesthetic

Treat hypotension aggressively with fluid and ephedrine IV, 5–10 mg

Manifestations

Depressed ventilation

Normally, the functional residual capacity is established with the first breath as the fetus makes the transition to neonate

Regular, rhythmic ventilation is established typically within the first 60–90 seconds

Decreased oxygenation

The arterial pO_2 decreases rapidly from 25–40 mm Hg in the fetus to less than 5 mm Hg

Anaerobic metabolism quickly follows, with a dramatic decrease in pH

Bradycardia

The Apgar score remains the most generally accepted index of neonatal well-being and need for resuscitation in the delivery room. Severe asphyxia results in an Apgar score of 0–2 at 1 minute.

The Apgar Scoring System

Sign	0	1	2
Heart rate	Absent	<100 bpm	>100 bpm
Respiratory effort	Absent	Slow, irregular	Good, crying
Color	Blue, pale	Body pink, extremities blue (acrocyanosis)	Completely pink
Reflex irritability (response to insertion of a nasal catheter)	Absent	Grimace	Cough, sneeze
Muscle tone	Limp	Some flexion of extremities	Active motion

Similar Events

Congenital abnormalities of the airways that interfere with adequate ventilation and gas exchange
Congenital cardiovascular anomalies characterized by right-to-left shunting (venous admixture)
Persistent pulmonary hypertension of the newborn
Pneumothorax

Management

General Principles
The restoration of airway patency and ventilation of the lungs with 100% O_2 is the principal goal in managing neonatal asphyxia
> Most pediatric cardiopulmonary arrests are the result of loss of airway patency or ventilatory inadequacy and hypoxia
> Open the airway using mandibular displacement, extension at the atlanto-occipital joint, or an oral airway
>> Neonates with micrognathia should be placed in the lateral or prone position to improve airway patency
> Administer 100% O_2
> Institute bag-mask-controlled ventilation and/or secure the airway by endotracheal intubation when necessary

Pharmacologic management and volume administration should be according to neonatal ACLS and PALS protocols

For Neonates with Apgar Scores of 0–2 (Severe Depression)
The trachea should be intubated immediately and positive pressure ventilation begun
> Confirm endotracheal intubation by multiple modalities since "breath sounds" may be easily heard over the entire body of a neonate
> The adequacy of ventilation should initially be determined by excursion of the chest wall, while examining carefully for symmetry and uniformity of chest rising.
> Most neonates do not require inflation pressures greater than 25–30 cm H_2O

Chest compression should be instituted for impaired circulation according to ACLS and PALS protocols
Vascular access should be established peripherally or through the umbilical artery for resuscitation
> If vascular access cannot be obtained, administer resuscitation medications directly through the ETT

For Neonates with Apgar Scores of 3–4 (Moderate Depression)
Ventilate the patient with O_2 by bag and mask
> If the neonate has not yet breathed or is breathing ineffectively, an ETT should be inserted before ventilating the lungs
> Gas may enter the stomach and interfere with ventilation; the stomach should be decompressed if necessary

For Neonates Born with Meconium Staining
The oropharynx should be suctioned while the baby is on the perineum (vaginal delivery) or within the surgical field (for operative delivery)
> The bulb syringe is as effective as the De Lee suction for intrapartum removal of nasopharyngeal meconium

This practice has been shown to improve the outcome with regard to meconium aspiration
Meconium should be suctioned from the lung using an ETT as a suction catheter before breathing is established
The absence of meconium in the pharynx does not guarantee lack of aspiration

Complications

Hyperinflation of the stomach, causing impairment of ventilation and oxygenation
Pharyngeal lacerations
Subglottic injury due to an inappropriately large ETT
Pneumothorax
Retinopathy of prematurity
Intraventricular hemorrhage

Suggested Readings

Brion LP, Goyal M, Suresh BR: Sudden deterioration of intubated newborn: four steps to the differential diagnosis and initial management. J Perinatol 12:281, 1992
Emergency Cardiac Care Committee and Subcommittees, American Heart Association: Guidelines for cardiopulmonary resuscitation and emergency cardiac care. Part VII. Neonatal resuscitation. JAMA 268:2276, 1992
Goddard-Finegold J, Mizrahi EM: Understanding and preventing perinatal, intracerebral, peri- and intraventricular hemorrhage. J Child Neurol 2:170, 1987
Gregory GA: Resuscitation of the newborn. In Miller RD (ed): Anesthesia. 3rd Ed. Churchill Livingstone, New York, 1990
Hird MF, Greenough A, Gamsu HR: Inflating pressures for effective resuscitation of preterm infants. Early Hum Dev 26:69, 1991
Jain L, Ferre C, Vidyasagar D et al: Cardiopulmonary resuscitation of apparently stillborn infants: survival and long-term outcome. J Pediatr 118:778, 1991
Kresch MJ, Brion LP, Fleischman AR: Delivery room management of meconium-stained neonates. J Perinatol 11:46, 1991
McKlveen RE, Ostheimer GW: Resuscitation of the newborn. Clin Obstet Gynecol 30:611, 1987
Milner AD: Resuscitation of the newborn. Arch Dis Child 66:66, 1991
Wiswell TE, Tuggle JM, Turner BS: Meconium aspiration syndrome: have we made a difference? Pediatrics 85:715, 1990

83 POSTEXTUBATION CROUP

Definition

Postextubation croup is stridor following removal of an ETT.

Etiology

Inflammation and edema of the subglottic region due to mechanical irritation by the ETT

Typical Situations

In patients 1–4 years of age after extubation of the trachea
> Stridor after short-term intubation in children has been reported with a frequency of 1–6%; this can be as high as 40% with long-term intubation
> Subglottic edema may occur when too large an ETT has been used in a child
>> Correct size is indicated by an air leak around the ETT
> Stridor is more common after there has been more than one attempt at endotracheal intubation or when the ETT or the patient's head has been manipulated during surgery

In patients who have a history of congenital or acquired subglottic stenosis
> These may not cause symptoms under ordinary conditions

In patients with a history of croup during upper respiratory tract infections

Prevention

Use an uncuffed ETT of appropriate size in children, using the following rules of thumb
> ETT size (mm) = 4 + age (years)/4
> ETT should be approximately the same diameter as the patient's fifth finger

Confirm that a leak around the ETT is present with an inspiratory pressure of 20–25 cm H_2O
Minimize manipulation of the ETT or the patient's head
Avoid anesthesia and surgery in patients with upper respiratory tract infections who have croup

Manifestations

Following extubation, stridor typically occurs within 1 to 2 hours, although severe respiratory obstruction can occur almost immediately.

High-pitched, noisy respiration (stridor) at the level of the trachea or larynx
> Stridor may be inspiratory, expiratory, or biphasic
> Inspiratory stridor is usually associated with extrathoracic airway obstruction
>> Postextubation croup occurs in the subglottic region and thus is extrathoracic
> Expiratory stridor is usually associated with an intrathoracic obstruction (see Event 75, *Aspiration of a Foreign Body* and Event 24, *Bronchospasm*)

Respiratory distress
> Dyspnea
> Tachypnea
> Retraction of the chest wall during inspiration

Hypoxemia
> May be manifested by restlessness in children

Increase in pulmonary secretions because of impaired ability to clear lung volumes
Tachycardia

Similar Events

Extrathoracic respiratory tract obstruction from other causes
Subglottic hemangioma
Intratracheal foreign bodies (see Event 75, *Aspiration of a Foreign Body*)
Webs

Vocal cord dysfunction or tumor
Arytenoid dislocation from intubation trauma
Pharyngeal edema or abcess
Laryngospasm
Angioneurotic edema
Pneumothorax or pneumomediastinum (see Event 28, *Pneumothorax*)

Management

For the Patient with Croup
Ensure adequate oxygenation and ventilation
    Administer O_2 as a cool mist
    Maintain airway patency
    Institute CPAP using a bag and mask if necessary
        Continue spontaneous ventilation
        CPAP decreases stridor by lowering the pressure gradient across the obstructed segment and possibly by stenting open the constricted segment
    Prepare for more invasive maneuvers to establish an airway
        Reintubation
        Cricothyrotomy with transtracheal jet ventilation
        Tracheostomy
Administer inhaled racemic epinephrine 2.25%, 0.5 ml in 2–4 ml NS, delivered by nebulizer
    Do not administer more frequently than q30min
    In equipotent doses racemic epinephrine has the same efficacy and adverse effects as the *l*-isomer alone
Administer dexamethasone IV, 0.5–1 mg/kg
    Corticosteroids are most effective when given prior to intubation, but may have some benefit if given after extubation
If stridor continues and helium or heliox is available, consider ventilating the patient with a helium and O_2 mixture
    Helium/O_2 mixtures have a lower density than O_2 alone
    During turbulent flow, gas density determines flow characteristics
If respiratory failure occurs despite these interventions, endotracheal intubation will be necessary
    Use an ETT one-half size (0.5 mm) smaller than typically calculated for age
    A leak should occur with an inspiratory pressure of 20–25 cm H_2O
Readiness for extubation may be evaluated by direct examination of the airway or by the "leak test"
    The leak test is a weak predictor of successful extubation

Complications

Hypoxemia
Hypercarbia
Arrhythmias
Aspiration of gastric contents
Cardiac arrest

Suggested Readings

Adderley RJ, Mullins GC: When to extubate the croup patient the "leak" test. Can J Anaesth 34:304, 1987

Diaz JH: Croup and epiglottitis in children: the anesthesiologist as diagnostician. Anesth Analg 64:621, 1985

Freezer N, Butt W, Phelan P: Steroids in croup: do they increase the incidence of successful extubation? Anaesth Intensive Care 18:224, 1990

Holzman RS: Advances in pediatric anesthesia implications for otolaryngology. Ear Nose Throat J 71:99, 1992

Koka BV, Jeon IS, Andre JM et al: Postintubation croup in children. Anesth Analg 56:501, 1977

Mesrobian RB: Stridor in the recovery room. p. 189. In Stehling L (ed): Common Problems in Pediatric Anesthesia. 2nd Ed. Mosby-Year Book, St. Louis, 1992

Motoyama EK: Recovery from anesthesia. p. 322. In Motoyama EK, Davis PJ (eds): Smith's Anesthesia for Infants and Children. 5th Ed. CV Mosby, St. Louis, 1990

Tibballs J, Shann FA, Landau LI: Placebo-controlled trial of prednisolone in children intubated for croup. Lancet 340:745, 1992

Index